Thyroid Cancer: Diagnosis, Prognosis and Treatment

Thyroid Cancer: Diagnosis, Prognosis and Treatment

Guest Editors

Luca Giovanella
Petra Petranović Ovčariček

MDPI

Basel • Beijing • Wuhan • Barcelona • Belgrade • Novi Sad • Cluj • Manchester

Guest Editors

Luca Giovanella
Clinic for Nuclear Medicine
and Intedisciplinary Thyroid
Centre
University Hospital of Zurich
Zurich
Switzerland

Petra Petranović Ovčariček
Department of Oncology and
Nuclear Medicine
University Hospital Center
Sestre Milosrdnice
Zagreb
Croatia

Editorial Office
MDPI AG
Grosspeteranlage 5
4052 Basel, Switzerland

This is a reprint of the Special Issue, published open access by the journal *Cancers* (ISSN 2072-6694), freely accessible at: https://www.mdpi.com/journal/cancers/special_issues/57624JGNGB.

For citation purposes, cite each article independently as indicated on the article page online and as indicated below:

Lastname, A.A.; Lastname, B.B. Article Title. *Journal Name* **Year**, *Volume Number*, Page Range.

ISBN 978-3-7258-6976-3 (Hbk)
ISBN 978-3-7258-6977-0 (PDF)
https://doi.org/10.3390/books978-3-7258-6977-0

Cover image courtesy of Petra Petranović Ovčariček

Contents

About the Editors

Luca Giovanella

Luca Giovanella, Clinic for Nuclear Medicine and Intedisciplinary Thyroid Centre, University Hospital of Zurich, 8091 Zurich, Switzerland. Luca Giovanella is an experienced and established nuclear medicine physician and endocrinologist. He leads the nuclear medicine department and the thyroid and parathyroid clinical unit at the Clinica Moncucco, Lugano, Switzerland, and serves as Professor of nuclear medicine at the University of Zurich, Switzerland. He has served as the Chair of the EANM Thyroid Committee since 2021, previously serving as the Deputy Chair (2014-2020). He is the author of more than 500 peer-reviewed papers, with a particular focus on thyroid disease. He is the co-author of several guidelines dedicated to thyroid and parathyroid diseases.

Petra Petranović Ovčariček

Petra Petranović Ovčariček, Department of Oncology and Nuclear Medicine, University Hospital Center Sestre Milosrdnice, Zagreb, Croatia. Petra Petranović Ovčariček is an experienced nuclear medicine physician currently employed at the University Hospital Center Sestre Milosrdnice, Zagreb, Croatia, and serves as Assistant Professor at the University of Zagreb, School of Medicine, Zagreb, Croatia. She is particularly dedicated to the study of thyroid and parathyroid diseases. She has been a member of the EANM Thyroid Committee since 2019, and has served as their guidelines representative since 2021. She is the co-author of several guidelines dedicated to thyroid and parathyroid diseases.

cancers

MDPI

Article

Relationship between the Expression of CHK2 and p53 in Tumor Tissue and the Course of Papillary Thyroid Cancer in Patients with *CHEK2* Germline Mutations

Danuta Gąsior-Perczak [1,2,*], Artur Kowalik [3,4], Janusz Kopczyński [5], Paweł Macek [1,6], Kornelia Niemyska [5], Agnieszka Walczyk [1,2], Krzysztof Gruszczyński [3], Monika Siołek [7], Tomasz Dróżdż [1,8], Marcin Kosowski [1], Iwona Pałyga [1,2], Piotr Przybycień [2], Olga Wabik [5], Stanisław Góźdź [1,9] and Aldona Kowalska [1,2]

1 Collegium Medicum, Jan Kochanowski University, 25-317 Kielce, Poland; pawel.macek@onkol.kielce.pl (P.M.); a.walczyk@post.pl (A.W.); tomasz.drozdz@ujk.edu.pl (T.D.); markos86@vp.pl (M.K.); iwonapa@tlen.pl (I.P.); stanislawgo@onkol.kielce.pl (S.G.); aldonako@onkol.kielce.pl (A.K.)
2 Endocrinology Clinic, Holycross Cancer Centre, S. Artwińskiego St. 3, 25-734 Kielce, Poland; przybycien.piotr@o2.pl
3 Department of Molecular Diagnostics, Holycross Cancer Centre, S. Artwińskiego Str. 3, 25-734 Kielce, Poland; artur.kowalik@onkol.kielce.pl (A.K.); gruszczynski.k@wp.pl (K.G.)
4 Division of Medical Biology, Institute of Biology, Jan Kochanowski University, Uniwersytecka 7, 25-406 Kielce, Poland
5 Surgical Pathology, Holycross Cancer Centre, S. Artwińskiego Str. 3, 25-734 Kielce, Poland; januszko@onkol.kielce.pl (J.K.); kornelia.niemyska@wp.pl (K.N.)
6 Department of Epidemiology and Cancer Control, Holycross Cancer Center S. Artwińskiego St. 3, 25-734 Kielce, Poland
7 Genetic Clinic, Holycross Cancer Centre, 25-734 Kielce, Poland; monika.siolek@wp.pl
8 Department of Radiology, Holycross Cancer Centre, S. Artwińskiego Str. 3, 25-734 Kielce, Poland
9 Clinical Oncology, Holycross Cancer Centre, S. Artwińskiego Str. 3, 25-734 Kielce, Poland
* Correspondence: danutagp@o2.pl

Simple Summary: CHK2 has functions in DNA damage repair. Germline *CHEK2* mutations impair these functions, increasing the risk of PTC. The aim of this study was to determine whether CHK2 and p53 expression in patients with a germline *CHEK2* mutation in tumor tissue can serve as a prognostic marker for papillary thyroid cancer (PTC), and whether copy number aberrations in *CHEK2* and *TP53* correlate with the course of PTC. This study included 156 patients with PTC who had been selected from a group of 1547 people previously tested for the presence of *CHEK2* mutations in their peripheral blood. Higher CHK2 expression was associated with poorer treatment responses and disease outcomes in PTC patients. Higher CHK2 expression and positive p53 together with a *TP53* deletion could have potential as a prognostic marker of unfavorable disease outcomes in patients with germline truncating mutations in *CHEK2*.

Abstract: The aim of this study was to determine whether the expression of CHK2 and p53 in tumor tissue in carriers of germline *CHEK2* mutations can serve as a prognostic marker for PTC, and whether *CHEK2* and *TP53* copy numbers correlates with the course of PTC disease. This study included 156 PTC patients previously tested for the presence of *CHEK2*. Clinicopathological features, treatment response, disease outcome, and germline mutation status of the *CHEK2* gene were assessed with respect to CHK2 and p53 expression, and *CHEK2* and *TP53* gene copy statuses. In patients with and without a germline mutation in *CHEK2* and with higher CHK2 expression, the chances of an excellent treatment response and no evidence of disease were lower than in patients without or with lower CHK2 expression. *TP53* deletion was associated with angioinvasion. In patients with a truncating mutation, the chance of a *CHEK2* deletion was higher than in patients with WT *CHEK2* alone or those with WT *CHEK2* and with the missense I157T mutation. Higher CHK2 expression was associated with poorer treatment responses and disease outcomes. Higher CHK2 expression and positive p53 together with a *TP53* deletion could be a prognostic marker of unfavorable disease outcomes in patients with germline truncating mutations in *CHEK2*.

Keywords: papillary thyroid cancer; *CHEK2* mutation; checkpoint kinase 2; p53; *TP53* gene; immunohistochemistry; fluorescence in situ hybridization

1. Introduction

In recent years, there has been a steady increase in the incidence of papillary thyroid cancer (PTC) worldwide, mainly due to improved diagnostic technologies and increased awareness of screening tests. Most new cases are cancers at a low clinical stage [1–3]. PTC currently has an excellent prognosis [4]. However, in some patients, PTC can lead to metastases and death of the patient. The mortality of patients with differentiated thyroid cancer is approximately 1–2% [5]. The molecular mechanisms determining this mortality are still largely unknown. Thus, it is extremely important to identify molecular markers not only in tumor tissue after surgery but, more importantly, in peripheral blood before surgery to select for patients in need of aggressive treatment. Mutations in DNA repair pathway genes (ATM/CHK2/p53) represent one potential source of markers. The checkpoint kinase 2 gene (*CHEK2*) is involved in DNA repair and is activated by DNA damage, especially double-strand breaks. It is also a tumor suppressor gene. It is located on the long arm of human chromosome 22 at position q12.1 and encodes a protein (CHK2, checkpoint kinase 2) with serine-threonine kinase activity. CHK2 regulates the cell cycle and prevents uncontrolled cell division. In response to a double-stranded DNA break, the serine- threonine kinase ATM (ataxia-telangiectasia mutated gene) is activated and phosphorylates and activates CHK2, which then phosphorylates proteins involved in the DNA damage response, such as p53, Cdc25A, Cdc25C, and BRCA1, which leads to cell cycle arrest in the G1, S, and G2 phases and initiation of DNA damage repair. However, if the DNA damage is irreparable, the cells undergo cell death in a process termed apoptosis. These observations suggest that CHK2 is regulated at sites of double-stranded DNA breaks and plays an important role in the DNA damage response. Therefore, an efficient signaling ATM/CHK2/p53 pathway is essential for the coordination of DNA repair, cell cycle progression, and apoptosis in response to DNA damage [6–8].

Mutations in the genes encoding DNA repair proteins may affect their stability and activity, which can lead to the development of cancer. Carriers of mutations in genes encoding tumor suppressor proteins, such as CHK2 and p53, are genetically predisposed to certain cancers. The expression of DNA repair pathway genes is increased in patients with malignant tumors, and this is associated with unfavorable disease outcomes in these patients. DNA repair pathway genes are also expressed at significantly higher levels in patients with melanoma metastases, suggesting that CHK2 may also mediate tumor progression [9]. A study by Zhao et al. reported that high CHK2 expression may be associated with PTC progression [10]. Increased CHK expression is also observed in most cases of diffuse large B-cell lymphoma (DLBCL), bladder cancer, and ovarian cancer, and is associated with poor clinical courses in these patients [11–13].

Like the *CHEK2* gene, the tumor suppressor gene *TP53* is important for maintaining genome integrity. It is referred to as the "guardian of the genome", not alone because it is involved in the control of cell growth and division [14,15], but also because mutations in this gene commonly occur in a wide range of malignant tumors, suggesting that it suppresses cancer formation [14]. Mutations that functionally impair p53 seriously compromise the cells' ability to repair DNA and result in apoptosis if the genetic defect is not repaired [16]. *TP53* mutations block inhibition of the G1 phase of cell cycle progression and deregulate apoptosis, resulting in the malignant transformation and proliferation of damaged cells [17–19].

Germinal *CHEK2* truncating mutations (1100delC, IVS2 + 1G > A, del5395) increase the risk of thyroid cancer by approximately 6-fold [20,21], and missense mutations such as I157T increase the risk by about 2–3 fold [20–23]. According to The Cancer Genome Atlas

Research, in addition to hereditary predisposition to the development of PTC, somatic mutations occur in the *CHEK2* gene, which may contribute to PTC tumor progression [24].

We have previously shown that *CHEK2* truncating mutations, rather than missense mutations, are significantly associated with angioinvasion and an intermediate or high initial risk of recurrent/persistent PTC [21]. However, that study did not assess the expression of CHK2 and p53 in tumor tissues in carriers of *CHEK2* germline mutations with PTC.

To learn more about the role of CHK2 and p53 in PTC and determine whether they have potential as diagnostic and prognostic markers of PTC, we measured the expression of the unphosphorylated forms of CHK2 and p53 using immunohistochemistry (IHC) and determined whether their expression levels correlated with disease progression in PTC patients. Furthermore, we used fluorescence in situ hybridization (FISH) to analyze copy number aberrations of *CHEK2* and *TP53* and determine whether they correlated with disease progression in PTC patients.

2. Materials and Methods

2.1. Patients

The study included 156 PTC patients who were selected from a group of 1547 PTC patients who had previously been tested for the presence of mutations in the *CHEK2* gene in DNA isolated from peripheral blood [21]. In 43 of 51 patients from the previous study with a truncating mutation in the *CHEK2* gene, it was possible to obtain archival paraffin-embedded blocks containing fixed tissues of the primary tumor for IHC and FISH testing. Seven patients were excluded from the study due to degraded DNA. One patient with a truncating mutation in the *CHEK2* gene, who underwent thyroid surgery after 2020, from whom archival blocks were also obtained, was included in the study. A total of 44 patients with a truncating mutation were included in the study. Archival blocks containing fixed tissues of the primary tumor were obtained from 7 out of 7 patients with the I157T homozygous mutation in the *CHEK2* gene. Fifty-three of 182 patients with the I157T heterozygous mutation in the *CHEK2* gene and 52 of 1307 patients without a mutation in the *CHEK2* gene from a previous study were randomly selected according to the procedure described below.

2.2. Description of the Test Procedure

Patients were ordered by medical history number (in ascending order) and each patient was assigned a unique number (between 1 and 1547). Of the patients assigned to the missense mutation group, 53 were randomly selected with the use of a random number generator (R software). Of the patients assigned to the no-mutation group, 52 were randomly selected. Number 182 (the number of all patients in the missense mutation group) was selected as a setting for the random number generator in the statistical software R (open source statistical software [25]) when drawing from the group with missense mutations. The number 1307 (the number of all patients in the no-mutation group) was selected as the random number generator setting when drawing from no-mutation group in the R program.

No additional randomization was performed because it was possible to obtain archival blocks containing fixed tissues of the primary tumor from all randomly selected patients.

All study procedures were approved by the Institutional Review Board of Jan Kochanowski University, Kielce, Poland (approval number: 31/2021). All patients gave written informed consent to participate in the study. All patients were informed about the nature, objectives, and methods of the study. All patients included in the study were Caucasian. Detailed data on *CHEK2* germline mutations have been reported previously [26]. Samples of archival paraffin-embedded tumor blocks after thyroid surgery were used for immunohistochemical (IHC) analysis of *CHEK2* and p53 expression as well as for analysis of *CHEK2* and *TP53* gene copy numbers via FISH. Clinicopathological data were available for all analyzed cases and were analyzed retrospectively. All PTCs were graded histopathologically according to the 8th edition of the American Joint Committee on Cancer (AJCC) thyroid cancer staging system (AJCC/Union for International Cancer Control (UICC) TNM staging system and American Thyroid Association (ATA) modified initial risk stratification system (low, intermediate, and high risk of recurrence)) [27,28]. All patients included in the study underwent primary surgical treatment (lobectomy, total thyroidectomy, or total thyroidectomy with central or central and lateral compartment lymphadenectomy). The scope of surgery and surgical procedure have been described previously [29]. Response to therapy was assessed 1 year after initial treatment. Response to initial treatment was classified into four categories: excellent, indeterminate, biochemically incomplete, and structurally incomplete [27]. Response to treatment after thyroidectomy and I-131 radiotherapy was assessed according to Tuttle's criteria [30], while response to treatment after thyroidectomy without I-131 radiotherapy or lobectomy was assessed according to Momesso's criteria [31].

All procedures for monitoring the course of the disease after surgery, assessing the response to treatment, and further follow-up, as well as treatment assessment, have been described previously [32,33]. Relapse was defined as the detection of biochemical or structural disease after a period of NED (no evidence of disease at least 12 months after initial therapy) and no symptoms of the disease [27,31].

Clinical observation was completed on 30 November 2022. Patients were classified into one of the following groups based on medical records in accordance with ATA recommendations [27]: NED, indeterminate response, biochemically and structurally chronic disease, deaths from cancer, and deaths from other causes.

2.3. Detection of CHEK2 Mutation

DNA was isolated from whole blood samples (100 μL), collected in EDTA tubes, within 12 h of collection, using the Maxwell® RSC Blood DNA Kit (Promega, Madison, WI, USA). DNA samples were eluted in 120 μL of buffer E. Genotyping and the diagnostic algorithm of molecular tests in our center have been described in detail in our previous work [21,26].

2.4. Fluorescence In Situ Hybridization (FISH)

CHEK2 and *TP53* copy number determination via FISH was performed on PTC tissue fixed in 10% buffered formalin and embedded in paraffin. Four-micrometer thick paraffin sections were placed on the positively charged side of an organosilane-coated slide to minimize tissue detachment from the slide during FISH. The sections were baked for 1 h on a hot plate at 56 °C and then subjected to the protocol recommended by the probe manufacturer (CytoTest, Washington, DC, USA).

After incubation overnight, the sections were immersed twice in xylene for 10 min each and then passed through a series of decreasing alcohol concentrations (100%, 96%) for 5 min each. After rinsing twice in purified water for 5 min, the sections were immersed in pretreatment solution at 95 °C for 30 min, passed through washing buffer twice for 5 min each, and then immersed in a protease solution at 37 °C for 30 min. After washing the sections twice in washing buffer, the sections were dried at room temperature. Two probes (10 μL each) were used in parallel: the *CHEK2*/CCP22 FISH Probe (CytoTest) and the *TP53*/CCP17 FISH Probe (CytoTest). The sections of the slides were covered with coverslips and sealed with rubber glue. The probe and DNA in the sections were denatured in a ThermoBrite apparatus for 5 min at 75 °C, and then allowed to hybridize at 37 °C overnight. The cover slip was removed and the excess of non-hybridized and non-specifically bound probe was removed by washing the sections twice for 2 min each in post-hybridization washing buffer (2 × SSC/03% NP-40). After drying at room temperature, 10 μL of DAPI Solution was applied to the sections and the sections were covered again with a coverslip. The preparations were stored in a dark place until signal counting.

CHEK2/CCP22 and *TP53*/CCP17 gene copy numbers were counted in 100 cell nuclei in non-overlapping fields of view containing cancer cells using a fluorescence microscope equipped with a double Orange/Green filter at 100× magnification with oil immersion. Hybridization with the *CHEK2*/CCP22 probe was confirmed by observing two red signals for the *CHEK2* and two green signals for the centromere of chromosome 22. Hybridization with the *TP53*/CCP17 probe was confirmed by observing two red signals for *TP53* and two green signals for the centromere of chromosome 17. The exact number of copies of each gene in each nucleus was recorded. When the copy number in more than 20% of the nuclei in each section exceeded the DNA ploidy number, this was considered gene amplification, whereas when the copy number in more than 30% of the nuclei was below the ploidy number, this was considered a gene deletion (Figure 1) [34].

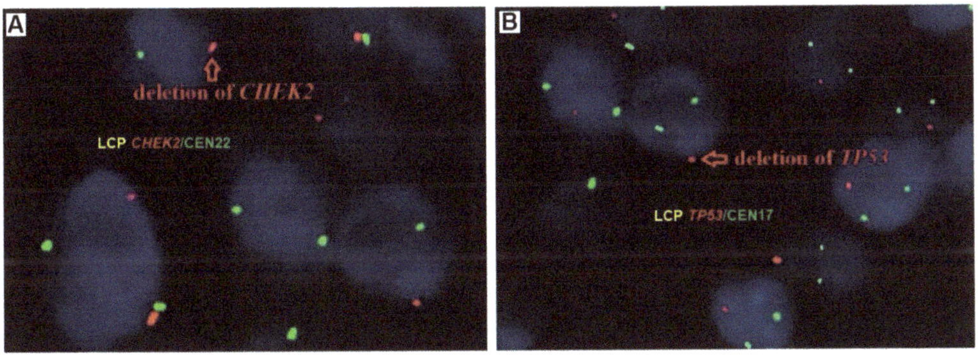

Figure 1. Gene status in PTC tumors samples examined by fluorescence in situ hybridization (FISH) using the probes LCP *CHEK2*/CEN22 and LCP *TP53*/CEN17; (**A**) detection of *CHEK2* (red signal indicates deletion of one copy of the *CHEK2* gene), and (**B**) detection of *TP53* (red signal indicates deletion of one copy of the *TP53* gene), magnification ×100.

2.5. Immunohistochemistry (IHC)

IHC Staining

Chk2(A-12) mouse monoclonal antibody from Santa Cruz Biotechnology (sc-5278) was used. Staining with this antibody was performed in an OMNIS staining device (Dako). Antigen unmasking was performed with EnV Flex TRS high pH reagent no. REF GV804 (Dako) at 97 °C for 20 min. The sections were incubated for 30 min with the primary antibody diluted 1:50 with EnV Flex/HRP polymer (Dako, REF GV800).

For p53 mouse monoclonal antibody (DO7) (Cell Marque; REF 453M-95, catalog number CM-453M-95), staining was performed in an OMNIS staining device (Dako). Antigen unmasking was performed with EnV Flex TRS high pH reagent (Dako; no. REF GV804) at 97 °C for 20 min. The sections were incubated for 30 min with the primary antibody at a dilution of 1:500 with EnV Flex/HRP polymer (Dako, REF GV800).

2.6. Analysis of Immunohistochemical Results

Immunohistochemical evaluation of CHK2 and p53 expression was performed by two pathologists specialized in PTC. The age of the tissue block had no effect on immunohistochemical staining. *CHEK2* staining was scored to evaluate the intensity of nuclear staining and determine the percentage of positive cells. Criteria for assessing the number of tumor cells were as follows: 0, no staining; 1, weak staining (≤10% of cells); 2, moderate staining (10–50% of cells); and 3, strong staining (>50% cancer cells). For statistical analysis, scores of 0 and 1 were classified as low CHK2 staining and scores of 2 and 3 as high staining. The following scoring system was also used for p53. Cases scored as positive showed strong nuclear staining in >30% of the cells, whereas normal thyroid follicular cells showed little staining. The CHK2 expression patterns revealed by IHC staining are shown in Figure 2.

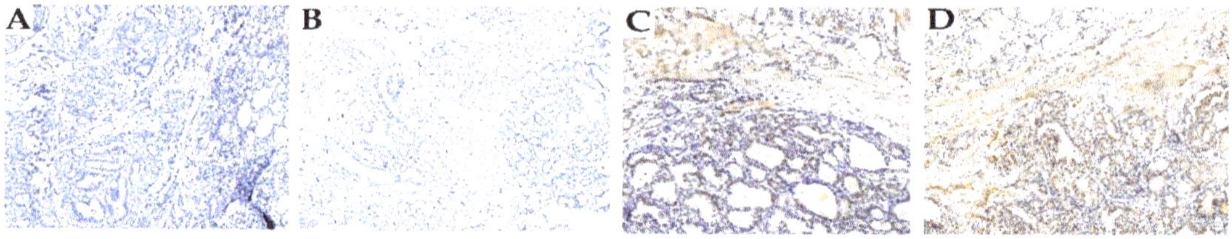

Figure 2. Detection of CHK2 expression by immunohistochemistry in PTC tumor samples. Representative staining intensities were scored as 0 (negative) (**A**), 1+ (weak) (**B**), 2+ (moderate) (**C**), and 3+ (strong) (**D**). Magnification ×200.

2.7. Statistical Analyses

Continuous data are presented as the mean (standard deviation) and median (lower/upper quartiles and ranges (minimum and maximum)). Categorical data are presented as numbers and percentages. Odds ratio (OR) and 95% confidence intervals (95% CI) were calculated using logistic regression models. A two-tailed p-value < 0.05 was considered statistically significant. Two binomial proportions (e.g., CHK2 frequency in patients with and without vascular invasion) were compared using a Bayesian A/B test. The predictive performances of three competing hypotheses were examined. The first, the null hypothesis (H0), which was assigned a prior probability model (P(M)) of 0.50, predicted the equality of the tested binomial proportions and had a log OR = 0. The second, one-sided alternative hypothesis with an assigned P(M) of 0.25 predicted a higher percentage of results defined as "categories of interest" in the group of patients with the tested feature present (e.g., a higher percentage of patients without vascular invasion in the group of patients with the CHK2 present). The hypothesis with a log OR > 0 predicted a clinically beneficial effect of the tested feature. The third, complementary alternative hypothesis (log OR < 0 and P(M) = 0.25) predicted fewer successes in the selected group of patients, i.e., a clinically unfavorable impact of the tested feature. The results of testing the hypothesis are presented in the form of the Bayes factor (BF). The BF defines the ratio of two competing statistical models represented by their marginal probability. The BF was used to quantify the support for one model over another. The subscript used in BF notation indicated which hypothesis was supported by the data. BF_{10} indicated a BF that was more in favor of the alternative hypothesis than the H0 hypothesis. BF assumed that any positive value was qualitatively interpreted in accordance with the classification proposed by Jeffreys, modified by Lee et al. [35]. The prior and posterior densities of the log OR for the quantity of interest were plotted. A standard normal prior distribution ($\mu = 0$ and $\sigma = 1$) on the log OR scale was adopted. The results were expressed as medians with 95% credible intervals (95% CI). For simplicity, descriptions of the results in the text were expressed as medians of the OR (anti-logarithm of log OR). A sequential analysis was performed to consider the results as a function of the total number of observations. The reproducibility of the estimates was determined by setting an initial random seed value (set seed = 123). All statistical analyses were performed using JASP (Version 16.0.0).

3. Results

3.1. Baseline Characteristics

Clinicopathological features of patients with PTC, molecular status of *CHEK2* mutation, primary treatment response categories, and disease outcomes for all 156 cases are presented in Table 1. In the study group of 156 Caucasian patients (median age was 49.5, range 39–59), the majority were women 138 (88.5%) and 98 patients were under 55 years of age (62.8%). The mean and standard deviation of tumor diameter for all patients was 13.1 ± 13.0 (range 1.0–84.0 mm). The stage of the primary lesion was pT1a in 94 (60.3%) patients, the dominant classic subtype was found in 107 (68.6%), gross extrathyroidal extension in two (1.3%), vascular invasion in 11 (7.1%), R1 surgical margin in 19 (12.2%), histologically verified lymph node metastases in 35 (22.4%), distant metastases in one (0.6%), and multifocality in 50 (32.1%) patients. Mutations in the *CHEK2* gene were found in 104 (66.7%) patients, including the I157T missense mutation in 60 (38.5%) and a truncating mutation (1100delC, IVS2 + 1G > A, del5395) in 38 (24.4%). No mutations in the *CHEK2* gene were found in 52 (33.3%) patients. Thirty-four patients (21.8%) were classified as intermediate risk and 25 patients (16.0%) as high risk according to ATA guidelines [27]. I-131 radiotherapy was administered to 111 (71.2%) patients, and 1100–3700 MBq of I-131 was used depending on cancer stage according to the TNM classification. Eighteen (11.5%) patients received I-131 radiotherapy more than once. The remaining 45 patients (28.9%) with a single PTC focus (≤1 cm in diameter) limited to the thyroid gland, without nodal and distant metastases (pT1aN0-xM0), did not receive I-131 treatment. In the entire study group, a very good response to primary treatment was observed in 127 (81.4%) patients. The median follow-up of the study group was 7 years (range 1–23). There were no cases of death due to cancer. However, deaths from other causes were recorded in five (3.2%) patients. At the end of follow-up, seven (4.5%) patients had an indeterminate response, one (0.6%) had biochemically persistent disease, and three (1.9%) had structurally persistent disease. Recurrence after a disease-free period (NED) occurred in five patients (3.2%).

Table 1. Basic characteristics of 156 patients with papillary thyroid carcinoma.

Characteristic	Total n = 156 (100%)
Sex	
Female	138 (88.5%)
Male	18 (11.5%)
Age at diagnosis (years)	
<55	98 (62.8%)
≥55	58 (37.2%)
Mean (SD)	48.5 (13.6)
Median (Q1–Q3)	49.5 (39.0–59.0)
Range	18.0–73.0
Tumor diameter (mm)	
Mean (SD)	13.1 (13.0)
Median (Q1–Q3)	8.0 (5.0–16.5)
Range	1.0–84.0
Tumor diameter (mm)	
≤10	94 (60.3%)
>10–20	32 (20.5%)
>20–40	25 (16.0%)
>40	5 (3.2%)
Papillary cancer histologic variant	
Classic	107 (68.6%)
Follicular	35 (22.4%)
Oxyphilic	3 (1.9%)
Diffuse sclerosing	3 (1.9%)
Tall cell	1 (0.6%)
Other *	7 (4.5%)
Surgical treatment	
Total thyroidectomy	152 (97.4%)
Lobectomy	4 (2.6%)
Nodal dissection	
Central	94 (60.3%)
Lateral	17 (10.9%)
No dissection	45 (28.8%)

Table 1. *Cont.*

Characteristic	Total n = 156 (100%)
Multifocality	
No	106 (68.0%)
Yes	50 (32.1%)
Lymph node metastases **	
N0a	76 (48.7%)
N0b	45 (28.9%)
N1a	18 (11.5%)
N1b	17 (10.9%)
Distant metastases	
M0	155 (99.4%)
M1	1 (0.6%)
Extrathyroidal extension	
Negative	124 (79.5%)
Microscopic	30 (19.2%)
Gross	2 (1.3%)
Vascular invasion	
No	145 (93%)
Yes	11 (7.1%)
Margin status	
R0	137 (87.8%)
R1	19 (12.2%)
Tumor stage	
pT1a	94 (60.3%)
pT1b	32 (20.5%)
pT2	23 (14.7%)
pT3a	5 (3.2%)
pT3b	2 (1.3%)
CHEK2 mutation status	
CHEK2 WT	52 (33.3%)
CHEK2 mutation any	104 (66.7%)
CHEK2 I157T missense mutation (any)	60 (38.5%)
I157T heterozygous	53 (34.0%)
I157T homozygous	7 (4.5%)
CHEK2 truncating heterozygous mutation (any)	38 (24.4%)
IVS2 + 1G > A	16 (10.3%)
Del5395	10 (6.4%)
1100delC	12 (7.7%)
Coexistence of two heterozygous *CHEK2* mutations	6 (3.8%)
I157T and IVS2 + 1G > A	3 (1.9%)
I157T and Del5395	1 (0.6%)
IVS2 + 1G > A and Del5395	2 (1.3%)
TNM (8th edition)	
I	144 (92.3%)
II	12 (7.7%)
ATA initial risk stratification system	
Low	97 (62.2%)
Intermediate	34 (21.8%)
High	25 (16.0%)
Radioactive iodine (I-131) therapy	
No	45 (28.9%)
Yes	111 (71.2%)

Table 1. Cont.

Characteristic	Total n = 156 (100%)
More than one course of radioactive iodine therapy (I-131)	
No	138 (88.5%)
Yes	18 (11.5%)
Response to therapy	
Excellent	127 (81.4%)
Indeterminate	24 (15.4%)
Biochemically incomplete	2 (1.3%)
Structurally incomplete	3 (1.9%)
Final follow-up (disease outcome)	
NED	145 (93.0%)
Indeterminate	7 (4.5%)
Biochemically persistent	1 (0.6%)
Structurally persistent	3 (1.9%)
Follow-up, recurrence	
No	151 (96.8%)
Yes	5 (3.2%)
Death	
No	151 (96.8%)
Yes	5 (3.2%)
Follow-up (years)	
Median (range)	7.0 (1.0–23.0)

* Warthin-like (n = 2); mixed variant (classic and follicular) (n = 5). ** N0a, one or more cytologically or histologically confirmed benign lymph nodes; N0b, no radiologic or clinical evidence of locoregional lymph node metastasis; N1a–N1b, metastasis to regional lymph nodes; R1, microscopically positive margin (resection); ATA, American Thyroid Association, determined according to the 8th edition of the American Joint Committee on Cancer/Union for International Cancer Control (tumor-node-metastasis) TNM staging system; *CHEK2* WT (wild type), cases without the following mutations: I157T, 1100delC, IVS2 + 1G > A, del5395; SD, standard deviation; NED, no evidence of disease.

3.1.1. CHK2 and p53 Expression: Impact on Clinicopathological Features, Treatment Response and Outcomes in PTC Patients with and without *CHEK2* Mutations

The relationship between CHK2 and p53 expression levels and clinicopathological features, response to treatment, and disease outcomes in 156 patients with PTC is presented in Table 2. There were no significant associations between CHK2 and p53 expression levels and sex, age at diagnosis, tumor size, histopathological subtypes, multifocality, lymph node (LN) metastases, distant metastases, extrathyroidal extension, vascular invasion, margin status, higher clinical stage of cancer, and intermediate and high recurrence or I-131 treatment. Patients with high CHK2 expression had a 70% and 80% lower chance of excellent and NED responses, respectively, than patients with no or lower CHK2 expression (OR, 0.28; 95% CI, 0.11–0.72; p = 0.009 and OR, 0.17; 95% CI, 0.05–0.62; p = 0.007). No such relationship was observed in patients who were positive for p53 expression.

Table 2. Relationship between clinicopathological characteristics and p53 expression, CHK2 expression, *CHEK2* gene copy deletion, *TP53* deletion, and p53 expression together with *TP53* deletion in the tumor tissues of patients with and without germline *CHEK2* mutations.

Variable	p53, n = 156 (100%)		CHK2, n = 156 (100%)		*CHEK2* (FISH), n = 151 (100%)		*TP53* (FISH), n = 151 (100%)		Positive p53 with *TP53* Deletion (FISH)	
	Positive n = 8 (5.1%)		High Expression n = 23 (14.7%)		Deletion n = 44 (29.1%)		Deletion n = 7 (4.6%)		n = 15 out of 151 (9.9%)	
	OR (95% CI)	p	OR (95% CI)	p	OR (95% CI)	p	OR (95% CI)	p	OR (95% CI)	p
Sex										
Female vs. male	NA (0 in cell)		1.44 (0.31–6.71)	0.645	1.08 (0.36–3.23)	0.892	1.09 (0.13–9.24)	0.938	NA (0 in cell)	
Age group										
≥55 years vs. <55 years	2.99 (0.69–13.00)	0.145	0.55 (0.20–1.49)	0.238	0.75 (0.36–1.58)	0.451	3.92 (0.94–16.35)	0.061	3.03 (1.02–9.05)	0.047
Tumor stage										
pT1a vs. pT1b, pT2, pT3a, pT3b	NA (0 in cell)		0.96 (0.11–8.38)	0.972	0.97 (0.18–5.21)	0.973	0.81 (0.21–3.16)	0.766	0.99 (0.33–2.93)	0.982
TNM (8th edition)										
TNM II vs. TNM I	NA (0 in cell)		1.17 (0.24–5.73)	0.845	0.52 (0.11–2.50)	0.414	1.65 (0.19–14.54)	0.652	0.90 (0.11–7.56)	0.923
Multifocality										
Yes vs. no	0.69 (0.14–3.57)	0.662	0.92 (0.35–2.39)	0.857	1.00 (0.47–2.13)	0.996	0.62 (0.12–3.08)	0.555	0.52 (0.14–1.95)	0.334
Lymph node metastasis *										
N1a, N1b vs. N0b, N0a	NA (0 in cell)		0.95 (0.33–2.78)	0.931	1.02 (0.44–2.35)	0.968	0.40 (0.05–3.29)	0.392	0.21 (0.03–1.69)	0.144
Distant metastasis										
M1 vs. M0	NA (0 in cell)		NA (0 in cell)		NA (0 in cell)		NA (0 in cell)	0.993	NA (0 in cell)	
Tumor diameter										
>10 and ≤20 mm vs. ≤10 mm	1.84 (0.41–8.18)	0.422	2.80 (1.00–7.88)	0.051	0.78 (0.31–1.95)	0.592	1.84 (0.41–8.21)	0.422	1.75 (0.54–5.70)	0.351
>20 and ≤40 mm vs. ≤10 mm	NA (0 in cell)		2.10 (0.65–6.83)	0.217	1.31 (0.52–3.34)	0.568	0.72 (0.08–6.43)	0.766	0.38 (0.05–3.15)	0.370
>40 mm vs. ≤10 mm	NA (0 in cell)		NA (0 in cell)		NA (0 in cell)		NA (0 in cell)		NA (0 in cell)	
Papillary cancer histologic variant										
Follicular vs. Classic	1.24 (0.23–6.68)	0.805	1.02 (0.34–3.05)	0.969	1.24 (0.54–2.86)	0.618	0.44 (0.05–3.69)	0.447	0.95 (0.25–3.68)	0.941
Other ** aggressive vs. Classic	NA (0 in cell)		6.13 (0.80–46.91)	0.081	0.86 (0.09–8.63)	0.900	4.67 (0.43–50.91)	0.206	3.17 (0.30–33.37)	0.337
Other *** non-aggressive vs. Classic	2.27 (0.24–21.56)	0.476	0.68 (0.08–5.77)	0.725	1.29 (0.30–5.52)	0.728	NA (0 in cell)		1.19 (0.13–10.49)	0.877
Extrathyroidal extension										
Micro and gross vs. negative	1.31 (0.25–6.83)	0.748	1.09 (0.37–3.20)	0.875	1.45 (0.63–3.35)	0.385	1.11 (0.22–5.65)	0.897	0.68 (0.20–2.31)	0.537
Vascular invasion										
Yes vs. no	NA (0 in cell)		1.31 (0.27–6.50)	0.739	2.62 (0.72–9.53)	0.145	8.38 (1.76–39.80)	0.008	4.00 (0.94–17.10)	0.061
Margin status										
R1 vs. R0	NA (0 in cell)		0.65 (0.14–3.02)	0.583	0.85 (0.29–2.53)	0.772	0.92 (0.11–7.81)	0.938	0.50 (0.06–4.05)	0.516
ATA										
Low vs intermediate, high	1.01 (0.23–4.41)	0.985	0.62 (0.25–1.50)	0.287	1.05 (0.50–2.17)	0.906	0.72 (0.19–2.81)	0.639	1.55 (0.53–4.54)	0.421

Table 2. *Cont.*

Variable	p53, *n* = 156 (100%)		CHK2, *n* = 156 (100%)		*CHEK2* (FISH), *n* = 151 (100%)		*TP53* (FISH), *n* = 151 (100%)		Positive p53 with *TP53* Deletion (FISH)	
	Positive *n* = 8 (5.1%)		High Expression *n* = 23 (14.7%)		Deletion *n* = 44 (29.1%)		Deletion *n* = 7 (4.6%)		*n* = 15 out of 151 (9.9%)	
	OR (95% CI)	*p*	OR (95% CI)	*p*	OR (95% CI)	*p*	OR (95% CI)	*p*	OR (95% CI)	*p*
Response to therapy Excellent vs. others	NA (0 in cell)		0.28 (0.11–0.72)	0.009	0.85 (0.34–2.14)	0.731	1.63 (0.19–13.61)	0.653	0.33 (0.04–2.66)	0.300
Radioactive iodine (I-131) therapy Yes vs. no	0.66 (0.15–2.89)	0.581	2.12 (0.68–6.61)	0.197	0.72 (0.34–1.53)	0.391	3.48 (0.42–28.64)	0.247	1.15 (0.34–3.81)	0.824
Number of I-131 courses 2–9 courses vs. 0–1 course	2.75 (0.51–14.79)	0.239	0.70 (0.15–3.25)	0.646	2.16 (0.79–5.89)	0.134	0.92 (0.11–7.81)	0.938	2.02 (0.51–7.97)	0.317
Final follow-up NED vs. others	NA (0 in cell)		0.17 (0.05–0.62)	0.007	0.96 (0.24–3.88)	0.951	0.54 (0.06–4.82)	0.582	0.99 (0.12–8.42)	0.994
Follow-up recurrence Yes vs. no	NA (0 in cell)		1.47 (0.16–13.74)	0.738	NA (0 in cell)		NA (0 in cell)		NA (0 in cell)	
Death Yes vs. no	NA (0 in cell)		NA (0 in cell)		0.60 (0.07–5.51)	0.651	4.31 (0.43–43.20)	0.214	2.36 (0.25–22.58)	0.457

* N0a, one or more cytologically or histologically confirmed benign lymph nodes; N0b, no radiologic or clinical evidence of locoregional lymph node metastasis; N1a–N1b, metastasis to regional lymph nodes; **diffuse sclerosing (n = 3); tall cell variant (n = 1); *** oxyphilic, Warthin-like (n = 2); mixed variant (classic and follicular) (n = 5); R1-microscopically positive margin (resection); ATA, American Thyroid Association, determined according to the 8th edition of the American Joint Committee on Cancer/Union for International Cancer Control (tumor-node-metastasis) TNM staging system; NED, no evidence of disease.

3.1.2. Impact of *CHEK2* and *TP53* Gene Status, and p53 Expression on Clinicopathological Features, Treatment Response and Outcomes in PTC Patients with and without *CHEK2* Mutations

The relationships between clinicopathological features, response to treatment, and disease outcome in 151 patients with PTC (five patients were not included in the analysis due to degraded histopathological material) and *CHEK2* gene copy number, *TP53* gene copy number, and p53 expression together with *TP53* gene copy status are presented in Table 2. Positive p53 together with a *TP53* gene copy deletion was significantly associated with older patient age (≥55 years) at diagnosis ($p = 0.047$). A significant relationship was found between a *TP53* gene copy deletion and angioinvasion ($p = 0.008$). However, there was no significant relationship between *CHEK2* gene copy number, *TP53* gene copy number, and positive p53 together with a *TP53* gene copy deletion and clinicopathological features, response to treatment, and disease outcome.

3.1.3. Prognostically Favorable and Predictive Results Defined as Categories of Interest in Groups of PTC Patients with and without *CHEK2* Mutations

In the analyses described above, the associations between clinicopathological features (tumor diameter, papillary cancer histologic variant, vascular invasion, and age), response to therapy, and final follow-up and CHK2 expression, *TP53* gene copy number, p53 expression, and p53 expression together with *TP53* gene copy number were either statistically significant or borderline significant. These associations were further explored using Bayesian A/B testing (Table 3). Excellent response, NED in final follow-up, tumor size ≤10 mm (vs. >10 mm and ≤20 mm), and classic cancer subtype (vs. other aggressive subtypes) were ~1.4-fold, ~1.2-fold, ~1.4-fold, and ~1.1-fold higher, respectively, in patients with low CHK2 expression than in those with high CHK2 expression. In patients with no loss of a *TP53* gene copy and negative p53 together with no loss of a *TP53* gene copy, the absence of vascular invasion was ~1.4-fold and ~1.2-fold higher, respectively, than in patients with a *TP53* gene copy deletion and positive p53 together with a *TP53* gene copy deletion. In patients under 55 years of age, no loss of a *TP53* gene copy and negative p53 together with no loss of a *TP53* gene copy were observed ~2.0 and ~1.7 times more often, respectively.

3.1.4. Predictive Value of Clinicopathological Features, Treatment Response, and Outcome Correlations with CHK2, *TP53* Status, and p53 Expression in PTC Patients with and without *CHEK2* Mutations

For all tested relationships (Table S1), H0 and the hypothesis predicting an increased frequency of categories defined as "categories of interest" in patients with high CHK2 expression, *TP53* gene copy deletion, and positive p53 together with a *TP53* gene copy deletion, the probability of the posterior model was reduced and these hypotheses were not consistent with the data. A third hypothesis predicting a reduced excellent response (compared to H0), NED in final follow-up, tumor size ≤10 mm (compared with >10 mm and ≤20 mm), classic cancer subtype (compared with other aggressive tumors), absence of vascular invasion, and age <55 years in patients with higher CHK2 expression, *TP53* gene copy deletion, and positive p53 together with a *TP53* gene copy deletion was qualitatively consistent with the data. The prior probability model of 0.25 was increased in all models from ~2-fold for positive p53 together with deletion of a *TP53* gene copy and age, and ~4-fold for higher CHK2 expression, treatment response, deletion of a *TP53* gene copy, and vascular invasion. In summary, the analyses provided strong or moderate evidence supporting the alternative hypothesis (compared with H0) predicting a lower prevalence of excellent response, NED in final follow-up, tumor size ≤10 mm (compared with >10 mm and ≤20 mm), classic cancer subtype (compared with other aggressive) in patients with higher CHK2 expression, lower prevalence of absence of vascular invasion, and age <55 years, in patients with deletion of the *TP53* gene copy and positive p53 together with deletion of the *TP53* gene copy. The accumulated evidence was 17,031, 20,554, 4,766, and 4,646 times more likely to support the hypothesis that excellent response, NED in final follow-up, tumor size ≤10 mm, and classic cancer subtype, respectively, occur less frequently in patients with higher CHK2 expression. The evidence was also 18,553 and 5,713 times more likely to support the hypothesis that the absence of vascular invasion is less common in patients with a *TP53* gene copy deletion and positive p53 together with a *TP53* gene copy deletion, respectively. In patients with a *TP53* gene copy deletion and positive p53 together with a *TP53* gene copy deletion, the probability of being <55 years old was 4,280 and 4,962 times less likely than for patients without a *TP53* gene copy deletion and negative p53 together with no loss of *TP53* gene copy (Table S1).

Table 3. The prevalence of prognostically favorable and predictive results, defined as category of interest in groups of PTC patients with and without *CHEK2* germline mutations.

Group	Category of Interest	Counts	Total	Proportion
Response to therapy	Excellent			
Low CHK2		113	133	0.850
High CHK2		14	23	0.609
Final follow-up	NED			
Low CHK2		127	133	0.955
High CHK2		18	23	0.783
Tumor diameter	≤10 mm			
Low CHK2		84	108	0.788
High CHK2		10	18	0.556
Papillary cancer histologic variant	Classic			
Low CHK2		92	94	0.979
High CHK2		15	17	0.882
Age	<55 years			
No loss of *TP53*		94	142	0.662
Deletion of *TP53*		3	9	0.333
Vascular invasion	No			
No loss of *TP53*		134	142	0.944
Deletion of *TP53*		6	9	0.667
Age	<55 years			
Negative p53 + no loss of *TP53*		91	136	0.669
Positive p53 + Deletion of *TP53*		6	15	0.400
Vascular invasion	No			
Negative p53 + no loss of *TP53*		128	136	0.941
Positive p53 + Deletion of *TP53*		12	15	0.800

CHK2 loss/low/high, CHK2 loss/low/high expression as determined by IHC on tumor tissue; IHC, immunohistochemistry; no loss of *TP53*/deletion of *TP53*, no loss/deletion of gene copy in tumor tissue as determined by FISH; FISH, fluorescence in situ hybridization; NED, no evidence of disease.

3.1.5. Posterior Distribution of Odds Log Ratio for Clinicopathological Correlations with CHK2, *TP53* Status, and p53 Expression in PTC Patients with and without *CHEK2* Mutations

Based on the median posterior distribution of the log OR, we found that in patients with high CHK2 expression compared with patients with low CHK2 expression, the probabilities of an excellent response, NED in final follow-up, tumor size ≤10 mm, and classic cancer subtype were 0.34 to 1, 0.27 to 1, 0.43 to 1, and 0.34 to 1, respectively. In patients with a *TP53* gene copy deletion and positive p53 together with a *TP53* gene copy deletion, the probabilities of not having vascular invasion were 0.23 to 1 and 0.35 to 1, respectively, compared with patients without these features. The probabilities of being <55 years of age in patients with a *TP53* gene copy deletion and positive p53 together with a *TP53* gene copy deletion were 0.39 to 1 and 0.42 to 1, respectively, compared with patients without this feature (Figure S1).

3.1.6. Sequential Analysis of Clinicopathological Correlations with CHK2, *TP53* Status, and p53 Expression in PTC Tumors with and without *CHEK2* Mutations

All panel figures (Figure S2) indicated an increase in the likelihood of the alternative hypothesis predicting a reduced excellent response, NED in final follow-up, tumor size ≤10 mm, and classic cancer subtype in patients with higher CHK2 expression, lower absence of vascular invasion, and age <55 years in patients with *TP53* gene deletion and positive p53 together with *TP53* gene deletion.

3.1.7. Correlation of Germline *CHEK2* Mutation with p53 and CHK2 Expression, and *CHEK2* and *TP53* Gene Statuses in PTC Patients with and without *CHEK2* Mutations

Table 4 shows the association between the germline *CHEK2* mutation and p53 expression, CHK2 expression, *CHEK2* and *TP53* gene statuses, and p53 expression together with *TP53* gene status. The association between germline heterozygous truncating *CHEK2* mutation variants (1100delC, IVS2 + 1G > A, del5395) with a *CHEK2* gene copy deletion and positive p53 together with deletion of a *TP53* gene copy was statistically significant. The chance of finding the *CHEK2* gene copy deletion in patients with germline heterozygous truncating *CHEK2* mutation variants (1100delC, IVS2 + 1G > A, del5395) was 62- and 57-fold higher than in patients with the WT *CHEK2* or WT *CHEK2* and patients with the missense I157T mutation, respectively. The chance of finding positive p53 together with a *TP53* gene copy deletion in patients with germline heterozygous truncating *CHEK2* mutation variants (1100delC, IVS2 + 1G > A, del5395) was more than 3-fold higher than in patients with WT *CHEK2* and the missense I157T mutation combined. Other associations between germline *CHEK2* mutations and p53 expression, CHK2 expression, *CHEK2* gene copy status, p53 expression together with *TP53* gene copy status, and *TP53* gene copy status alone were not statistically significant.

Table 4. Relationships between the germline *CHEK2* mutation and p53 expression, CHK2 expression, *CHEK2* and *TP53* gene statuses, and p53 expression together with *TP53* gene status (FISH) in tumor tissues from PTC patients with and without *CHEK2* germline mutations.

Variable	*CHEK2* Truncating vs. WT		*CHEK2* Missense vs. WT		*CHEK2* Truncating vs. WT + Missense I157T	
	OR (95% CI)	*p*	OR (95% CI)	*p*	OR (95% CI)	*p*
p53 expression Positive vs. negative	0.42 (0.04–4.19)	0.459	1.17 (0.25–5.47)	0.845	0.35 (0.04–2.92)	0.331
CHK2 expression High vs. low	3.48 (0.99–12.30)	0.052	2.12 (0.61–7.33)	0.236	2.24 (0.90–5.58)	0.083
CHEK2 gene status Deletion vs. no loss of gene copy	62.67 (16.37–239.93)	<0.001	1.31 (0.35–4.91)	0.693	57.23 (19.36–169.24)	<0.001
TP53 gene status Deletion vs. no loss of gene copy	NA (0 in cell)		NA (0 in cell)		NA (0 in cell)	
p53 expression and *TP53* gene status Positive vs. negative and deletion vs. no loss of gene copy	3.47 (0.84–14.37)	0.087	1.17 (0.25–5.47)	0.845	3.33 (1.13–9.84)	0.029

Abbreviations: *CHEK2* truncating, germline heterozygous truncating *CHEK2* mutation variants (1100delC, IVS2 + 1G > A, del5395); WT, wild type.

3.1.8. The Incidence of Unfavorable Prognostic Factors Linked to *CHEK2* and *TP53* Gene Alterations, CHK2 and p53 Expression in PTC Patients with and without *CHEK2* Mutations

The analyses described above examined the associations between germline heterozygous truncating *CHEK2* mutation variants (1100delC, IVS2 + 1G > A, del5395) and *CHEK2* gene status, CHK2 expression, and p53 expression together with *TP53* gene status. We decided to examine further the associations that were significant or marginally significant. We tested the equality of following two binomial proportions: *CHEK2* gene copy deletion/no deletion; higher/lower CHK2 expression, and positive/negative p53 together with *TP53* gene copy deletion/no deletion in patients with *CHEK2* truncating mutations (1100delC, IVS2 + 1G > A, del5395), and in patients with WT *CHEK2* or WT *CHEK2* and the missense I157T mutation using the Bayesian A/B test. In the compared groups, categories of interest were defined as *CHEK2* gene copy deletion, higher CHK2 expression, and positive p53 together with a *TP53* gene copy deletion. The results are presented in Table 5. Among patients with germline heterozygous truncating *CHEK2* mutation variants (1100delC, IVS2 + 1G > A, del5395) the percentages of cases with a *CHEK2* gene copy deletion, higher CHK2 expression, and positive p53 together a *TP53* gene copy deletion were ~10-, ~3-, and ≈3-fold higher than in those with WT *CHEK2*, respectively. Among patients with germline heterozygous truncating *CHEK2* mutation variants (1100delC, IVS2 + 1G > A, del5395) and the missense I157T mutation, the percentages of cases with a *CHEK2* gene copy deletion, higher CHK2 expression, and positive p53 together with a *TP53* gene copy deletion were ~10-, ~2-, and ~3-fold higher, respectively, than in those with WT *CHEK2* or the missense I157T mutation (Table 5).

Table 5. The incidence of unfavorable prognostic factors, such as deletion of the *CHEK2* gene copy, higher CHK2 expression, and p53 expression together with deletion of the *TP53* gene copy by FISH, in tumor tissues from PTC patients with and without the *CHEK2* germline mutations.

Variable		***CHEK2* Truncating and WT**			***CHEK2* Truncating and WT + Missense I157T**		
	Group	**Counts**	**Total**	**Proportion**	**Counts**	**Total**	**Proportion**
CHEK2 deletion	No mutation	4	51	0.078	10	111	0.090
	Mutation	32	38	0.842	34	40	0.850
High expression of CHK2	No mutation	4	52	0.077	13	112	0.116
	Mutation	9	40	0.225	10	44	0.227
Positive p53 and *TP53* deletion	No mutation	3	51	0.059	7	111	0.063
	Mutation	7	38	0.184	8	40	0.200

Abbreviations: *TP53* deletion, deletion of a *TP53* gene copy in tumor tissue as determined by FISH; FISH, fluorescence in situ hybridization; positive p53, p53 expression as determined by IHC; IHC, immunohistochemistry; *CHEK2* truncating, germline heterozygous truncating *CHEK2* mutation variants (1100delC, IVS2 + 1G > A, del5395); WT, wild type.

3.1.9. Predictive Value of *CHEK2* and *TP53* Gene Status, CHK2 and p53 Expression in PTC Patients with WT and/or I157T *CHEK2* Mutations

Table S2 shows the predictive value of the three competing hypotheses. For H0 and the hypothesis predicting no *CHEK2* gene copy deletion, low CHK2 expression, and negative p53 together with no loss of *TP53* gene copy in patients with germline heterozygous *CHEK2* truncating mutations (1100delC, IVS2 + 1G > A, del5395) compared with those with WT *CHEK2* or WT *CHEK2* and those with the missense I157T mutation, posterior model probabilities were reduced (compared to prior model probabilities) and these hypotheses were not consistent with the data. The third hypothesis predicted higher probabilities of a *CHEK2* gene copy deletion, high CHK2 expression, and positive p53 together with deletion of the *TP53* gene copy in patients with heterozygous *CHEK2* truncating germline mutations (1100delC, IVS2 + 1G > A, del5395) than in those with WT *CHEK2* or WT *CHEK2* and those with the missense I157T mutation. The predictions were qualitatively consistent with the data; the a priori model probability of 0.25 was increased by more than 4-fold in both tested models for the *CHEK2* gene copy deletion, 2-fold in both models for high CHK2 expression, and 2- and 3-fold in models for positive p53 together with deletion of the *TP53* gene copy. To sum up, the analyses provided high or moderate evidence supporting the alternative hypothesis (compared with H0) predicting higher probabilities of a *CHEK2* gene copy deletion, high CHK2 expression, and positive p53 together with a *TP53* gene copy deletion in patients with the heterozygous *CHEK2* truncating germline mutation (1100delC, IVS2 + 1G > A, del5395) than in those with WT *CHEK2* or WT *CHEK2* and those with the I157T missense mutation, with the accumulated evidence showing that the alternative hypothesis (log OR > 0) would predict that these features are 1,781 $\times$ 10^{10}, 4,215, and 3,194 times more likely, respectively, in patients with *CHEK2* truncating germline mutations (1100delC, IVS2 + 1G > A, del5395) than in those with WT *CHEK2*. The evidence also showed that it was 1,054 $\times$ 10^{15}, 3,058, and 9,999 times more likely that the alternative hypothesis (log OR > 0) would predict that the *CHEK2* gene copy deletion, high CHK2 expression, and positive p53 with a *TP53* gene copy deletion, respectively, occurs more often in patients with heterozygous *CHEK2* truncating germline mutations (1100delC, IVS2 + 1G > A, del5395) than in those with WT *CHEK2* and the missense I157T mutation.

3.1.10. Posterior Odds Log Ratio Distribution for *CHEK2* and *TP53* Gene Status, CHK2 and p53 Expression in PTC Patients with and without *CHEK2* Mutations

Based on the median posterior distribution for the log OR, we found that the probability of a *CHEK2* gene copy deletion in patients with germline heterozygous *CHEK2* truncating mutations (1100delC, IVS2 + 1G > A, del5395) was ~22 to 1 and ~26 to 1, respectively, compared with patients with WT *CHEK2* and WT *CHEK2* with the missense I157T mutation. The probabilities of higher CHK2 and positive p53 in the presence of *TP53* gene copy deletion in patients with a *CHEK2* truncating germline mutation (1100delC, IVS2 + 1G > A, del5395) were ~2.5 to 1 and ~2 to 1, respectively, compared with patients with WT *CHEK2*, whereas the probabilities were ~2 to 1 and ~3 to 1 compared with patients with WT *CHEK2* and WT *CHEK2* with the missense I157T mutation, respectively (Figure S3).

3.1.11. Sequential Analysis of Associations Involving *CHEK2* and *TP53* Gene Status, CHK2 and p53 Expression in PTC Patients with and without *CHEK2* Mutations

Based on the sequential analysis, the obtained results were considered as a function of the total number of observations. The panels in Figure S4 depict two circles visualizing the prior and posterior probabilities of the tested hypotheses based on all available data. All the panels in the figures indicate an increase in the probability of the alternative hypothesis that *CHEK2* gene copy deletion, higher CHK2 expression, or positive p53 together with the *TP53* gene copy deletion occur more frequently in patients with a germline heterozygous *CHEK2* truncating mutation (1100delC, IVS2 + 1G > A, del5395) (Figure S4).

4. Discussion

Cell cycle checkpoints induced by DNA mutations play a key role in maintaining genome stability. Tumor suppressors associated with DNA damage responses and the regulation of cell cycle checkpoints include checkpoint kinase 2 (*CHEK2* gene, CHK2) and p53. Due to defects in the function of suppressor genes involved in the DNA repair pathway, genome instability and a predisposition to cancer development may occur [6, 36]. Depending on the nature of the damage, the type and function of the damaged cell, and other factors, CHK2 can phosphorylate over 20 different proteins involved in the regulation of cellular responses, including p53 and BRCA1 [37]. The association between germline mutations in the *CHEK2* gene and the development of various types of cancer, including PTC, has been reported in numerous case-control studies [20,38–46]. To date, the mechanism responsible for the increased CHK2 levels in PTC patients remains poorly understood. The data in this study identified CHK2 expression as an independent prognostic parameter of PTC. Patients expressing CHK2 had a 70% and 80% lower chance of an excellent response and NED, respectively, than patients not expressing or expressing lower amounts of CHK2. Tumor size, histological subtype of the cancer (features that were of borderline statistical significance), response to treatment, and final disease status (features that were statistically significant) were further explored using the Bayesian A/B test.

Excellent response to primary treatment, final follow-up NED, tumor size ≤ 10 mm (compared with >10 mm and ≤20 mm), and classic cancer type (compared with other aggressive subtypes) were from 10% to 40% higher in patients without CHK2 expression than in those with CHK2 expression. In a study by Zhao W et al. 2018 [10], it was found that CHK2 expression levels and phosphorylated CHK2 (p-CHK2) were significantly higher in most PTCs than in tumor-adjacent thyroid tissues. They also reported that high p-CHK2 expression, male sex, classical variant, stage N, and LN metastasis were associated with cancer aggressiveness. In the present study, we did not evaluate p-CHK2 expression. However, CHK2 expression in the study by Zhao W et al. 2018 correlated significantly and negatively with multifocality [10], but we were unable to evaluate this in the present study. Zhao W et al. 2018 also found that CHK2 and p-CHK2 expression were significantly downregulated in LN metastasis compared with matched primary PTC tumors and suggested that CHK2 levels may be negatively associated with circulating tumor cell survival and metastatic behavior [10]. In the current study, we also analyzed CHK2 expression in all 35 patients with LN metastasis, but found that CHK2 expression in LN metastasis tumors was not higher than that in matched primary tumors (Figure S5).

Similarly, increased CHK2 expression has been observed in other human malignancies, such as melanoma metastases, most cases of DLBCL [11], bladder cancer, and ovarian cancer [13]. However, other studies on the prognostic value of CHK2 expression revealed low CHK2 expression was associated with poor prognosis in 918 cases of gastric cancer. These differences in patient outcomes may be because CHK2 has multiple and diverse functions and interacts with a wide variety of key cancer genes, each of which can cause CHK2 overexpression under certain conditions [47,48].

The molecular database employed in the present study allowed us to examine the association between CHK2 expression and molecular features of interest. We selected patients with germline mutations in the *CHEK2* gene (truncating 1100delC, IVS2 + 1G > A, del5395, and missense I157T mutations) and patients without a mutation in the *CHEK2* gene (*CHEK2* WT). In our previous work, we showed that truncating mutations, but not missense mutations, in the *CHEK2* gene are significantly associated with angioinvasion and an intermediate or high initial risk of recurrent/persistent disease in PTC patients [21]; however, we did not evaluate CHK2 and p53 expression in tumor tissues. Therefore, in the current study, we performed IHC analysis of CHK2 and p53 expression in tumors to assess the value of the ATM/CHK2/p53 pathway as a prognostic marker. In addition, we used FISH to analyze for *CHEK2* and *TP53* copy number aberrations and correlate these aberrations with the course of PTC disease. Positive p53 expression together with *TP53* gene deletion was significantly associated with older (≥55 years) patient age at diagnosis. This can be attributed to the decrease in p53 pathway activity with age, which is associated with an increased mutation rate (due to impaired DNA repair) and mutation fixation (due to a decrease in p53-mediated apoptosis) in older people. The decline in p53 function with age may result in the accumulation of *TP53* mutations, which is probably why older people have lower rates of cell division fidelity, higher DNA replication error rates, and a higher incidence of cancer [49]. In this study, we found a significant association between angioinvasion and *TP53* gene copy deletion, but this association lost statistical significance when we examined the association between angioinvasion and positive p53 expression together with a *TP53* gene copy deletion. These associations were further explored using a Bayesian A/B test, where patients with no loss of a *TP53* gene copy together with negative p53 expression and patients with no loss of a *TP53* gene copy alone had a 20% to 40% lower prevalence of vascular invasion than patients with no loss of a *TP53* gene copy together with positive p53 expression and patients with a *TP53* gene copy deletion alone. So far, angioinvasion is thought to be associated with an unfavorable clinical course and poor prognosis, which has important consequences for cancer treatment [50]. Moreover, in accordance with the ATA Management Guidelines criteria, vascular invasion is a key feature that is absent from low-risk PTC patients [27]. Mutations in the *TP53* gene, in addition to poorly differentiated and anaplastic thyroid cancer, where such mutations occur most frequently, have also been found in some well-differentiated cancers, including PTC [51]. It is also likely that well-differentiated cancers with a *TP53* mutation are more inclined to undergo tumor dedifferentiation and result in a more aggressive clinical course [52].

To the best of our knowledge, no previous studies have assessed CHK2 and p53 expression by IHC and *CHEK2* and *TP53* gene statuses by FISH in a large group of PTC patients with germline mutations in the *CHEK2* gene. The only study to have evaluated patients with a germline *CHEK2* mutation in PTC patients was a paper by Zhao Y et al. [53], which reported a Chinese family with a germline *CHEK2* mutation c.417C > A. Molecular analysis showed that the 417C > A substitution created a premature stop codon (Y139X). Tumor tissue analysis showed that two patients with the loss-of-function Y139X variant exhibited lower mRNA expression of the mutant allele, lower CHK2 expression, and lower p53 and phosphorylated p53 expression than in patients with sporadic PTC (WT *CHEK2*). The molecular database employed in the present study comprised patients with truncating mutations (1100delC, IVS2 + 1G > A, and del5395) and a I157T missense mutation, but no patients with a nonsense mutation [53].

The association between CHK2 expression and mutation of the *CHEK2* gene was clear in patients with truncating mutations (1100delC, IVS2 + 1G > A, and del5395). In patients with *CHEK2* truncating mutations, one copy of the *CHEK2* gene remains intact (in the FISH method in this study, all detected deletions had only one damaged copy of the gene) while the other is truncated. The intact copy can synthesize a sufficient amount of CHK2, or in some cases produce larger amounts of CHK2 than cells with two normal copies of *CHEK2*. Complete loss of CHK2 function only occurs when the remaining intact copy is mutated or deleted, termed loss of heterozygosity, but we did not test for this in our study.

On the other hand, higher CHK2 expression may be due to impaired degradation of CHK2, the mechanism of which is not fully understood in cancer cells. It is possible that the ubiquitin-proteasome pathway was disturbed in the tumor cells. The ubiquitin-proteasome pathway is crucial for the expression and control of the activity of proteins involved in cell cycle regulation and the DNA damage response. It is known that interactions between proteins may change in response to DNA damage [54].

Increased expression of CHK2 may also be attributed to impaired ubiquitination caused by aberrations in p53. Bohgaki et al. demonstrated that, in mice, CHK2 phosphorylated at S460 (which corresponds to S456 in humans) undergoes ubiquitination that is facilitated by the p53-induced RING-H2 protein (PIRH2) and subsequent degradation by the proteasome [55].

Our study has several strengths. First, the study examined a large homogeneous group of Caucasian patients from one center in Poland. Second, to our knowledge, there have been no studies in the literature assessing CHK2 and p53 expression in a large number of PTC patients with a germline mutation in the *CHEK2* gene. Third, there have been no studies assessing the statuses of the *CHEK2* and *TP53* genes by FISH in patients with PTC.

Our study has some limitations. First, the study mainly included low-risk tumors (62.2%), with a high number of microcarcinomas ($\leq$1 cm, 60.3%), and this could have influenced the results. Second, the number of patients with advanced clinical disease was relatively small. Third, the follow-up period was short (7 years). Follow-up periods beyond 7 years could reveal more information about PTC-related recurrence or death and improve understanding of the roles of CHK2 and p53. Due to financial constraints, we were unable to examine the tumor tissues for phosphorylated CHK2 and p53 or sequence both genes (*CHEK2*, *TP53*) in the tumor tissues, which could have improved the risk stratification. It will be interesting to evaluate p-CHK2 and p53 expression and sequence both genes in future studies.

5. Conclusions

High CHK2 expression is associated with poor treatment response and outcomes in patients with PTC. Increased expression of CHK2 and positive p53 expression together with deletion of a *TP53* gene copy in patients with a truncating mutation in the *CHEK2* gene could have potential as a prognostic marker for an unfavorable disease course in this group of patients. Therefore, further studies will be required using larger patient groups with germline mutations, in particular those with a truncating mutation in the *CHEK2* gene, to assess whether patients with increased expression of CHK2 and p53 in cancer cells, especially their phosphorylated forms, require different treatment regimens or oncological follow-up protocols from those of patients with tumors that do not express these genes.

Supplementary Materials: The following supporting information can be downloaded at: https://www.mdpi.com/article/10.3390/cancers16040815/s1, Figure S1: Posterior distribution of the odds log ratio for the relationships between clinicopathological features and CHK2 expression, *TP53* gene status, and p53 expression together with *TP53* gene status in tumor tissues from PTC patients with and without *CHEK2* germline mutations; Figure S2: Sequential analysis for the relationships between clinicopathological features and CHK2 expression, *TP53* gene status, and p53 expression together with *TP53* gene status in the tumor tissues of PTC patients with and without *CHEK2* germline mutations; Figure S3: Posterior distribution of the odds log ratio for the association between *CHEK2* gene status, CHK2 expression, and the p53 expression together with *TP53* gene status in tumor tissues from PTC patients with and without the *CHEK2* germline mutations; Figure S4: Sequential analysis of the associations between *CHEK2* gene status, CHK2 expression as determined by IHC, and p53 expression together with *TP53* gene status as determined by FISH in tumor tissues from PTC patients with and without the *CHEK2* germline mutations; Figure S5: CHK2 expression levels in primary papillary thyroid cancer tissue and lymph node metastases; Table S1: Predictive values of the tested hypotheses for the relationships between clinicopathological features, treatment response, and disease outcome and level of CHK2 expression and *TP53* gene status, and p53 expression together with *TP53* status in tumor tissues from PTC patients with and without *CHEK2* germline mutations; Table S2: Predictive value of tested hypotheses for the association between *CHEK2* gene status, CHK2 expression, and p53 expression together with *TP53* gene status in PTC patients with and without the *CHEK2* germline mutations.

Author Contributions: Conceptualization, D.G.-P.; methodology, D.G.-P., A.K. (Artur Kowalik), J.K., O.W., P.M., K.G., K.N. and T.D.; software, P.M.; validation, M.K.; formal analysis, D.G.-P., A.K. (Artur Kowalik), P.M. and A.K. (Aldona Kowalska); investigation, D.G.-P.; resources, D.G.-P., P.P., M.S., A.W. and I.P.; data curation, D.G.-P. and A.K. (Aldona Kowalska); writing—original draft preparation, D.G.-P.; writing—review and editing, D.G.-P., A.K. (Artur Kowalik) and P.M.; visualization, D.G.-P. and P.P.; supervision, D.G.-P. and S.G.; project administration, D.G.-P.; funding acquisition, D.G.-P. and S.G. All authors have read and agreed to the published version of the manuscript.

Funding: This research was funded by grants from the Minister of Education and Science termed "Regional Initiative of Excellence" in the years 2019–2023 (project no. 024/RID/2018/19; amount of financing, 11,999,000.00 PLN).

Institutional Review Board Statement: This study was conducted according to the guidelines of the Declaration of Helsinki and approved by the Ethics Committee of the Institutional Review Board of Jan Kochanowski University, Kielce, Poland (approval number: 31/2021).

Informed Consent Statement: Informed consent was obtained from all subjects involved in the study.

Data Availability Statement: Data are available on reasonable request.

Conflicts of Interest: The authors declare no conflicts of interest.

References

1. Davies, L.; Welch, H.G. Increasing incidence of thyroid cancer in the United States, 1973–2002. *JAMA* **2006**, *295*, 2164–2167. [CrossRef]
2. Davies, L.; Welch, H.G. Current thyroid cancer trends in the United States. *JAMA Otolaryngol. Head Neck Surg.* **2014**, *140*, 317–322. [CrossRef] [PubMed]
3. Ahn, H.S.; Kim, H.J.; Welch, H.G. Korea's thyroid-cancer "epidemic"—Screening and overdiagnosis. *N. Engl. J. Med.* **2014**, *371*, 1765–1767. [CrossRef] [PubMed]
4. Carling, T.; Udelsman, R. Thyroid cancer. *Annu. Rev. Med.* **2014**, *65*, 125–137. [CrossRef]
5. Cady, B.; Rossi, R. An expanded view of risk-group definition in differentiated thyroid carcinoma. *Surgery* **1988**, *104*, 947–953.
6. Bartek, J.; Falck, J.; Lukas, J. CHK2 kinase—A busy messenger. *Nat. Rev. Mol. Cell. Biol.* **2001**, *2*, 877–886. [CrossRef] [PubMed]

7. Ahn, J.; Urist, M.; Prives, C. The Chk2 protein kinase. *DNA Repair* **2004**, *3*, 1039–1047. [CrossRef]
8. Bahassi, E.M.; Ovesen, J.L.; Riesenberg, A.L.; Bernstein, W.Z.; E Hasty, P.; Stambrook, P.J. The checkpoint kinases Chk1 and Chk2 regulate the functional associations between hBRCA2 and Rad51 in response to DNA damage. *Oncogene* **2008**, *27*, 3977–3985. [CrossRef]
9. Kauffmann, A.; Rosselli, F.; Lazar, V.; Winnepenninckx, V.; Mansuet-Lupo, A.; Dessen, P.; Oord, J.J.v.D.; Spatz, A.; Sarasin, A. High expression of DNA repair pathways is associated with metastasis in melanoma patients. *Oncogene* **2007**, *27*, 565–573. [CrossRef]
10. Zhao, W.; Chen, S.; Hou, X.; Chen, G.; Zhao, Y. CHK2 Promotes Anoikis and is Associated with the Progression of Papillary Thyroid Cancer. *Cell. Physiol. Biochem.* **2018**, *45*, 1590–1602. [CrossRef]
11. Dai, B.; Zhao, X.F.; Mazan-Mamczarz, K.; Hagner, P.; Corl, S.; Bahassi, E.M.; Lu, S.; Stambrook, P.J.; Shapiro, P.; Gartenhaus, R.B. Functional and molecular interactions between ERK and CHK2 in diffuse large B-cell lymphoma. *Nat. Commun.* **2011**, *2*, 402. [CrossRef]
12. Bartkova, J.; Guldberg, P.; Grønbæk, K.; Koed, K.; Primdahl, H.; Møller, K.; Lukas, J.; Ørntoft, T.F.; Bartek, J. Aberrations of the Chk2 tumour suppressor in advanced urinary bladder cancer. *Oncogene* **2004**, *23*, 8545–8551. [CrossRef]
13. Davidson, B.; Bjørnerem, M.; Holth, A.; Hellesylt, E.; Falkenthal, T.E.H.; Flørenes, V.A. Expression, activation and clinical relevance of CHK1 and CHK2 in metastatic high-grade serous carcinoma. *Gynecol. Oncol.* **2018**, *150*, 136–142. [CrossRef]
14. Barnoud, T.; Parris, J.L.D.; Murphy, M.E. Common genetic variants in the *TP53* pathway and their impact on cancer. *J. Mol. Cell. Biol.* **2019**, *11*, 578–585. [CrossRef]
15. Bell, D.W.; Varley, J.M.; Szydlo, T.E.; Kang, D.H.; Wahrer, D.C.R.; Shannon, K.E.; Lubratovich, M.; Verselis, S.J.; Isselbacher, K.J.; Fraumeni, J.F.; et al. Heterozygous Germ Line *hCHK2* Mutations in Li-Fraumeni Syndrome. *Science* **1999**, *286*, 2528–2531. [CrossRef]
16. Soussi, T. The p53 tumor suppressor gene: From molecular biology to clinical investigation. *Ann. N. Y. Acad. Sci.* **2000**, *910*, 121–137, discussion 137–139. [CrossRef]
17. Levine, A.J. p53, the cellular gatekeeper for growth and division. *Cell* **1997**, *88*, 323–331. [CrossRef]
18. Levine, A.J.; Momand, J.; Finlay, C.A. The p53 tumour suppressor gene. *Nature* **1991**, *351*, 453–456. [CrossRef] [PubMed]
19. el-Deiry, W.S.; Harper, J.W.; O'Connor, P.M.; Velculescu, V.E.; Canman, C.E.; Jackman, J.; Pietenpol, J.A.; Burrell, M.; Hill, D.E.; Wang, Y.; et al. WAF1/CIP1 is induced in p53-mediated G1 arrest and apoptosis. *Cancer Res.* **1994**, *54*, 1169–1174. [PubMed]
20. Siolek, M.; Cybulski, C.; Gąsior-Perczak, D.; Kowalik, A.; Kozak-Klonowska, B.; Kowalska, A.; Chłopek, M.; Kluźniak, W.; Wokołorczyk, D.; Pałyga, I.; et al. *CHEK2* mutations and the risk of papillary thyroid cancer. *Int. J. Cancer* **2015**, *137*, 548–552. [CrossRef] [PubMed]
21. Gasior-Perczak, D.; Kowalik, A.; Gruszczyński, K.; Walczyk, A.; Siołek, M.; Pałyga, I.; Trepka, S.; Mikina, E.; Trybek, T.; Kopczyński, J.; et al. Incidence of the *CHEK2* Germline Mutation and Its Impact on Clinicopathological Features, Treatment Responses, and Disease Course in Patients with Papillary Thyroid Carcinoma. *Cancers* **2021**, *13*, 470. [CrossRef]
22. Kaczmarek-Ryś, M.; Ziemnicka, K.; Hryhorowicz, S.T.; Górczak, K.; Hoppe-Gołębiewska, J.; Skrzypczak-Zielińska, M.; Tomys, M.; Gołąb, M.; Szkudlarek, M.; Budny, B.; et al. The c.470 T > C *CHEK2* missense variant increases the risk of differentiated thyroid carcinoma in the Great Poland population. *Hered. Cancer Clin. Pract.* **2015**, *13*, 8. [CrossRef] [PubMed]
23. Wójcicka, A.; Czetwertyńska, M.; Świerniak, M.; Długosińska, J.; Maciąg, M.; Czajka, A.; Dymecka, K.; Kubiak, A.; Kot, A.; Płoski, R.; et al. Variants in the *ATM-CHEK2-BRCA1* axis determine genetic predisposition and clinical presentation of papillary thyroid carcinoma. *Genes Chromosom. Cancer* **2014**, *53*, 516–523. [CrossRef] [PubMed]
24. The Cancer Genome Atlas Research Network. Integrated genomic characterization of papillary thyroid carcinoma. *Cell* **2014**, *159*, 676–690. [CrossRef]
25. R Core Team. (2020). R: A Language and Environment for Statistical Computing. Vienna, Austria: R Foundation for Statistical Computing. Available online: https://www.R-project.org/ (accessed on 30 January 2024).
26. Gąsior-Perczak, D.; Kowalik, A.; Walczyk, A.; Siołek, M.; Gruszczyński, K.; Pałyga, I.; Mikina, E.; Trybek, T.; Kopczyński, J.; Mężyk, R.; et al. Coexisting Germline *CHEK2* and Somatic BRAF(V600E) Mutations in Papillary Thyroid Cancer and Their Association with Clinicopathological Features and Disease Course. *Cancers* **2019**, *11*, 1744. [CrossRef]
27. Haugen, B.R.; Alexander, E.K.; Bible, K.C.; Doherty, G.M.; Mandel, S.J.; Nikiforov, Y.E.; Pacini, F.; Randolph, G.W.; Sawka, A.M.; Schlumberger, M.; et al. 2015 American Thyroid Association Management Guidelines for Adult Patients with Thyroid Nodules and Differentiated Thyroid Cancer: The American Thyroid Association Guidelines Task Force on Thyroid Nodules and Differentiated Thyroid Cancer. *Thyroid* **2016**, *26*, 1–133. [CrossRef] [PubMed]
28. Tuttle, M.L.; Morris, L.F.; Haugen, B.; Shah, J.; Sosa, J.A.; Rohren, E.; Subramaniam, R.M.; Hunt, J.L.; Perrier, N.D. *AJCC Cancer Staging Manual*; Springer: New York, NY, USA, 2017; Volume 8, pp. 1–19.
29. Gąsior-Perczak, D.; Pałyga, I.; Szymonek, M.; Kowalik, A.; Walczyk, A.; Kopczyński, J.; Lizis-Kolus, K.; Trybek, T.; Mikina, E.; Szyska-Skrobot, D.; et al. The impact of BMI on clinical progress, response to treatment, and disease course in patients with differentiated thyroid cancer. *PLOS ONE* **2018**, *13*, e0204668. [CrossRef]
30. Tuttle, R.M.; Tala, H.; Shah, J.; Leboeuf, R.; Ghossein, R.; Gonen, M.; Brokhin, M.; Omry, G.; Fagin, J.A.; Shaha, A. Estimating Risk of Recurrence in Differentiated Thyroid Cancer After Total Thyroidectomy and Radioactive Iodine Remnant Ablation: Using Response to Therapy Variables to Modify the Initial Risk Estimates Predicted by the New American Thyroid Association Staging System. *Thyroid®* **2010**, *20*, 1341–1349. [CrossRef]

31. Momesso, D.P.; Vaisman, F.; Yang, S.P.; Bulzico, D.A.; Corbo, R.; Vaisman, M.; Tuttle, R.M. Dynamic Risk Stratification in Patients with Differentiated Thyroid Cancer Treated Without Radioactive Iodine. *J. Clin. Endocrinol. Metab.* **2016**, *101*, 2692–2700. [CrossRef]
32. Kowalska, A.; Walczyk, A.; Pałyga, I.; Gąsior-Perczak, D.; Gadawska-Juszczyk, K.; Szymonek, M.; Trybek, T.; Lizis-Kolus, K.; Szyska-Skrobot, D.; Mikina, E.; et al. The Delayed Risk Stratification System in the Risk of Differentiated Thyroid Cancer Recurrence. *PLOS ONE* **2016**, *11*, e0153242. [CrossRef]
33. Gąsior-Perczak, D.; Pałyga, I.; Szymonek, M.; Kowalik, A.; Walczyk, A.; Kopczyński, J.; Lizis-Kolus, K.; Słuszniak, A.; Słuszniak, J.; Łopatyński, T.; et al. Delayed risk stratification system in pT1aN0/Nx DTC patients treated without radioactive iodine. *Endocr. Connect.* **2017**, *6*, 522–527. [CrossRef] [PubMed]
34. Li, C.; Bai, J.; Hao, X.; Zhang, S.; Hu, Y.; Zhang, X.; Yuan, W.; Hu, L.; Cheng, T.; Zetterberg, A.; et al. Multi-gene fluorescence in situ hybridization to detect cell cycle gene copy number aberrations in young breast cancer patients. *Cell Cycle* **2014**, *13*, 1299–1305. [CrossRef] [PubMed]
35. Lee, M.D.; Wagenmakers, E.J. *Bayesian Cognitive Modeling: A Practical Course*; Cambridge University Press: Cambridge, UK, 2013.
36. Stolarova, L.; Kleiblova, P.; Janatova, M.; Soukupova, J.; Zemankova, P.; Macurek, L.; Kleibl, Z. *CHEK2* Germline Variants in Cancer Predisposition: Stalemate Rather than Checkmate. *Cells* **2020**, *9*, 2675. [CrossRef] [PubMed]
37. Ertych, N.; Stolz, A.; Valerius, O.; Braus, G.H.; Bastians, H. *CHK2 – BRCA1* tumor-suppressor axis restrains oncogenic Aurora-A kinase to ensure proper mitotic microtubule assembly. *Proc. Natl. Acad. Sci. USA* **2016**, *113*, 1817–1822. [CrossRef] [PubMed]
38. Cybulski, C.; Górski, B.; Huzarski, T.; Masojć, B.; Mierzejewski, M.; Dębniak, T.; Teodorczyk, U.; Byrski, T.; Gronwald, J.; Matyjasik, J.; et al. *CHEK2* Is a Multiorgan Cancer Susceptibility Gene. *Am. J. Hum. Genet.* **2004**, *75*, 1131–1135. [CrossRef] [PubMed]
39. Cybulski, C.; Masojć, B.; Oszutowska, D.; Jaworowska, E.; Grodzki, T.; Waloszczyk, P.; Serwatowski, P.; Pankowski, J.; Huzarski, T.; Byrski, T.; et al. Constitutional *CHEK2* mutations are associated with a decreased risk of lung and laryngeal cancers. *Carcinog.* **2008**, *29*, 762–765. [CrossRef]
40. Brennan, P.; McKay, J.; Moore, L.; Zaridze, D.; Mukeria, A.; Szeszenia-Dabrowska, N.; Lissowska, J.; Rudnai, P.; Fabianova, E.; Mates, D.; et al. Uncommon *CHEK2* mis-sense variant and reduced risk of tobacco-related cancers: Case–control study. *Hum. Mol. Genet.* **2007**, *16*, 1794–1801. [CrossRef]
41. Szymanska-Pasternak, J.; Szymanska, A.; Medrek, K.; Imyanitov, E.; Cybulski, C.; Gorski, B.; Magnowski, P.; Dziuba, I.; Gugala, K.; Debniak, B.; et al. *CHEK2* variants predispose to benign, borderline and low-grade invasive ovarian tumors. *Gynecol. Oncol.* **2006**, *102*, 429–431. [CrossRef]
42. Wang, Y.; McKay, J.D.; Rafnar, T.; Wang, Z.; Timofeeva, M.N.; Broderick, P.; Zong, X.; Laplana, M.; Wei, Y.; Han, Y.; et al. Rare variants of large effect in BRCA2 and *CHEK2* affect risk of lung cancer. *Nat. Genet.* **2014**, *46*, 736–741. [CrossRef]
43. Rudd, M.F.; Sellick, G.S.; Webb, E.L.; Catovsky, D.; Houlston, R.S. Variants in the ATM-BRCA2-*CHEK2* axis predispose to chronic lymphocytic leukemia. *Blood* **2006**, *108*, 638–644. [CrossRef]
44. Złowocka, E.; Cybulski, C.; Górski, B.; Dębniak, T.; Słojewski, M.; Wokołorczyk, D.; Serrano-Fernández, P.; Matyjasik, J.; van de Wetering, T.; Sikorski, A.; et al. Germline mutations in the *CHEK2* kinase gene are associated with an increased risk of bladder cancer. *Int. J. Cancer* **2007**, *122*, 583–586. [CrossRef] [PubMed]
45. Teodorczyk, U.; Cybulski, C.; Wokołorczyk, D.; Jakubowska, A.; Starzyńska, T.; Ławniczak, M.; Domagała, P.; Ferenc, K.; Marlicz, K.; Banaszkiewicz, Z.; et al. The risk of gastric cancer in carriers of *CHEK2* mutations. *Fam. Cancer* **2013**, *12*, 473–478. [CrossRef] [PubMed]
46. Havranek, O.; Spacek, M.; Hubacek, P.; Mocikova, H.; Markova, J.; Trneny, M.; Kleibl, Z. Alterations of *CHEK2* forkhead-associated domain increase the risk of Hodgkin lymphoma. *Neoplasma* **2011**, *58*, 392–395. [CrossRef] [PubMed]
47. Abdel-Fatah, T.M.; Arora, A.; Alsubhi, N.; Agarwal, D.; Moseley, P.M.; Perry, C.; Doherty, R.; Chan, S.Y.; Green, A.R.; Rakha, E.; et al. Clinicopathological Significance of ATM-Chk2 Expression in Sporadic Breast Cancers: A Comprehensive Analysis in Large Cohorts. *Neoplasia* **2014**, *16*, 982–991. [CrossRef] [PubMed]
48. Eichenauer, T.; Federlein, F.; Möller, K.; Chirico, V.; Kind, S.; Lennartz, M.; Lutz, F.; Hube-Magg, C.; Höflmayer, D.; Fisch, M.; et al. High CHK2 protein expression is a strong and independent prognostic feature in ERG negative prostate cancer. *Pathology* **2020**, *52*, 421–430. [CrossRef]
49. Feng, Z.; Hu, W.; Teresky, A.K.; Hernando, E.; Cordon-Cardo, C.; Levine, A.J. Declining p53 function in the aging process: A possible mechanism for the increased tumor incidence in older populations. *Proc. Natl. Acad. Sci. USA* **2007**, *104*, 16633–16638. [CrossRef] [PubMed]
50. Cipriani, N.A. Prognostic Parameters in Differentiated Thyroid Carcinomas. *Surg. Pathol. Clin.* **2019**, *12*, 883–900. [CrossRef]
51. Nikiforova, M.N.; Wald, A.I.; Roy, S.; Durso, M.B.; Nikiforov, Y.E. Targeted Next-Generation Sequencing Panel (ThyroSeq) for Detection of Mutations in Thyroid Cancer. *J. Clin. Endocrinol. Metab.* **2013**, *98*, E1852–E1860. [CrossRef]
52. Hsiao, S.J.; Nikiforov, Y.E. Molecular approaches to thyroid cancer diagnosis. *Endocr. Relat. Cancer* **2014**, *21*, T301–T313. [CrossRef]
53. Zhao, Y.; Yu, T.; Chen, L.; Xie, D.; Wang, F.; Fu, L.; Cheng, C.; Li, Y.; Zhu, X.; Miao, G. A Germline *CHEK2* Mutation in a Family with Papillary Thyroid Cancer. *Thyroid®* **2020**, *30*, 924–930. [CrossRef] [PubMed]

54. García-Limones, C.; Lara-Chica, M.; Jiménez-Jiménez, C.; Pérez, M.; Moreno, P.; Muñoz, E.; A Calzado, M. CHK2 stability is regulated by the E3 ubiquitin ligase SIAH2. *Oncogene* **2016**, *35*, 4289–4301. [CrossRef] [PubMed]
55. Bohgaki, M.; Hakem, A.; Halaby, M.J.; Bohgaki, T.; Li, Q.; A Bissey, P.; Shloush, J.; Kislinger, T.; Sanchez, O.; Sheng, Y.; et al. The E3 ligase PIRH2 polyubiquitylates CHK2 and regulates its turnover. *Cell Death Differ.* **2013**, *20*, 812–822. [CrossRef] [PubMed]

cancers

MDPI

Article

Differentiating Benign from Malignant Thyroid Tumors by Kinase Activity Profiling and Dabrafenib BRAF V600E Targeting

Riet Hilhorst [1], Adrienne van den Berg [1], Piet Boender [1], Tom van Wezel [2], Tim Kievits [1,†], Rik de Wijn [1], Rob Ruijtenbeek [1,‡], Willem E. Corver [2,*] and Hans Morreau [2]

1 PamGene International BV, 5211 HH 's-Hertogenbosch, The Netherlands; rhilhorst@pamgene.com (R.H.)
2 Leiden University Medical Center, 2333 ZA Leiden, The Netherlands; j.morreau@lumc.nl (H.M.)
* Correspondence: w.e.corver@lumc.nl
† Current address: Precision Medicine Lab, 5349 AE Oss, The Netherlands.
‡ Current address: GenMab, 3584 CT Utrecht, The Netherlands.

Simple Summary: Recurrent non-medullary thyroid cancer (NMTC) is difficult to treat and therapy options are limited. Of the available compounds, serine/threonine kinase (STK) inhibitors are currently widely used. However, this form of targeted therapy is not always effective and additional response-related biological information may improve both accuracy and efficacy. Using in-depth STK activity profiling, in this study, we aimed to determine whether benign and malignant thyroid tumors can be differentiated based on these profiles. In addition, we analyzed the impact of the BRAF V600E-specific inhibitor dabrafenib, as well as the generic RAF inhibitors sorafenib and regorafenib, in a subgroup of BRAF V600E and non-BRAF V600E papillary thyroid carcinomas. We demonstrate that STK activity profiling can differentiate benign from malignant thyroid tumors. Furthermore, the BRAF V600E-specific inhibitor dabrafenib can distinguish BRAF V600E from non-BRAF V600E papillary thyroid carcinomas. We conclude that STK activity profiling is beneficial when the goal is to differentiate benign from malignant thyroid tumors. In addition, this approach aids in the selection of likely effective (novel) kinase inhibitors for treatment of recurrent thyroid and other cancers.

Abstract: Differentiated non-medullary thyroid cancer (NMTC) can be effectively treated by surgery followed by radioactive iodide therapy. However, a small subset of patients shows recurrence due to a loss of iodide transport, a phenotype frequently associated with BRAF V600E mutations. In theory, this should enable the use of existing targeted therapies specifically designed for BRAF V600E mutations. However, in practice, generic or specific drugs aimed at molecular targets identified by next generation sequencing (NGS) are not always beneficial. Detailed kinase profiling may provide additional information to help improve therapy success rates. In this study, we therefore investigated whether serine/threonine kinase (STK) activity profiling can accurately classify benign thyroid lesions and NMTC. We also determined whether dabrafenib (BRAF V600E-specific inhibitor), as well as sorafenib and regorafenib (RAF inhibitors), can differentiate BRAF V600E from non-BRAF V600E thyroid tumors. Using 21 benign and 34 malignant frozen thyroid tumor samples, we analyzed serine/threonine kinase activity using PamChip®peptide microarrays. An STK kinase activity classifier successfully differentiated malignant (26/34; 76%) from benign tumors (16/21; 76%). Of the kinases analyzed, PKC (theta) and PKD1 in particular, showed differential activity in benign and malignant tumors, while oncocytic neoplasia or Graves' disease contributed to erroneous classifications. Ex vivo BRAF V600E-specific dabrafenib kinase inhibition identified 6/92 analyzed peptides, capable of differentiating BRAF V600E-mutant from non-BRAF V600E papillary thyroid cancers (PTCs), an effect not seen with the generic inhibitors sorafenib and regorafenib. In conclusion, STK activity profiling differentiates benign from malignant thyroid tumors and generates unbiased hypotheses regarding differentially active kinases. This approach can serve as a model to select novel kinase inhibitors based on tissue analysis of recurrent thyroid and other cancers.

Keywords: thyroid; *BRAF* mutation; dabrafenib; kinase activity profiling; peptide microarray

1. Introduction

Non-medullary thyroid cancer (NMTC) accounts for 97% of all thyroid cancers and is the most common endocrine cancer worldwide. NMTC is currently the ninth most frequent cancer worldwide, with over a half million new cases annually, notably in Asia (GLOBOCAN 2020: http://globocan.iarc.fr/Pages/factsheetspopulation.aspx (accessed on 19 January 2023)).

Several types of thyroid lesions can be distinguished using routine microscopic examination. Benign thyroid lesions are typically classified as hyperplasia (HP), follicular adenoma (FA) or oncocytic adenoma (OA) [1,2]. Among the NMTCs, papillary thyroid cancer (PTC) and follicular thyroid cancer (FTC) are the most common. PTC and FTC comprise approximately 81% and 12% of all NMTC, respectively, which include variants of PTC. Oncocytic carcinoma of the thyroid (OCA) [2] (previously known as Hürthle cell carcinoma (HCC) or oncocytic variant of follicular thyroid carcinoma (FTC-OV)) [3,4] comprises around 3–4% of all NMTC and has been recognized by the WHO as a distinct subvariant. Anaplastic thyroid carcinoma (ATC) is the most aggressive form but accounts for less than 1% of all NMTC [5,6]. Well-differentiated NMTC can be curatively treated by surgery, with or without adjuvant radioactive iodide therapy. However, a subset of patients shows recurrence due to a loss of sodium iodide transport [7], with two forms primarily seen: OCA and PTC with the *BRAF* V600E variant.

Recurrent OCA is mainly characterized by a near-homozygous genome [3] and diverse DNA variants with or without mitochondrial DNA mutations [4,8,9], while recurrent PTC is typically associated with somatic *BRAF* V600E mutations (with increased frequencies of *hTERT* alterations) or gene fusions involving *ALK* or *NTRK*. The involvement of individual signaling pathways in recurrent iodide refractory thyroid cancer cases increases therapeutic options, such as the increasingly used VEGF pathway inhibitors. Another example is the serine/threonine protein kinase BRAF, a component of the MAPK signaling pathway [10]. Several drugs have been developed that interact with the serine/threonine kinase activity of BRAF or the BRAF V600E variant. The multi-kinase inhibitor sorafenib has been proven to be beneficial in the treatment of recurrent NMTC, despite its low affinity for BRAF V600E [11,12]. Furthermore, vemurafenib and dabrafenib were specifically designed to target this mutant and are effective against BRAF V600E-positive thyroid cancer [13,14]. Both inhibitors stimulate radioactive iodide uptake [15,16], and the results of a phase I trial in *BRAF* V600E-positive cancers have been published recently [17–19].

Next generation sequencing (NGS) revolutionized the detection of genetic variants suitable for targeted therapy, and has become an indispensable tool in daily diagnostic settings. While targeted therapy is often beneficial, it is also clear that is it is not a panacea.

Additional tools to better characterize tumors and improve understanding of underlying molecular biology might also be helpful. We propose that serine/threonine kinase (STK) activity profiling could be a rich source of biological information.

The aim of this study was therefore two-fold. First, we asked whether benign thyroid abnormalities and NMTC can be classified based on STK activity profiles, and whether these profiles can provide new insights concerning the differential activity of kinases between groups. Second, we investigated whether the BRAF V600E-specific inhibitor dabrafenib, as well as the RAF inhibitors sorafenib and regorafenib, induce differences in kinase inhibition between BRAF V600E and non-BRAF V600E thyroid tumors, and between recurrent and non-recurrent tumors. In order to address the first question, we used peptide microarrays to measure STK activity in lysates from 55 primary clinical tissue samples from benign and malignant thyroid tumors [20]. We demonstrate that STK activity profiling correctly differentiates benign and malignant thyroid tumors in 76% of cases. We also identified putative upstream kinases that are differentially active in benign and malignant tumors.

Ex vivo spiking of PTC thyroid tumor lysates with the specific kinase inhibitor dabrafenib achieved partial differential inhibition of somatic *BRAF* V600E-positive versus non-*BRAF* V600E thyroid tumors and of recurrent versus non-recurrent tumors, which was not the case with regorafenib and sorafenib.

2. Materials and Methods

2.1. Patient Material

Patient material was processed immediately after surgery. A piece of fresh tumor was cut in half, one part was snap frozen and the second part was formalin-fixed and paraffin-embedded (FFPE). From the FFPE blocks and the fresh frozen tissue, 4 μm sections were cut and hematoxylin/eosin stained. An experienced pathologist (HM) performed morphological evaluation on both FFPE and fresh frozen tissue sections (see Supplementary Table S1 for histology). All samples were processed in concurrence with the medical ethical guidelines as described in the Code Proper Secondary Use of Human Tissue (Dutch Federation of Medical Sciences, www.federa.org (accessed on 28 November 2022)). That Code has a system of 'opt-out' for further use in scientific research of coded human tissue, unless there are special circumstances. The current study, including the used 'opt-out' policy, was approved by the Medical Ethical Committee of the Leiden University Medical Centre, protocol no. B16.012.

2.2. Nucleic Acid Isolation, DNA Variant, and Fusion Analysis

Isolation of total nucleic acids was performed as described earlier [21]. In short, total nucleic acid (DNA and RNA) was isolated from 0.6 mm FFPE tissue cores (tissue microarrayer, Estigen OÜ, Tartu, Estonia) using a fully automated extraction procedure [22]. DNA variant analysis (e.g., *BRAF*, *NRAS*, *HRAS*, and *KRAS*) was performed using either a customized AmpliSeq Cancer Hotspot Panel or with Sanger sequencing, depending on the time period as previously described [3,23]. Additional *TERT* promoter variant (NM_198253.2; c.-57A>C, c.-124C>T, and c.-146C>T) analysis was performed by Sanger sequencing. The 8 non-tested HP cases did not significantly differ based on age of onset, gender, histological subtype, and genetic alterations distribution from 47 tested cases (Supplementary Table S1). Gene fusion analysis was performed as described earlier [21] on selected DNA-variant negative cases. Data analysis was performed using the online Archer Analysis software version 5.0 (http://analysis.archerdx.com (accessed on 4 September 2023)). Only 'strong-evidence' fusions within the software annotation were reported. Furthermore, *BRAF*/*RAS* point mutations were reported based on DNA/RNA reads. The total number of reads and the fractions of unique reads/RNA reads were documented for all samples as possible quality indicators.

Allelic state analysis, providing chromosomal copy number and loss of heterozygosity information, was performed as described earlier [24].

2.3. Materials

Mammalian Protein Extraction Reagent (M-PER^{TM}, Cat. No. 78503), Halt^{TM} protease inhibitor cocktail EDTA free (Cat. No. 78437), and Halt^{TM} phosphatase inhibitor cocktail (Cat. No. 78420) were from ThermoFisher Scientific (Waltham, MA, USA). Dabrafenib (GSK2118436, Cat. No. S2807), regorafenib hydrochloride (Cat. No. S4947), and sorafenib tosylate (BAY 43-9006, Cat. No. S1040) were from SelleckChem (Houston, TX, USA). Stock solutions were prepared in 100% DMSO and stored at −20 °C prior to use.

Protein serine/threonine kinase peptide microarrays and reagents were obtained from PamGene International BV ('s-Hertogenbosch, The Netherlands). The PamChip® peptide microarrays used for this study contained either 240 or 140 substrate peptides. Experiments were performed with 96-array plates on a PamStation 96^{TM}.

2.4. Preparation of Lysates

Cryo-sections of 10 μm thickness were cut (Leica Frigocut, 2800E, Wetzlar, Germany), collected in a pre-cooled (−20 °C) polypropylene tube, and stored at −80 °C until further use.

The 10 μm sections were lysed in M-PER lysis buffer (100 μL in the first lysis batch (55 samples), 20 μL in second and third lysis batches (PCTs only)), supplemented with protease and phosphatase inhibitor cocktail (1/100 diluted) as described by Hilhorst et al. [20]. The supernatants were aliquoted and stored at −80 °C until use. For every experiment, a new aliquot was used. The protein content of the lysates was determined with the Bradford protein assay (Bio-Rad, Hercules, CA, USA).

2.5. Kinase Activity Assays

For 55 thyroid samples, kinase activity was determined at 30 °C with 10 μL of lysate in the presence of both primary and secondary antibodies on 96-array plates in the presence or absence of 400 μM ATP (Sigma, Cat. No. A2383, St. Louis, MO, USA) on a peptide microarray with 240 peptides, as described by Hilhorst et al. [20]. Benign and malignant samples were equally distributed over the plates. Each sample was tested in duplicate with ATP and once without ATP on a 96-array plate. For each sample, this test was repeated on a second plate, in an independent experiment. Incubations without ATP were performed to correct for non-specific binding of proteins or antibodies to peptides.

For 13 samples, i.e., 10 PTC and 3 FVPTC (Th-50, Th-52, and Th-53), the effect of kinase inhibitors on STK activity was additionally determined using 0.5 μg of protein and 100 μM of ATP on 96-array plates comprising 140 peptides per array, in the presence of primary antibodies (PamGene International BV, 's-Hertogenbosch, The Netherlands), followed by visualization of the signal for 60 min with FITC labeled secondary antibody (PamGene International BV, 's-Hertogenbosch, The Netherlands), after washing of the arrays. Incubations were either without inhibitor or in the presence of regorafenib ($n = 3$), sorafenib ($n = 3$) or dabrafenib ($n = 3$). In the experimental design, incubations without and with inhibitor were performed on adjacent arrays on the same strip on 96-array plates (each 96-array plate comprises 24 strips). Final concentrations of regorafenib, sorafenib, and dabrafenib were 50, 10, and 10 μM, respectively. Concentrations were chosen to yield 25% to 50% inhibition of the basal profiles, since these concentrations have proven to be most discriminative. Final DMSO content in the assays was 0.5%.

2.6. Data Quantification

After a visual check of all arrays and grids for correct spot finding, signals for each peptide at multiple CCD exposure times were quantified with BioNavigator version 6.3.67 software (PamGene International BV, 's-Hertogenbosch, The Netherlands). For each spot on the array, signal intensity after subtraction of local background was used for further analysis. All data processing, statistical analyses, and visualizations were performed using BioNavigator version 6.3.67 software (PamGene International BV, 's-Hertogenbosch, The Netherlands).

Signals measured at the end of the incubation were used for analysis. Signals from multiple exposure times were integrated into one value. For the 55 basal profiles, signal intensity was corrected for the signals in the absence of ATP on that 96-array plate and averaged, followed by ^{2}log transformation and normalization per 96-array plate to correct for systematic differences between different 96-array plates. After this step, values for replicates obtained on different 96-array plates, were averaged. Only peptides that showed an ATP-dependent signal and an increase in signal intensity in >30% of the arrays with ATP were included in the analysis, resulting in 123 peptides.

For the analysis of the measurements with inhibitors, the same peptide selection was used. Ninety-two of these were present on the 140 peptide arrays used for these experiments. For these samples, an inhibition ratio (log fold change, LFC) was calculated for each peptide by subtracting the ^{2}log value without inhibitor from the ^{2}log value with inhibitor for the incubations on the same strip. The LFC values of the technical replicates were averaged. The value is equal to zero for peptides for which no changes occur, and <0 for peptides for which inhibition of the relevant kinase activity occurs in the presence of inhibitor.

2.7. Classification of Benign and Malignant Samples

Based on the basal profiles of the 55 samples, a class prediction model was built in MATLAB using partial least squares discriminant analysis (PLS-DA) [25] without prior selection of discriminative peptides; coefficients assigned to the peptides reflect the individual contribution of a peptide to the classification model. The performance of the class prediction model was estimated by leave-one-out-cross-validation (LOOCV), ensuring that for each iteration of the cross validation, the model was built independent of the left out sample [26]. Application of this class prediction model to the left out sample results in a prediction score, where prediction score >0 means that the sample is predicted to be benign, and with prediction score <0, the sample is predicted to be malignant. A permutation test was run in which the full 10-fold cross validation procedure was repeated 500 times, but with the 'benign' and 'malignant' class labels randomly re-assigned to the samples. A detailed description of the method is given in Supplementary Information by Arni et al. [27].

2.8. Statistical Analysis

The two-sample two-tailed Student's *t*-test was used to compare signal intensities per peptide for two group comparisons. The false discovery rate (FDR) was calculated with the Benjamini–Hochberg correction for multiple testing [28]. The statistical analysis was performed with Bionavigator version 6.3.67 software (PamGene International BV).

2.9. Upstream Kinase Analysis

In upstream kinase analysis, the phosphorylation changes in peptides on the peptide microarray between two groups are compared and linked to kinases that are known to phosphorylate these sites using several databases and theoretical interactions (PhosphoNet), as described by Chirumamilla et al. [29]. As the peptide sequences on the peptide microarray may be present in multiple proteins, the peptide sequences were blasted in UniProt against human proteins using the PAM30 substitution matrix [30]. Similarity was defined as the ratio of the PAM30 score for a retrieved sequence and the original sequence. Peptides with a similarity score equal to 1 were included. The upstream kinase algorithm provides a list of kinases that might be differentially active between the two groups as described by the kinase statistic, indicating the size and direction of the change, and the kinase score. The ranking of the kinases is based on the kinase score, resulting from the addition of mean significance score and mean specificity score. The mean significance score gives the significance of the change represented by the normalized kinase statistic (direction and size of change in signal) between two groups (using 500 permutations across sample labels), whereas the mean specificity score indicates the specificity of the mean kinase statistic with respect to the number of peptides used for predicting the corresponding kinase (using 500 permutations across target peptides) [29]. The predicted kinases were projected on a phylogenetic tree of the human protein kinase family (courtesy Cell Signaling Technologies, Danvers, MA, USA), using CORAL (http://phanstiel-lab.med.unc.edu/CORAL/ (accessed on 16 January 2023)) [31]. Branch and node color reflect the kinase statistic, node size, and kinase score.

2.10. Network Analysis

Protein Atlas (https://www.proteinatlas.org (accessed on 18 January 2023)) was used to check the mRNA and protein presence in both normal and malignant thyroid tissues for the 40 kinases with the highest kinase score. Kinases with a low RNA or protein presence in normal and tumor tissues were excluded, resulting in 29 kinases to build the network. STRING v12.0 (https://string-db.org (accessed on 19 January 2023)) was used to create networks.

3. Results

3.1. Patient Characteristics

Fifty-five thyroid samples, collected between 2001 and 2010, were included in the study. Histological classifications determined on FFPE sections were confirmed using sections of fresh frozen material. One case (Th-46) judged FVPTC based on the FFPE section, but HP (with Graves' disease) was based on the fresh frozen section. Since the current work used fresh frozen material, this sample was considered benign. Twenty-one cases were classified as benign, i.e., hyperplasia (HP), follicular adenoma (FA) or oncocytic adenoma (OA), while thirty-four cases were classified as malignant with various histology (Figure 1A).

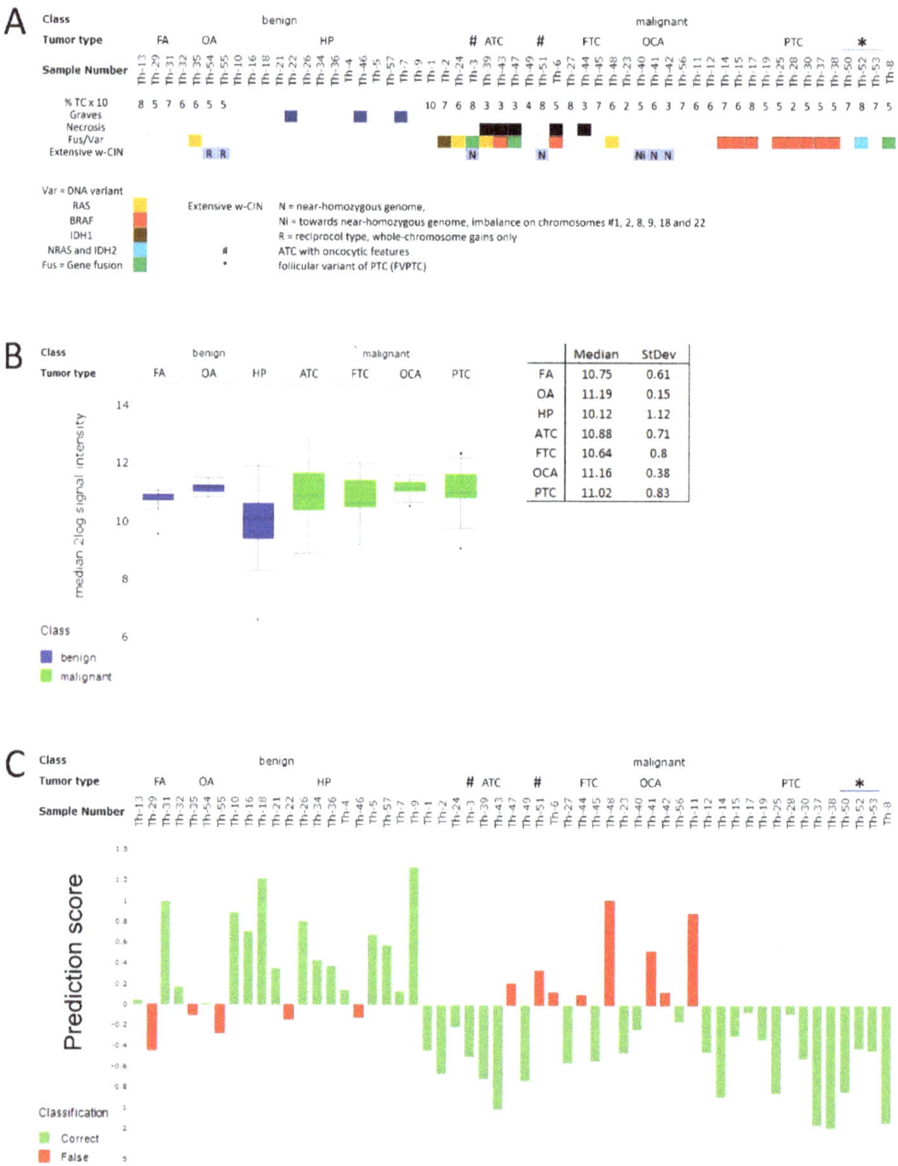

Figure 1. Synopsis of patient cohort and serine/threonine kinase activity profiles and classification of thyroid tumors. (**A**) Benign and malignant thyroid tumor samples of this study were arranged by histological subtype based on the evaluation of formalin-fixed, paraffin-embedded HE sections. Percentage tumor cells (% TC), whether it concerned a patient with Graves' disease, presence of necrosis,

a fusion or DNA variant (Fus/Var), and extensive whole chromosome instability (w CIN) were annotated: the near-homozygous genome type (N) or the reciprocal type (R) [32,33]. (**B**) Box plot showing the median ^{2}log signal intensity and upper and lower quartiles per sample (median value of 123 peptides), grouped per tumor type. Note the relatively low activity in HP compared to FA, OA, and thyroid cancers (ATC, FTC, OCA, and PTC). The median activity in HP is significantly lower than in ATC, OCA, and PTC (p-values 0.008, 0.021, and 0.001, respectively). (**C**) Classification of benign or malignant thyroid tumor samples using a PLS-DA classifier and Leave-One-Out-Cross-Validation. Samples are colored by their classification. The prediction score indicates their classification. A positive value for the prediction score implies a benign tumor, a negative value a malignant tumor. Eight malignant tumors were misclassified as benign, whereas five benign samples were misclassified as malignant. FA: follicular adenoma; HP: hyperplasia; OA: oncocytic adenoma; ATC: anaplastic thyroid carcinoma; FTC: follicular thyroid carcinoma; OCA: oncocytic carcinoma of the thyroid; PTC: papillary thyroid carcinoma. * FVPTC subtype, # Oncocytic features.

In summary, the following genetic alterations were found:

OA (1/3) NRAS Q61R, FTC (1/4) NRAS Q61R, FVPTC (1/3) NRAS Q61R and IDH2 I170T, PTC (8/12) BRAF V600E and ATC (2/10) BRAF V600E, ATC (1/10) HRAS G13R, ATC (1/10) NRAS Q61R, ATC (1/10) IDH1 Q185R, ATC (1/10) fusion HSPA8 (e9)—MET (i3-e4) and ATC (1/10) IDH1 q185r, AQP4 (e1)—RAF1 (i8-e9); FGFR3 (e17-i17)—LCN2 (e7). In three ATC, of which one showed oncocytic characteristics, no genetic alterations were detected. This was also the case for FA (four cases) and OCA (five cases), using targeted sequencing for RAS, RAF, and PIK3CA (Figure 1A).

Seven out of ten lesions with oncocytic characteristics showed extensive whole-chromosome copy number changes, ranging from massive gains (Th-54 and Th-55, OA) to whole-chromosome losses (Th-40, Th-41, Th-42 (OCA), Th-3, and Th-51 (ATC)). Th-35 showed loss of chromosome 22 (Figure 1A). These findings have been reported previously [32]. Relevant clinical and other detailed information, histology, and molecular typing can be found in Supplementary Table S1.

3.2. Kinase Activity Profiling Classifies Benign and Malignant Thyroid Tumors

Aberrant kinase activity is frequently observed in thyroid tumors, suggesting to us that kinase activity might be able to differentiate aggressive from benign tumors. STK activity was therefore determined in 55 samples, as described in Materials and Methods. HP showed a lower overall STK activity (Figure 1B and Supplementary Figure S1) compared with various tumor types, and was significantly lower than ATC ($p = 0.008$), PTC ($p = 0.001$), and OCA ($p = 0.02$). The activity found in other benign tumor types (FA, OA) more closely resembled thyroid cancer (Supplementary Table S2).

Statistical analysis (Student's t-test) revealed a signal intensity for 82 peptides that was significantly ($p < 0.05$, FDR 8%) different between benign and malignant samples, but a full separation between the benign and malignant groups was not observed using principal component analysis (PCA). While basal signals showed many intra-group commonalities, subtle differences were also observed (see heatmap in Supplementary Figure S1A).

A class prediction model was built using partial least squares discriminant analysis (PLS-DA), while leave-one-out-cross-validation (LOOCV) was used to classify samples and evaluate classification performance.

The model correctly classified 26 of 34 (76%) malignant and 16 of 21 (76%) benign samples (Figure 1C). Of the thirty-four malignant lesions, eight (3/10 ATCs, 2/4 FTCs, 2/5 OCAs, 1/12 PTCs, and 0/3 FVPTCs) were misclassified, with prediction scores ranging between 0.096 and 1.005. Prediction scores for the correctly classified malignant samples ranged from −1.190 to −0.070 (see Supplementary Table S1 for details). Of the twenty-one benign lesions, five samples (1/4 FA, 2/3 OCA, and 2/14 HP) were misclassified, with prediction scores between −0.103 and −0.442. The correctly classified samples had prediction scores ranging from 0.010 to 1.326.

In addition, 5/10 oncocytic lesions were misclassified, of which four showed extensive chromosomal copy number changes.

The classification accuracy for all samples was 76%, the positive predictive value (PPV) was 72%, and the negative predictive value (NPV) was 87%. A permutation test, where the labels 'benign' and 'malignant' were repeatedly randomly assigned to the samples, gave a misclassification rate of less than 30% in less than 1% of the permutations. This shows that the obtained classifier has a significant prediction performance ($p < 0.01$).

3.3. Molecular Interpretation of Differences between Benign and Malignant Samples

We found that STK activity is increased in malignant tumors (Figure 1B and Supplementary Figure S1A,B), and using upstream kinase analysis, we identified kinases that are potentially responsible for the differences in peptide phosphorylation between benign and malignant tumors. When the kinases were assigned to a kinome tree, as shown in Figure 2A, an increased activity of members of the ACG kinase family was suggested, which includes cyclic nucleotide binding kinases like PKA, PKG, PRKX, and PRKY, several members of the PKC family, kinases in the mTOR pathway, such as AKT1, AKT2, mTOR, as well as the ribosome-associated kinases, such as p70S6K, RSK, and MSK.

Table 1. Kinases, differentially active in benign vs. malignant tumors, ranked by kinase score after upstream kinase analysis. The presence of RNA and protein in normal and tumor thyroid tissues and the quality assessment of protein presence as checked from Protein Atlas (www.proteinatlas.org (accessed on 19 January 2023)). Kinases are indicated by their UniProt names and ID.

					Thyroid Presence			
Rank	Kinase	Gene Name	UniProt ID	Kinase Score	Normal Tissue	Cancer	Reliability Score *	Remarks
1	RSK2	RPS6KA3	P51812	5.09	yes	yes	approved	
2	MSK1	RPS6KA5	O75582	4.74	yes	yes	approved	
3	PKC[epsilon]	PRKCE	Q02156	4.46	yes	yes	enhanced	
4	PKA[alpha]	PRKACA	P17612	4.66	yes	yes	approved	
5	Pim1	PIM1	P11309	4.38	low	low	uncertain	
6	SGK2	SGK2	Q9HBY8	3.82	low	low	uncertain	
7	ANP[alpha]	NPR1	P16066	3.98	yes	yes	na	Has kinase-like homology domain
8	p70S6K[beta]	RPS6KB2	Q9UBS0	3.90	yes	yes	approved	
9	PKC[gamma]	PRKCG	P05129	3.89	low	low	enhanced	
10	Pim3	PIM3	Q86V86	4.06	yes	yes	na	
11	PRKX	PRKX	P51817	3.96	yes	yes	supported	Thyroid cancer enhanced
12	AurA/Aur2	AURKA	O14965	3.77	low	low	enhanced	
13	Pim2	PIM2	Q9P1W9	3.71	low	low	na	
14	MSK2	RPS6KA4/RSKB	O75676	3.70	yes	yes	approved	
15	CHK2	CHEK2	O96017	3.64	yes	yes	enhanced	
16	GSK3[beta]	GSK3B	P49841	3.66	yes	yes	approved	
17	PKC[theta]	PRKCQ	Q04759	3.62	yes	yes	na	Unfavorable prognostic marker
18	PKD1	PRKD1	Q15139	3.62	yes	yes	uncertain	Unfavorable prognostic marker

Table 1. *Cont.*

Rank	Kinase	Gene Name	UniProt ID	Kinase Score	Thyroid Presence Normal Tissue	Thyroid Presence Cancer	Reliability Score *	Remarks
19	PKC[delta]	PRKCD	Q05655	3.74	yes	yes	enhanced	
20	Akt1/PKB[alpha]	PKB (alpha)	P31749	3.61	yes	yes	supported	
21	Akt2/PKB[beta]	PKB (beta)	P31751	3.58	yes	yes	uncertain	
22	CDKL5	CDKL5	O76039	3.59	yes	yes	approved	
23	GSK3[alpha]	GSK3A	P49840	3.45	yes	yes	approved	
24	AurB/Aur1	AURKB	Q96GD4	3.49	low	low	enhanced	
25	p70S6K	RPS6KB1	P23443	3.45	yes	yes	approved	
26	RSKL2	RPS6KL1	Q9Y6S9	3.49	low	low	approved	
27	TBK1	TBK1	Q9UHD2	3.36	yes	yes	uncertain	
28	PKC[alpha]	PRKCA	P17252	3.47	low	low	enhanced	
29	PKC[beta]	PRKCB	P05771	3.46	yes	yes	approved	
30	CaMK4	CAMK4	Q16566	3.49	low	low	approved	
31	PRKY	PRKY	O43930	3.28	na	na	na	
32	PKC[zeta]	PRKCZ	Q05513	3.40	yes	yes	enhanced	
33	ADCK3	COQ8A	Q8NI60	3.27	na	na	na	
34	PKG1	PRKG1	Q13976	3.48	yes	yes	enhanced	
35	PKN1/PRK1	PKN1	Q16512	3.38	yes	yes	approved	
36	PKC[eta]	PRKCH	P24723	3.30	yes	yes	approved	
37	mTOR/FRAP	FRAP	P42345	3.31	yes	yes	approved	
38	RSK3	RPS6KA1	Q15418	3.30	yes	yes	approved	
39	RSK1/p90RSK	RPS6KA2	Q15349	3.27	yes	yes	enhanced	Thyroid cancer enhanced
40	AlphaK1	ALPK3	Q96L96	3.25	low	yes	uncertain	

* Reliability score for protein presence in normal tissue, based on knowledge-based evaluation of available RNA-seq data, protein/gene characterization data, and immunohistochemical data from one or several antibodies designed towards non-overlapping sequences of the same gene. The reliability score is based on the 44 normal tissues analyzed (https://www.proteinatlas.org/about/assays+annotation#ih_reliability (accessed on 20 January 2023)). Reliability score from high to low: Enhanced, Supported, Approved, Uncertain; na: evidence based on RNA expression, no evidence for protein presence reported.

To further investigate these kinases, the presence of the forty kinases with the highest kinase score, i.e., those most likely to be differentially active, was analyzed in both normal and malignant thyroid (www.proteinatlas.org (accessed on 19 January 2023)) (Table 1). After exclusion of the lowest-expressed kinases, a network analysis was performed in STRING for the 29 remaining kinases (Figure 2B). This network contained six interconnected members of the PKC family, five of which link to mTOR. MTOR is the central hub that connects PKCs via AKT and GSK3β to several ribosomal protein kinases (RPS6KA and RPS6KB). PKA and PKG are also connected to GSK3β and the ribosomal protein kinases.

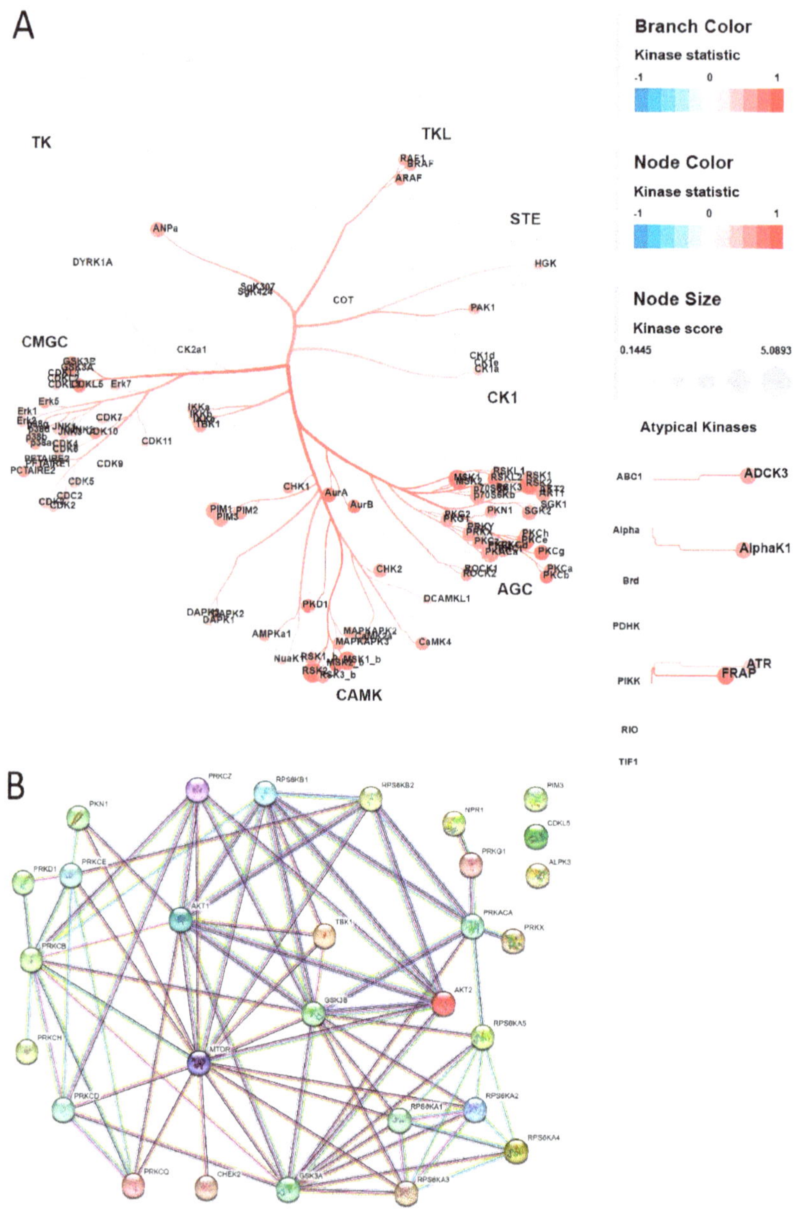

Figure 2. Upstream kinases and STRING Network analysis. (**A**) Results of upstream kinase analysis to identify kinases that may be differentially active between benign and malignant tumors. The kinases were mapped onto a phylogenetic tree of the human kinome using the CORAL application. The branches and nodes are colored by the kinase statistic (i.e., direction and size of the effect). The brighter red the color, the higher the likelihood of a kinase having increased activity in malignant samples. The size of the circle indicates the kinase score of the corresponding kinase (a higher score indicates a higher likelihood to contribute to the observed phosphorylation changes). (**B**) STRING Network analysis of 29 kinases with the highest kinase score for benign vs. malignant tumors (Table 1). Kinases were selected for expression in normal and malignant thyroid tissue using data from Protein Atlas.

3.4. Differentiating Non-BRAF V600E and BRAF V600E PTC Using RAF Inhibitors

We then asked whether ex vivo addition of a BRAF V600E-specific inhibitor to a tumor lysate could be used to distinguish between *BRAF* V600E and non-*BRAF* V600E thyroid tumors, as well as between recurrent and non-recurrent tumors. We compared kinase activity profiles in six non-*BRAF* V600E tumors, including three FVPTC (Th-50, Th-52, and Th-53, annotated as PTC), and seven *BRAF* V600E-mutant PTC (see Supplementary Table S1) without and with the *BRAF* V600E-specific inhibitor dabrafenib, and the low-affinity RAF inhibitors sorafenib and regorafenib. Owing to their different histology, the two *BRAF* V600E-positive ATCs were excluded from this experiment.

Basal kinase activity profiles of the *BRAF* V600E samples showed wide variation (median 2log signal intensity 8.27 ± 0.67 for *BRAF* V600E and 8.66 ± 0.35 for non-BRAF V600E tumors, $p = 0.31$) (Figure 3A and Supplementary Figure S2A).

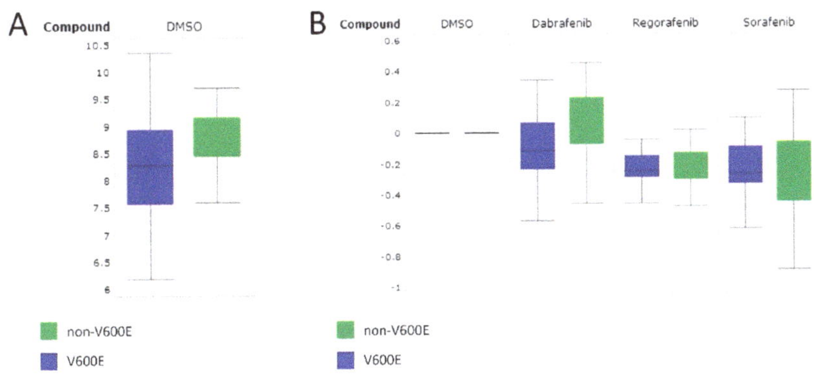

Figure 3. (**A**) Box plot of median ^{2}log signal intensity of 13 PTC samples, i.e., seven *BRAF* V600E-positive and six non-*BRAF* V600E (indicated by non-BRAF V600E) thyroid tumor lysates. (**B**) Median log fold changes (log ratio compared to the corresponding untreated sample) of the 13 PTC samples with addition of 10 µM dabrafenib, 50 µM regorafenib or 10 µM sorafenib in the assay. The log fold change for the DMSO controls is equal to 0. Th-50, Th-52, and Th-53 comprise the FVPTC subtype.

For the 13 PTC samples, the ratio of inhibited to non-inhibited signal (log fold change, LFC) was calculated and represented in heatmaps (Supplementary Figure S2B–D). Dabrafenib, regorafenib, and sorafenib showed inhibition of overall kinase activity in the tested samples, as demonstrated by altered LFCs of the peptides. However, in a global analysis, median inhibition by regorafenib and sorafenib in *BRAF* V600E and non-BRAF V600E samples was comparable (−0.25 ± 0.1 vs. −0.23 ± 0.08 and −0.27 ± 0.12 vs. −0.31 ± 0.15, respectively), while dabrafenib showed a greater average inhibition of *BRAF* V600E (−0.12 ± 0.2 vs. −0.001 ± 0.15).

(Figure 3B). Compared to regorafenib-treated or sorafenib-treated samples, dabrafenib resulted in more distinct differences between samples (Supplementary Figure S2B–D).

Statistical analysis of the basal profiles yielded five peptides (ADDB_696-708, ERF_519-531, GSUB_61-73, LMNB1_16-28, and PP2AB_297-309) that showed a significantly different signal ($p < 0.05$, FDR 76%) and was able to differentiate *BRAF* V600E from non-*BRAF* V600E thyroid cancers (Figure 4A). In particular, phosphorylation of the peptide LMNB1_16-28 differed significantly between thyroid cancers ($p = 0.0006$, FDR 6%), and analysis of the same 13 PTC samples from the previous experiment confirmed this finding (LMNB1_16-28: $p < 0.05$, FDR 25%). Since this peptide is a good substrate for several members of the MAPK family, this suggests higher MAPK activity in non-*BRAF* V600E tumors, contrary to the expected increase in MAPK activity in the *BRAF* V600E samples.

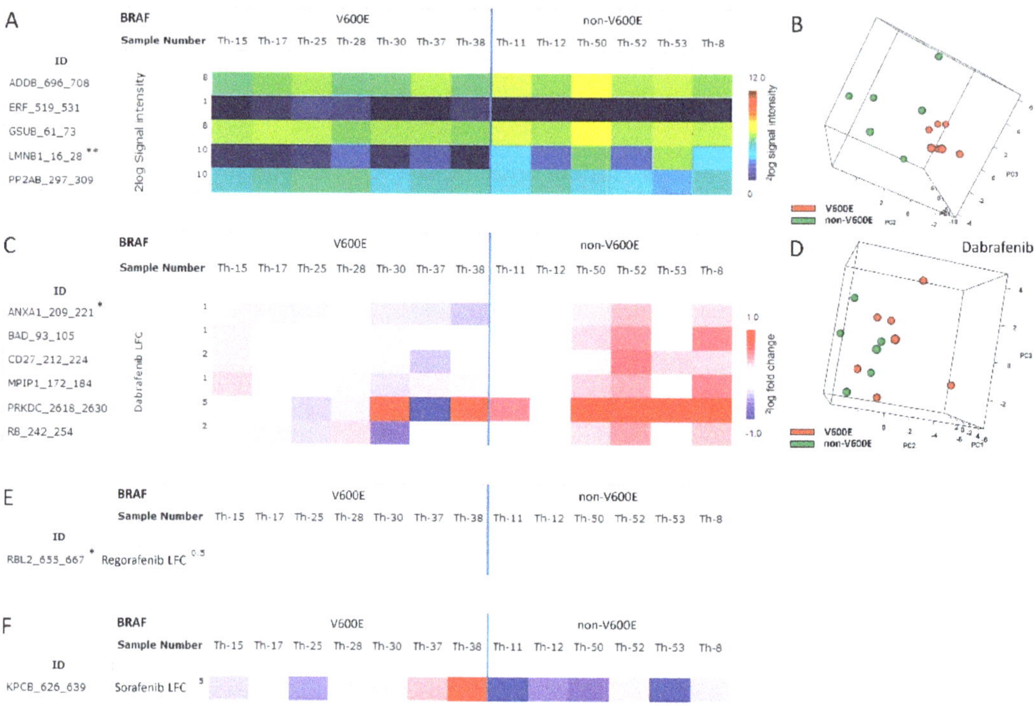

Figure 4. Peptides significantly different ($p < 0.05$) between *BRAF* V600E-positive and non-*BRAF* V600E. PTC samples for basal kinase activity profiles (**A**) or log fold changes (LFC) after ex vivo addition of dabrafenib (**C**), regorafenib (**E**) or sorafenib (**F**). * indicates $p < 0.01$, ** indicates $p < 0.001$. (**B**,**D**) Separation of *BRAF* V600E-positive and non-*BRAF* V600E PCT by basal kinase activity profiles (**B**) or LFC with dabrafenib (**D**) after principal component analysis (PCA).

Although the biological heterogeneity of *BRAF* V600E samples was substantial, PCA analysis of the basal kinase activity profiles of these PTCs allowed us to distinguish *BRAF* V600E and non-*BRAF* V600E samples (Figure 4B).

Statistical analysis of the LFC profiles with the *BRAF* V600E-specific inhibitor dabrafenib differentiated *BRAF* V600E and non-*BRAF* V600E thyroid cancers, with six peptides (BAD_93- 105, CD27_212-224, MPIP1_172-184, PRKDC_2618-2630, and RB_242-254) showing $p < 0.05$.

(FDR 62%) and one peptide (ANXA1_209_221, Annexin 1) showing $p < 0.01$ (FDR 45%) (Figure 4C). PCA analysis of the log fold change profiles of the PTC exposed to dabrafenib allowed for some distinction of *BRAF* V600E and non-*BRAF* V600E samples (Figure 4D).

In contrast, the low-affinity inhibitors regorafenib and sorafenib showed no significant differences in LFC between *BRAF* V600E and non-*BRAF* V600E PTCs (regorafenib, one peptide with $p < 0.01$, FDR 36%; sorafenib, one peptide with $p < 0.05$, FDR 99%) (Figure 4E and 4F, respectively).

The same data were then used to differentiate recurrent and non-recurrent samples. Using the *BRAF* V600E-specific inhibitor dabrafenib, six peptides (ACM1_421-433, CGHB_109-121, CREB1_126-138, H2B1B_27-40, LMNB1-16-28, and RB_242-254) differed significantly ($p < 0.05$, FDR 47%) between recurrent and non-recurrent samples. Of these six peptides, CGHB_109-121 and LMNB1_16-28 had $p < 0.01$ (FDR 43%). Basal profiles as well as LFC profiles obtained with RAF inhibitors were not able to differentiate these groups: sorafenib, basal, and LFC profiles revealed no significantly different peptides, and only two peptides (CDK7_163-175 and H32_3-18) had a $p < 0.05$ with regorafenib.

4. Discussion

4.1. Kinase Activity Profiling Correctly Classifies Benign and Malignant Thyroid Tumors

Targeted therapy, which is currently based on NGS, does not always guarantee success and may, in some cases, be accompanied by adverse side effects. Although the mechanisms responsible for failure of targeted therapy are still poorly understood, deregulated kinase activity is thought to play an important role. In many tumor types, deregulated kinase activity has been reported to be associated with DNA variants and tumorigenesis. For example, in non-small cell lung carcinoma (NSCLC), kinase activity profiling of tumor tissue has successfully differentiated short- from long-term survivors [27], and *BRAF* V600E from WT *BRAF* metastatic melanoma [34].

Here, we used serine/threonine (STK) activity profiling to characterize benign and malignant thyroid lesions. Based on our data, a classification model was developed which correctly classified 76% of samples. The misclassification of the remaining 24% of samples, consisting of five benign and eight malignant samples, can be partially explained by the presence of numerous inflammatory cells (Graves' disease, Th-22 and Th-46, false positive), oncocytic neoplasia (Th-41, Th-42, and Th-51, false negative) associated with reduced kinetic activity, and necrosis (Th-6, Th-47, and Th-44, poor sample quality). Collectively, these data show that increased STK activity is primarily associated with malignancy. As kinase activity profiling can correctly classify 76% of samples, it clearly shows promise as a tool to distinguish benign from malignant tumors in cases where current methods are inconclusive. To more firmly establish the potential of this method, the testing of larger numbers of samples will be needed. Furthermore, exclusion of samples showing necrosis or chromosomal instability will likely improve classification.

4.2. Molecular Interpretation of Differences between Benign and Malignant Samples

With a few exceptions, malignant thyroid tumors showed higher STK activity compared with benign lesions. This difference allows us to generate unbiased hypotheses about kinases that are differentially active between benign and malignant samples, irrespective of whether this increased activity is caused by overexpression, chromosomal rearrangements, fusions, mutations of kinases or by factors that modulate kinase activity. This approach could potentially provide new treatment targets for recurrent NMTC. Upstream kinase analysis suggested increased activity of numerous kinases, but only four kinases were associated with thyroid tumors. Mutations in RAF and RAS kinases are most frequent in PTC and FTC, respectively. However, BRAF, ARAF, and RAF1 were not among the top 40 hits in the upstream kinase analysis (ranked 49, 51, and 60, respectively) (see Table 1). Conversely, mutations in higher-ranked kinases such as CHK2 (Table 1, rank 15) or PKD1 (rank 18) are rare (less than 1% of the PTC cases) and do not seem to contribute to thyroid cancer [35]. By comparing the transcriptome of thyroid cancer to the transcriptome of 16 other cancer types, the Protein Atlas shows kinases upregulated in thyroid tumor tissue [36]. Among the 289 genes (of 20,090 human genes) included, three serine/threonine-protein kinases (RSK1, CAMK2B, and STK32A (YANK)) and four tyrosine-protein kinases (ALK, DAPK2, EPHA4, and NTRK2) show elevated expression in thyroid tumor tissue. Of these, only RSK1 was identified in our study (see Table 1). We found an increase in RSK1 (RPS6KA2, rank 39) and PRKX (rank 11) expression, but this was not related to prognosis. The unfavorable prognostic markers PKD1 (rank 18) and PKC (theta) (PRKCQ, rank 17) were not upregulated [37,38]. These observations suggest that modulation of kinase activity, rather than the simple presence of a kinase, is important in malignant tumors. Notably, kinases of the AGC family (i.e., several PKC family members) and PKA, PKG or PRKX, as well as kinases in the AKT/mTOR pathway, show elevated activity in malignant tissue. This same group of kinases was found to have increased activity in vemurafenib-resistant melanoma harboring *BRAF* V600E mutations [34]. Network analysis also pointed to a central role for mTOR/AKT and PKA in malignant samples, similar to the RAS-like PTC subtype as defined by the Cancer Genome Atlas Research Network [35]. A RAS-like subtype was expected, since 25/34 samples were non-*BRAF* V600E. Activation of these hubs occurs through two routes: via cyclic nucleotide second messengers and PIP3. The cyclic nucleotide second messengers, cAMP and cGMP, activate PKA, PKG1, and PKG2. PKA and cAMP seem to protect thyroid cells from apoptosis and support a contribution of p70S6K to viability [39–44].

Kinase activity profiling of tumor lysates with multiple drugs may reveal alternative treatment options. Recent work from Huo et al. [45] highlighted the utility of drug screening in PDXs carrying the BRAF G469V variant by identifying an unexpected therapeutic target for EGFR inhibitors. Our analysis (see Table 1 and Figure 2) suggests an important role for members of the PKC family, including the unfavorable prognostic marker PKC (theta) (PRKCQ, rank 17). PKC family members show a strong connection to PKC (epsilon) (PRKCE, rank 3) and PKC (beta) (PRKCB, rank 16). These network hubs, in addition to PKD1 and PKC (theta), merit further investigation and might provide new targets for treatment of NMTC. Inhibitors designed to target these kinases are at several stages of development, including a PKC (theta) inhibitor at the clinical stage [46] and several PKD inhibitors in preclinical development [47].

4.3. *Distinguishing Non-BRAF V600E from BRAF V600E PTC Using RAF Inhibitors*

New treatments are urgently needed for thyroid cancer patients with radioactive iodide refractory disease. While kinase inhibitors such as sorafenib, lenvatinib or cabozantinib can be beneficial, their use is limited owing to significant adverse side effects as well as the development of resistance. Treatment with *BRAF* V600E-specific inhibitors, alone or in combination with an MEK inhibitor, may be a viable alternative. BRAF V600E-targeted mono- and combination therapy is effective in *BRAF* V600E melanoma [17,48], but is ineffective against *BRAF* V600E colorectal cancer [49,50]. Dabrafenib has been approved for ATC thyroid tumors carrying this mutation [51], but not for PTC [15,16,19,52–54].

Using STK activity profiling and by spiking with dedicated *BRAF* V600E kinase inhibitor(s), we also investigated whether the effect of RAF inhibitors differs between non-BRAF V600E and *BRAF* V600E PTCs, and between recurrent and non-recurrent tumors. In a study of melanoma samples harboring the *BRAF* V600E mutation, this approach could distinguish responders and non-responders to dabrafenib monotherapy [34].

In our study, basal kinase activity profiles and LFC profiles with dabrafenib could distinguish *BRAF* V600E from non-*BRAF* V600E tumors based on differential phosphorylation. This was not the case for the kinase inhibitors sorafenib and regorafenib (see Figure 4E,F). Dabrafenib could also successfully distinguish refractive from non-refractive tumors. However, since in all cases the variation in profiles between groups was large and the aforementioned differences were due to a small number of peptides with low signal intensities, these results are unlikely to provide a robust biomarker to help differentiate these groups. However, differences in ex vivo inhibition by dabrafenib might reliably predict responders and non-responders to BRAF inhibitor therapy, as shown for melanoma [34]. This could be beneficial for a subgroup of PTC patients, because vemurafenib and dabrafenib have been shown to not only inhibit the RAF/MEK/ERK pathway in thyroid tumors, but also to induce redifferentiation and radioactive iodide restoration [15,16,19,52,53] via re-expression of the sodium/iodide symporter (NIS) [54].

In conclusion, as STK activity profiling allowed us to correctly classify 76% of thyroid tumor samples, this method appears to be able to differentiate benign from malignant thyroid tumors. Moreover, a plausible explanation was found for ten of the thirteen misclassified samples. Molecular interpretation of these differences prompted hypotheses concerning the differential activity of kinases in benign versus malignant tumors. Two of these kinases, PKC (theta) and PKD1, have been previously reported to be prognostic in thyroid cancer [35,55] and might represent new targets for treatment. In addition, ex vivo administration of dabrafenib showed increased inhibition of BRAF V600E in PTC.

We have shown that STK activity profiling can be a beneficial tool for differentiating benign and malignant thyroid tumors. In addition, our approach aids in the selection of (novel) kinase inhibitors for treatment of recurrent thyroid and other cancers.

Supplementary Materials: The following supporting information can be downloaded at: https://www.mdpi.com/article/10.3390/cancers15184477/s1, Figure S1: Heat map of basal serine/threonine kinase activity profiles; Figure S2: Kinase activity profiles of 13 PTC; Table S1: Information of all patients included in the study; Table S2: *p*-Values of the median serine/threonine kinase activity.

Author Contributions: Conception: T.K., R.R., H.M., W.E.C. and T.v.W.; Sample selection: W.E.C., H.M. and T.v.W.; Investigation: R.d.W., P.B., A.v.d.B., R.R., T.K., H.M., W.E.C. and R.H.; Experiments: P.B. and A.v.d.B.; Data Analysis: A.v.d.B., P.B., R.H. and R.d.W.; Data interpretation: T.K., R.R., H.M., W.E.C. and R.H.; Writing: R.H., W.E.C. and H.M.; Revisions: all authors; Final approval: all authors. All authors have read and agreed to the published version of the manuscript.

Funding: This research received no external funding.

Institutional Review Board Statement: Not applicable.

Informed Consent Statement: All samples were processed in concuR.R.ence with the medical ethical guidelines as de-scribed in the Code Proper Secondary Use of Human Tissue (Dutch Federation of Medical Sciences, www.federa.org.

Data Availability Statement: The data can be shared up on request.

Conflicts of Interest: RH and P.B. are retired and former employees of the biotech company PamGene. Prior to joining Genmab, R.R. was vice president R&D at PamGene. A.v.d.B., T.K. and R.d.W. are cuR.R.ently employed by PamGene. W.E.C., H.M. and T.v.W. are employed by the Leiden University Medical Center, The Netherlands, and don't have a conflict of interest.

References

1. Bai, Y.; Kakudo, K.; Jung, C.K. Updates in the Pathologic Classification of Thyroid Neoplasms: A Review of the World Health Organization Classification. *Endocrinol. Metab.* **2020**, *35*, 696–715. [CrossRef] [PubMed]
2. Christofer Juhlin, C.; Mete, O.; Baloch, Z.W. The 2022 WHO classification of thyroid tumors: Novel concepts in nomenclature and grading. *Endocr. Relat. Cancer* **2023**, *30*, e220293. [CrossRef] [PubMed]
3. Corver, W.E.; Ruano, D.; Weijers, K.; den Hartog, W.C.; van Nieuwenhuizen, M.P.; de Miranda, N.; van Eijk, R.; Middeldorp, A.; Jordanova, E.S.; Oosting, J.; et al. Genome haploidisation with chromosome 7 retention in oncocytic follicular thyroid carcinoma. *PLoS ONE* **2012**, *7*, e38287. [CrossRef] [PubMed]
4. Corver, W.E.; van Wezel, T.; Molenaar, K.; Schrumpf, M.; van den Akker, B.; van Eijk, R.; Ruano Neto, D.; Oosting, J.; Morreau, H. Near-haploidization significantly associates with oncocytic adrenocortical, thyroid, and parathyroid tumors but not with mitochondrial DNA mutations. *Genes Chromosomes Cancer* **2014**, *53*, 833–844. [CrossRef] [PubMed]
5. Bible, K.C.; Ryder, M. Evolving molecularly targeted therapies for advanced-stage thyroid cancers. *Nat. Rev. Clin. Oncol.* **2016**, *13*, 403–416. [CrossRef] [PubMed]
6. Cabanillas, M.E.; McFadden, D.G.; Durante, C. Thyroid cancer. *Lancet* **2016**, *388*, 2783–2795. [CrossRef]
7. Tesselaar, M.H.; Smit, J.W.; Nagarajah, J.; Netea-Maier, R.T.; Plantinga, T.S. Pathological processes and therapeutic advances in radioiodide refractory thyroid cancer. *J. Mol. Endocrinol.* **2017**, *59*, R141–R154. [CrossRef]
8. Ganly, I.; Makarov, V.; Deraje, S.; Dong, Y.; Reznik, E.; Seshan, V.; Nanjangud, G.; Eng, S.; Bose, P.; Kuo, F.; et al. Integrated Genomic Analysis of Hurthle Cell Cancer Reveals Oncogenic Drivers, RecuR.R.ent Mitochondrial Mutations, and Unique Chromosomal Landscapes. *Cancer Cell* **2018**, *34*, 256–270.e255. [CrossRef]
9. Valero, C.; Ganly, I.; Shah, J.P. Head and neck paragangliomas: 30-year experience. *Head Neck* **2020**, *42*, 10. [CrossRef]
10. Caronia, L.M.; Phay, J.E.; Shah, M.H. Role of BRAF in thyroid oncogenesis. *Clin. Cancer Res.* **2011**, *17*, 7511–7517. [CrossRef]
11. Schneider, T.C.; Abdulrahman, R.M.; Corssmit, E.P.; Morreau, H.; Smit, J.W.; Kapiteijn, E. Long-term analysis of the efficacy and tolerability of sorafenib in advanced radio-iodine refractory differentiated thyroid carcinoma: Final results of a phase II trial. *Eur. J. Endocrinol.* **2012**, *167*, 643–650. [CrossRef] [PubMed]
12. Brose, M.S.; Nutting, C.M.; Jarzab, B.; Elisei, R.; Siena, S.; Bastholt, L.; de la Fouchardiere, C.; Pacini, F.; Paschke, R.; Shong, Y.K.; et al. Sorafenib in radioactive iodine-refractory, locally advanced or metastatic differentiated thyroid cancer: A randomised, double-blind, phase 3 trial. *Lancet* **2014**, *384*, 319–328. [CrossRef] [PubMed]
13. Brose, M.S.; Cabanillas, M.E.; Cohen, E.E.; Wirth, L.J.; Riehl, T.; Yue, H.; Sherman, S.I.; Sherman, E.J. Vemurafenib in patients with BRAF(V600E)-positive metastatic or unresectable papillary thyroid cancer refractory to radioactive iodine: A non-randomised, multicentre, open-label, phase 2 trial. *Lancet Oncol.* **2016**, *17*, 1272–1282. [CrossRef]
14. Huillard, O.; Tenenbaum, F.; Clerc, J.; Goldwasser, F.; Groussin, L. Vemurafenib for BRAFV600E-positive metastatic papillary thyroid cancer. *Lancet Oncol.* **2016**, *17*, e468. [CrossRef]
15. Rothenberg, S.M.; McFadden, D.G.; Palmer, E.L.; Daniels, G.H.; Wirth, L.J. Redifferentiation of iodine-refractory BRAF V600E-mutant metastatic papillary thyroid cancer with dabrafenib. *Clin. Cancer Res.* **2015**, *21*, 1028–1035. [CrossRef]

16. Dunn, L.A.; Sherman, E.J.; Baxi, S.S.; Tchekmedyian, V.; Grewal, R.K.; Larson, S.M.; Pentlow, K.S.; Haque, S.; Tuttle, R.M.; Sabra, M.M.; et al. Vemurafenib Redifferentiation of BRAF Mutant, RAI-Refractory Thyroid Cancers. *J. Clin. Endocrinol. Metab.* **2019**, *104*, 1417–1428. [CrossRef]
17. Falchook, G.S.; Millward, M.; Hong, D.; Naing, A.; Piha-Paul, S.; Waguespack, S.G.; Cabanillas, M.E.; Sherman, S.I.; Ma, B.; Curtis, M.; et al. BRAF inhibitor dabrafenib in patients with metastatic BRAF-mutant thyroid cancer. *Thyroid* **2015**, *25*, 71–77. [CrossRef]
18. Fujiwara, Y.; Yamazaki, N.; Kiyohara, Y.; Yoshikawa, S.; Yamamoto, N.; Tsutsumida, A.; Nokihara, H.; Namikawa, K.; Mukaiyama, A.; Zhang, F.; et al. Safety, tolerability, and pharmacokinetic profile of dabrafenib in Japanese patients with BRAF V600 mutation-positive solid tumors: A phase 1 study. *Investig. New Drugs* **2017**, *36*, 10. [CrossRef]
19. Tchekmedyian, V.; Dunn, L.; Sherman, E.; Baxi, S.S.; Grewal, R.K.; Larson, S.M.; Pentlow, K.S.; Haque, S.; Tuttle, R.M.; Sabra, M.M.; et al. Enhancing Radioiodine Incorporation in BRAF- Mutant, Radioiodine-Refractory Thyroid Cancers with Vemurafenib and the Anti-ErbB3 Monoclonal Antibody CDX-3379: Results of a Pilot Clinical Trial. *Thyroid* **2022**, *32*, 273–282. [CrossRef] [PubMed]
20. Hilhorst, R.; Houkes, L.; Mommersteeg, M.; Musch, J.; van den Berg, A.; Ruijtenbeek, R. Peptide microaR.R.ays for profiling of serine/threonine kinase activity of recombinant kinases and lysates of cells and tissue samples. *Methods Mol. Biol.* **2013**, *977*, 259–271. [CrossRef]
21. van der Tuin, K.; Ventayol Garcia, M.; Corver, W.E.; Khalifa, M.N.; Ruano Neto, D.; Corssmit, E.P.M.; Hes, F.J.; Links, T.P.; Smit, J.W.A.; Plantinga, T.S.; et al. Targetable gene fusions identified in radioactive iodine refractory advanced thyroid carcinoma. *Eur. J. Endocrinol.* **2019**, *180*, 235–241. [CrossRef] [PubMed]
22. van Eijk, R.; Stevens, L.; Morreau, H.; van Wezel, T. Assessment of a fully automated high- throughput DNA extraction method from formalin-fixed, paraffin-embedded tissue for KRAS, and BRAF somatic mutation analysis. *Exp. Mol. Pathol.* **2013**, *94*, 121–125. [CrossRef]
23. Sibinga Mulder, B.G.; Mieog, J.S.D.; Handgraaf, H.J.M.; Farina Sarasqueta, A.; Vasen, H.F.A.; Potjer, T.P.; Swijnenburg, R.-J.; Luelmo, S.A.C.; Feshtali, S.; Inderson, A.; et al. Targeted next- generation sequencing of FNA-derived DNA in pancreatic cancer. *J. Clin. Pathol.* **2017**, *70*, 174–178. [CrossRef]
24. Corver, W.E.; Middeldorp, A.; Ter Haar, N.T.; Jordanova, E.S.; van Puijenbroek, M.; van Eijk, R.; Cornelisse, C.J.; Fleuren, G.J.; Morreau, H.; Oosting, J.; et al. Genome-wide allelic state analysis on flow-sorted tumor fractions provides an accurate measure of chromosomal abeR.R.ations. *Cancer Res.* **2008**, *68*, 10333–10340. [CrossRef] [PubMed]
25. Barker, M.; Rayens, W. Partial least squares for discrimination. *J. Chemometr.* **2003**, *17*, 166–173. [CrossRef]
26. Boulesteix, A.L.; Strobl, C.; Augustin, T.; Daumer, M. Evaluating microaR.R.ay-based classifiers: An overview. *Cancer Inform.* **2008**, *6*, 77–97. [CrossRef] [PubMed]
27. Arni, S.; Le, T.H.N.; de Wijn, R.; Garcia-Villegas, R.; Dankers, M.; Weder, W.; Hillinger, S. Ex vivo multiplex profiling of protein tyrosine kinase activities in early stages of human lung adenocarcinoma. *Oncotarget* **2017**, *8*, 68599–68613. [CrossRef]
28. Benjamini, Y.; Drai, D.; Elmer, G.; Kafkafi, N.; Golani, I. Controlling the false discovery rate in behavior genetics research. *Behav. Brain Res.* **2001**, *125*, 279–284. [CrossRef]
29. Chirumamilla, C.S.; Fazil, M.; Perez-Novo, C.; Rangarajan, S.; de Wijn, R.; Ramireddy, P.; Verma, N.K.; Vanden Berghe, W. Profiling Activity of Cellular Kinases in Migrating T-Cells. *Methods Mol. Biol.* **2019**, *1930*, 99–113. [CrossRef]
30. Pearson, W.R. Selecting the Right Similarity-Scoring Matrix. *Curr. Protoc. Bioinform.* **2013**, *43*, 9. [CrossRef]
31. Metz, K.S.; Deoudes, E.M.; Berginski, M.E.; Jimenez-Ruiz, I.; Aksoy, B.A.; Hammerbacher, J.; Gomez, S.M.; Phanstiel, D.H. Coral: Clear and Customizable Visualization of Human Kinome Data. *Cell Syst.* **2018**, *7*, 347–350.e341. [CrossRef] [PubMed]
32. Corver, W.; Demmers, J.; Oosting, J.; Sahraeian, S.; Boot, A.; Ruano, D.; van Wezel, T.; Morreau, H. ROS-induced near-homozygous genomes in thyroid cancer. *Endocr. Relat. Cancer* **2018**, *25*, 15. [CrossRef] [PubMed]
33. de Koster, E.J.; Corver, W.E.; de Geus-Oei, L.F.; Oyen, W.J.G.; Ruano, D.; Schepers, A.; Snel, M.; van Wezel, T.; Vriens, D.; Morreau, J. A clinically applicable molecular classification of Hürthle cell thyroid nodules. *Endocr. Relat. Cancer* **2023**, *30*, e230047. [CrossRef] [PubMed]
34. Krayem, M.; Aftimos, P.; Najem, A.; van den Hooven, T.; van den Berg, A.; Hovestad-Bijl, L.; de Wijn, R.; Hilhorst, R.; Ruijtenbeek, R.; Sabbah, M.; et al. Kinome Profiling to Predict Sensitivity to MAPK Inhibition in Melanoma and to Provide New Insights into Intrinsic and Acquired Mechanism of Resistance. *Cancers* **2020**, *12*, 512. [CrossRef] [PubMed]
35. Cancer Genome Atlas Research Network. Integrated genomic characterization of papillary thyroid carcinoma. *Cell* **2014**, *159*, 676–690. [CrossRef]
36. Cancer Tissue Specific Score. Available online: https://www.proteinatlas.org/search/cancercategoryrna%3Athyroid+cancer%3BCancer+enriched%2CGroup+enriched%2CCancer+enhanced+AND+sortby%3Atissue+specific+score/6 (accessed on 19 January 2023).
37. PRKCQ. Available online: https://www.proteinatlas.org/ENSG00000065675-PRKCQ (accessed on 19 January 2023).
38. Available online: https://www.proteinatlas.org/ENSG00000184304-PRKD1/pathology (accessed on 19 January 2023).
39. Saavedra, A.P.; Tsygankova, O.M.; Prendergast, G.V.; Dworet, J.H.; Cheng, G.; Meinkoth, J.L. Role of cAMP, PKA and Rap1A in thyroid follicular cell survival. *Oncogene* **2002**, *21*, 778–788. [CrossRef] [PubMed]
40. Nikiforova, M.N.; Wald, A.I.; Roy, S.; Durso, M.B.; Nikiforov, Y.E. Targeted next-generation sequencing panel (ThyroSeq) for detection of mutations in thyroid cancer. *J. Clin. Endocrinol. Metab.* **2013**, *98*, E1852–E1860. [CrossRef]
41. Salabe, G.B. Pathogenesis of thyroid nodules: Histological classification? *Biomed. Pharmacother.* **2001**, *55*, 39–53. [CrossRef]

42. Del Gobbo, A.; Peverelli, E.; Treppiedi, D.; Lania, A.; Mantovani, G.; Ferrero, S. Expression of protein kinase A regulatory subunits in benign and malignant human thyroid tissues: A systematic review. *Exp. Cell Res.* **2016**, *346*, 85–90. [CrossRef]
43. Kari, S.; Vasko, V.V.; Priya, S.; Kirschner, L.S. PKA Activates AMPK Through LKB1 Signaling in Follicular Thyroid Cancer. *Front. Endocrinol.* **2019**, *10*, 769. [CrossRef]
44. Miasaki, F.Y.; Fuziwara, C.S.; Carvalho, G.A.; Kimura, E.T. Genetic Mutations and Variants in the Susceptibility of Familial Non-Medullary Thyroid Cancer. *Genes* **2020**, *11*, 1364. [CrossRef] [PubMed]
45. Huo, K.G.; Notsuda, H.; Fang, Z.; Liu, N.F.; Gebregiworgis, T.; Li, Q.; Pham, N.A.; Li, M.; Liu, N.; Shepherd, F.A.; et al. Lung Cancer Driven by BRAF(G469V) Mutation Is Targetable by EGFR Kinase Inhibitors. *J. Thorac. Oncol.* **2022**, *17*, 277–288. [CrossRef] [PubMed]
46. Piperno-Neumann, S.; Carlino, M.S.; Boni, V.; Loirat, D.; Speetjens, F.M.; Park, J.J.; Calvo, E.; Carvajal, R.D.; Nyakas, M.; Gonzalez-Maffe, J.; et al. A phase I trial of LXS196, a protein kinase C (PKC) inhibitor, for metastatic uveal melanoma. *Br. J. Cancer* **2023**, *128*, 1040–1051. [CrossRef] [PubMed]
47. Lv, D.; Chen, H.; Feng, Y.; Cui, B.; Kang, Y.; Zhang, P.; Luo, M.; Chen, J. Small-Molecule Inhibitor Targeting Protein Kinase D: A Potential Therapeutic Strategy. *Front. Oncol.* **2021**, *11*, 680221. [CrossRef]
48. Long, G.V.; Stroyakovskiy, D.; Gogas, H.; Levchenko, E.; de Braud, F.; Larkin, J.; Garbe, C.; Jouary, T.; Hauschild, A.; Grob, J.J.; et al. Combined BRAF and MEK inhibition versus BRAF inhibition alone in melanoma. *N. Engl. J. Med.* **2014**, *371*, 1877–1888. [CrossRef]
49. Kopetz, S.; Desai, J.; Chan, E.; Hecht, J.R.; O'Dwyer, P.J.; Maru, D.; Morris, V.; Janku, F.; Dasari, A.; Chung, W.; et al. Phase II Pilot Study of Vemurafenib in Patients with Metastatic BRAF-Mutated Colorectal Cancer. *J. Clin. Oncol.* **2015**, *33*, 4032–4038. [CrossRef]
50. Corcoran, R.B.; Atreya, C.E.; Falchook, G.S.; Kwak, E.L.; Ryan, D.P.; Bendell, J.C.; Hamid, O.; Messersmith, W.A.; Daud, A.; Kurzrock, R.; et al. Combined BRAF and MEK Inhibition with Dabrafenib and Trametinib in BRAF V600-Mutant Colorectal Cancer. *J. Clin. Oncol.* **2015**, *33*, 4023–4031. [CrossRef]
51. Subbiah, V.; Kreitman, R.J.; Wainberg, Z.A.; Cho, J.Y.; Schellens, J.H.M.; Soria, J.C.; Wen, P.Y.; Zielinski, C.; Cabanillas, M.E.; Urbanowitz, G.; et al. Dabrafenib and Trametinib Treatment in Patients with Locally Advanced or Metastatic BRAF V600-Mutant Anaplastic Thyroid Cancer. *J. Clin. Oncol.* **2018**, *36*, 7–13. [CrossRef]
52. Iravani, A.; Solomon, B.; Pattison, D.A.; Jackson, P.; Ravi Kumar, A.; Kong, G.; Hofman, M.S.; Akhurst, T.; Hicks, R.J. Mitogen-Activated Protein Kinase Pathway Inhibition for Redifferentiation of Radioiodine Refractory Differentiated Thyroid Cancer: An Evolving Protocol. *Thyroid* **2019**, *29*, 1634–1645. [CrossRef]
53. Jafri, S.; Yaqub, A. Redifferentiation of BRAF V600E-Mutated Radioiodine Refractory Metastatic Papillary Thyroid Cancer After Treatment with Dabrafenib and Trametinib. *Cureus* **2021**, *13*, e17488. [CrossRef]
54. Ullmann, T.M.; Liang, H.; Moore, M.D.; Al-Jamed, I.; Gray, K.D.; Limberg, J.; Stefanova, D.; Buicko, J.L.; Finnerty, B.; Beninato, T.; et al. Dual inhibition of BRAF and MEK increases expression of sodium iodide symporter in patient-derived papillary thyroid cancer cells in vitro. *Surgery* **2020**, *167*, 56–63. [CrossRef] [PubMed]
55. Gopal, R.K.; Kubler, K.; Calvo, S.E.; Polak, P.; Livitz, D.; Rosebrock, D.; Sadow, P.M.; Campbell, B.; Donovan, S.E.; Amin, S.; et al. Widespread Chromosomal Losses and Mitochondrial DNA Alterations as Genetic Drivers in Hurthle Cell Carcinoma. *Cancer Cell* **2018**, *34*, 242–255.e245. [CrossRef] [PubMed]

cancers

MDPI

Article

Portrait of the Inflammatory Response to Radioiodine Therapy in Female Patients with Differentiated Thyroid Cancer with/without Type 2 Diabetes Mellitus

Adina Elena Stanciu [1,*], Anca Hurduc [2], Marcel Marian Stanciu [3], Mirela Gherghe [4,5,*], Dan Cristian Gheorghe [6,7], Virgiliu Mihail Prunoiu [8,9] and Adina Zamfir-Chiru-Anton [10]

1 Department of Carcinogenesis and Molecular Biology, Institute of Oncology Bucharest, 022328 Bucharest, Romania
2 Department of Radionuclide Therapy, Institute of Oncology Bucharest, 022328 Bucharest, Romania; ahurduc@yahoo.com
3 Electrical Engineering Faculty, University Politehnica of Bucharest, 060042 Bucharest, Romania; marcel.stanciu@upb.ro
4 Nuclear Medicine Department, Institute of Oncology Bucharest, 022328 Bucharest, Romania
5 Nuclear Medicine Department, University of Medicine and Pharmacy "Carol Davila" Bucharest, 050474 Bucharest, Romania
6 ENT Department, "Maria Sklodowska Curie" Children's Emergency Hospital, 077120 Bucharest, Romania; gheorghe.dancristian@gmail.com
7 ENT Department, University of Medicine and Pharmacy "Carol Davila" Bucharest, 050474 Bucharest, Romania
8 Oncological Surgery Department, Institute of Oncology Bucharest, 022328 Bucharest, Romania; virgiliu.prunoiu@umfcd.ro
9 Oncological Surgery Department, University of Medicine and Pharmacy "Carol Davila" Bucharest, 050474 Bucharest, Romania
10 ENT Department, "Grigore Alexandrescu" Children's Emergency Hospital, 011743 Bucharest, Romania; zamfiradina@yahoo.com
* Correspondence: adinaelenastanciu@yahoo.com (A.E.S.); mirela.gherghe@umfcd.ro (M.G.)

Simple Summary: No clinical studies have investigated the effect of radioiodine (^{131}I)-targeted therapy on the potential markers of ongoing inflammation in patients with DTC associated with T2DM and obesity. To our knowledge, this is the first study to report the relationship between prescribed ^{131}I activity, blood radioactivity, BMI, and neutrophil-to-lymphocyte and platelet-to-lymphocyte ratios measured three days after ^{131}I intake in DTC with/without T2DM patients. The strong correlation measured between blood radioactivity and high BMI, without a correlation between blood radioactivity and the ^{131}I dose, proves a possible connection between ^{131}I uptake in the bloodstream and chronic inflammation, the so-called "perfect storm", specific to T2DM. Considering the immune response to ^{131}I therapy, the two groups of patients can be seen as a synchronous portrait of two sides: in patients without T2DM, if ^{131}I therapy has immunosuppressive effects, in the chronic inflammation context of T2DM, ^{131}I therapy amplifies immune metabolism.

Abstract: No clinical studies have investigated the effect of radioiodine (^{131}I)-targeted therapy on the neutrophil-to-lymphocyte ratio (NLR) and platelet-to-lymphocyte ratio (PLR) as inflammatory response markers in patients with differentiated thyroid cancer (DTC) associated with type 2 diabetes mellitus (T2DM) and obesity. This study aimed to assess the relationship between blood radioactivity, body mass index (BMI), and peripheral blood cells three days after ^{131}I intake in 56 female patients without T2DM (DTC/−T2DM) vs. 24 female patients with T2DM (DTC/+T2DM). Blood radioactivity, measured three days after ^{131}I intake, was significantly lower in the DTC/+T2DM than in the DTC/−T2DM patients (0.7 mCi vs. 1.5 mCi, $p < 0.001$). The relationship between blood radioactivity and BMI (r = 0.83, $p < 0.001$), blood radioactivity and NLR (r = 0.53, $p = 0.008$), and BMI and NLR (r = 0.58, $p = 0.003$) indicates a possible connection between the bloodstream ^{131}I uptake and T2DM-specific chronic inflammation. In patients without T2DM, ^{131}I therapy has immunosuppressive effects, leading to increased NLR (19.6%, $p = 0.009$) and PLR (39.1%, $p = 0.002$). On the contrary, in the chronic inflammation context of T2DM, ^{131}I therapy amplifies immune metabolism, leading to a drop in NLR (10%, $p = 0.032$) and PLR (13.4%, $p = 0.021$). Our results show that, in DTC/+T2DM, the bidirectional crosstalk between neutrophils and obesity may limit ^{131}I uptake in the bloodstream. Considering the immune response to ^{131}I therapy, the two groups of patients can be seen as a synchronous portrait of two sides. The explanation could lie in the different radiosensitivity of T and B lymphocytes, with T lymphocytes being predominant in patients with DTC/−T2DM and, most likely, B lymphocytes being predominant in T2DM.

Keywords: differentiated thyroid cancer; type 2 diabetes mellitus; ^{131}I; BMI; blood radioactivity; NLR; PLR

1. Introduction

The International Diabetes Federation (IDF) Diabetes Atlas 10th edition estimates a continued global increase in the prevalence of diabetes mellitus (DM), from 537 million adults in 2021 to 643 million by 2030 and 783 million by 2045 [1]. The most frequent type of DM, type 2 diabetes (T2DM), is commonly associated with a high body mass index (BMI) (expressed by overweight and obesity) [2]. Previous studies and meta-analyses have provided substantial evidence of the associations between T2DM and an increased risk of liver, pancreas, gallbladder, colorectal, breast, thyroid, kidney, and bladder cancer [3]. Evidence suggests a strong underlying relationship between differentiated thyroid cancer (DTC), the most common endocrine malignancy, and T2DM [4]. Standard-of-care management for DTC includes risk-adapted surgery, postoperative radioiodine (^{131}I) therapy based on the individual risk assessment, and thyroid hormone therapy [5–9]. Post-thyroidectomy suppression of thyroid-stimulating hormone (TSH) by high-dose levothyroxine can harm glucose homeostasis by impacting pancreatic β-cell development and glucose metabolism. A retrospective population-based cohort study revealed a U-shaped dose-dependent relationship between the levothyroxine dosage and T2DM [10].

The thyroid gland concentrates iodine via a sodium–iodide symporter (NIS) [11]. NIS has a longer half-life (5 days) in the presence of a high TSH level than in its absence (3 days) [11]. This explains why ^{131}I requires a TSH level greater than 30 mIU/L to enhance iodine uptake by thyroid cancer cells. Moreover, the thyroid gland concentrates iodine by a factor of 20–40 times compared to plasma [12]. This characteristic is the basis for treating patients with thyroid cancers originating from cells that concentrate iodine. ^{131}I-targeted therapy is based on delivering cytotoxic radiation levels to thyroid cancer cells or their microenvironment (presumably benign residual thyroid tissue, suspected but not identified remaining disease, and/or known residual or recurrent disease). However, some studies indicate the organification of iodine in tissues other than the thyroid, with NIS expression even being detected in the pancreas (ductal cells, exocrine parenchymal cells, and islets of Langerhans) [13,14]. Very few studies have analyzed the relationship between ^{131}I and pancreatic function in DTC patients. The uptake of a large dose of ^{131}I by the pancreas may affect β-cells, especially in patients diagnosed with T2DM [14]. Even if the ^{131}I therapy has achieved its desired therapeutic success, there are still question marks related to cellular heterogeneity in the tumor mass and/or cellular radiobiological response in patients with DTC associated with T2DM (DTC/+T2DM).

T2DM, historically considered a metabolic disease, is characterized by chronic systemic inflammation promoted by age and obesity. Inflammageing, the long-term result of the chronic physiological stimulation of the innate immune system, and metaflammation, a chronic low-grade inflammatory state orchestrated by metabolic cells in response to excess nutrients and energy (high BMI), represent the yin and yang of the T2DM [15,16]. Inflammation is widely acknowledged to play a significant role in the onset and progression of both cancer and T2DM and can be considered a hallmark of both diseases [3]. Chronic inflammation, the so-called "perfect storm", is an extreme challenge that cancer and T2DM patients face. Growing evidence shows that chronic systemic inflammation and the patient's immune status are closely related. Even though the overall mechanisms are not fully understood, radiation exposure is believed to have an ambivalent role on the immune system, exerting both immunogenic antitumor and immunosuppressive effects. Unlike conventional radiation therapy, targeted radionuclide therapy has a more pronounced effect on the immune system [14,17–22]. Recent data provide valuable information on potential markers of ongoing inflammation, including neutrophil counts, platelet counts, lymphocyte counts, platelet-to-lymphocyte ratio (PLR), and neutrophil-to-lymphocyte ratio (NLR) [18–22] after ^{131}I therapy.

While the number of publications investigating the effect of targeted therapy with ^{131}I on these potential new indicators of chronic inflammation in patients with DTC is relatively limited [18–22], they are practically nonexistent in patients with DTC associated with T2DM. This study aims to strengthen the results obtained by us previously [21,23]. Based on our results showing a higher incidence of platelets and lymphocytes in DTC/+T2DM patients than in DTC/−T2DM [23], we hypothesized that the effect of ^{131}I therapy on the peripheral blood cells measured in the two groups should also differ. To our knowledge, this is the first study to report the relationship between the prescribed ^{131}I activity, whole-blood radioactivity, BMI, NLR, and PLR measured three days after ^{131}I intake in patients with DTC/+T2DM vs. DTC/−T2DM.

2. Materials and Methods

2.1. Patients and Study Protocol

This prospective study included 56 female patients with DTC/−T2DM (mean age, 57.3 ± 9.1 years) and 24 female patients with DTC/+T2DM (mean age, 61.6 ± 6.9 years) who were referred to the Department of Radionuclide Therapy of the Institute of Oncology Bucharest for targeted therapy with ^{131}I over a period of approximately two years between 2019 and 2020. The enrolled patients discontinued L-thyroxine treatment and followed a low-iodine diet for at least four weeks and two weeks, respectively, before the administration of ^{131}I sodium iodide ThyroTop, a radiopharmaceutical purchased from the Institute of Isotopes Co. Ltd. (Budapest, Hungary). For a strong uptake into the thyroid bed, ^{131}I sodium iodide ThyroTop was administered when the TSH level was higher than 30 IU/mL after fasting for more than 4 h and continuing to fast for another 2 h. The ^{131}I given activity in this patient cohort was based on the joint statement on the theranostic approaches in the management and therapy of DTC [5,6] by the European Thyroid Association (ETA), American Thyroid Association (ATA), Society of Nuclear Medicine and Molecular Imaging (SNMMI), and the European Association of Nuclear Medicine (EANM), as well as the recent SNMMI/EANM practice guideline [8] and ETA Consensus [9], in accordance with safety precautions [24]. Patients were instructed to maintain adequate hydration after receiving the therapeutic dose of ^{131}I to enable frequent urination and quickly eliminate the ^{131}I from the body.

The following were the exclusion criteria: (i) age under 18 years; (ii) acute or chronic infection (known to affect the NLR and PLR value); (iii) renal impairment (kidney function is involved in ^{131}I elimination) [21]; (iv) gastrointestinal disease (stool frequency); (v) ongoing diuretic treatment (urine frequency); (vii) ongoing treatment with steroidal or non-steroidal anti-inflammatory drugs (known to affect the NLR and PLR value) [25]; (vi) ongoing treatment with aspirin (known to affect the platelets and PLR value); (vii) a history of coronary heart disease, cerebral infarction, and blood system disease(s) that would possibly affect platelet- and PLR-related indices; (viii) poorly controlled diabetes (known to lead to insulin resistance and hyperinsulinemia, which causes thyroid tissue proliferation) [4]. Because antidiabetics such as sulfonylureas, pioglitazone, and thiazolidinediones can have a negative impact on thyroid disease [4], the DTC/+T2DM patients were treated with metformin, which is beneficial for both T2DM and DTC. To avoid intersex variations, only women were included in the study.

The medical and medication histories and demographic data (age, height, weight) of each enrolled patient were compiled. The serum TSH level measured upon admission to the Department of Radionuclide Therapy was collected from medical records. The blood volume and body mass index (BMI) of the recruited individuals were computed using their height (H) and weight (W). The Nadler equation for females was used to obtain the whole blood volume/patient: $Blood_{Volume} = (0.3561xH^3) + (0.03308xW) + 0.1833$. The patient's kilograms (kg) weight was divided by their height in meters squared (m^2) to calculate BMI. BMIs between 18.5 and 24.9 kg/m^2 are considered to be optimum. Overweight is defined as a BMI between 25 and 29.9 kg/m^2. In comparison, obesity is defined as a BMI equal to or greater than 30 kg/m^2 (obesity class I: BMI = 30 to 34.9 kg/m^2, obesity class II: BMI = 35 to 39.9 kg/m^2, and obesity class III: BMI greater than or equal to 40 kg/m^2) [26].

The study was conducted following the guiding principles of the Declaration of Helsinki and was approved by the local ethics committee of our institution (No.15140/10.09.2019). The research objectives and the medical procedure required for blood sampling were explained to each subject. At admission, each participant signed an informed consent form.

2.2. Blood Sampling and Radioactivity Quantification

Peripheral blood samples were extracted through intravenous puncture into BD Vacutainer EDTA tubes (purchased from Becton, Dickinson, and Company, Franklin Lakes, NJ, USA) with a draw volume of 2 mL before and three days after the therapeutic dose of ^{131}I administration (immediately before the patient's discharge from the isolation ward). As the blood samples collected after the ^{131}I intake were still radioactive, each tube was tagged with an international radioactivity symbol sticker. The radioactivity of each blood sample tube (2 mL) was measured three times in a dose calibrator (CURIEMENTOR^R 4 Isotope Calibrator, PTW Freiburg, Freiburg, Germany). The background count was assessed before each radioactivity measurement and then subtracted from the registered value. The measurements ranged from 0.01 µCi to 2486 mCi (or from 0.001 mBq to 92 GBq), with an accuracy of about 5%. The blood radioactivity per 1 mL was then calculated by dividing the average of the three radioactivity measurements per blood sample tube (2 mL) by 2. Then, the blood sample radioactivity per 1 mL was multiplied by the patient's blood volume to obtain each patient's whole blood radioactivity.

A procedure has been developed for collecting, transporting, processing, and disposing of radioactive blood tubes. This procedure adheres to the current recommendations issued by the European Association of Nuclear Medicine (EANM) Dosimetry Committee [27].

2.3. Biomarker Measurement

Blood cell analysis (blood-count parameters: neutrophils, platelets, and lymphocytes) was conducted using an ADVIA 2120i automatic Hematology System with an auto slide (Siemens, Munich, Germany). The PLR and NLR were computed by dividing the absolute platelet count by the absolute lymphocyte count and the absolute neutrophil count by the absolute lymphocyte count, respectively.

2.4. Statistics

Patient data were processed using Microsoft Office Excel 2007 SP2 (including Data Analysis Tools). Statistica software (version 8.0; StatSoft, Inc., Tulsa, OK, USA) was used for statistical analysis. Continuous variables were expressed as the means ± standard deviation or median value with interquartile range (IQR: 25–75%) when appropriate. The data acquired after preliminary analysis were verified using the Anderson–Darling, Shapiro–Wilk, and Kolmogorov–Smirnov tests. The non-parametric Kruskal–Wallis test was used to compare the distribution of continuous variables between different categories for independent samples (DTC/−T2DM vs. DTC/+T2DM groups), while the Wilcoxon test was used for paired samples (DTC/−T2DM group before and three days after ^{131}I intake and DTC/+T2DM before and three days after ^{131}I intake). The correlation between circulating biomarkers and their ratios was assessed using Pearson's correlation coefficient (r). For all tests, significance was set at a p-value < 0.05.

3. Results

3.1. Blood Parameters before the ^{131}I Intake

Several blood parameters measured in the two study groups before the ^{131}I sodium iodide ThyroTop intake are summarized in Table 1. Significant differences in absolute lymphocyte and platelet counts were observed among the DTC/−T2DM and DTC/+T2DM patients (1.6×10^9/L vs. 1.9×10^9/L, $p = 0.015$ and 233.5×10^9/L vs. 333×10^9/L, $p < 0.001$). Increased platelet and lymphocyte counts were reported in female patients with concomitant T2DM. The median TSH level, confirming the short hypothyroid state specific to the four weeks of thyroid hormone withdrawal, was comparable (81.2 mIU/L in DTC/−T2DM patients vs. 81.3 mIU/L in DTC/+T2DM patients), with no statistical significance between the two groups.

Table 1. Blood parameters measured before ^{131}I intake in the two study groups.

Variables	DTC/−T2DM	DTC/+T2DM	p-Value
	n = 56	n = 24	
Lymphocytes ($\times 10^9$/L) [a]	1.6 (1.3–1.9)	1.9 (1.3–2.2)	0.015
Neutrophils ($\times 10^9$/L) [a]	3.6 (3.1–4.5)	3.7 (3.0–4.6)	0.731
Platelets ($\times 10^9$/L) [a]	233.5 (199.0–273.0)	333.0 (312.0–378.0)	<0.001
NLR [a]	2.2 (1.7–2.9)	2.1 (1.7–2.8)	0.712
PLR [a]	143.1 (115.1–184.5)	177.5 (153.5–224.8)	0.035
TSH (mIU/L) [a]	81.2 (62.7–98.5)	81.3 (62.9–99.1)	0.752

DTC/−T2DM, differentiated thyroid cancer without type 2 diabetes mellitus; DTC/+T2DM, differentiated thyroid cancer with type 2 diabetes mellitus; NLR, neutrophil-to-lymphocyte ratio; PLR, platelet-to-lymphocyte ratio; ^{131}I, radioiodine; TSH, thyroid stimulating hormone; [a] Data are expressed as median and interquartile ranges (25–75%).

3.2. Characteristics of the Study Population with a Focus on Whole-Blood Radioactivity

There were no significant differences between the two groups (DTC/−T2DM and DTC/+T2DM) regarding age ($p = 0.153$). BMI analysis showed that, unlike the DTC/−T2DM patients who were overweight, DTC/+T2DM patients suffered from obesity (obesity class I), with a median BMI of 33.3 kg/m^2 ($p < 0.001$) (Table 2). Based on height and weight, the median volume of blood per patient was higher in the subjects with concomitant T2DM than in those without (4880.1 mL vs. 4363.1 mL, $p = 0.018$). Regarding whole-blood radioactivity, even though the administered median activity of ^{131}I was higher in the DTC/+T2DM group than in DTC/−T2DM (107.9 mCi vs. 88.7 mCi or 3.992 GBq vs. 3.282 GBq, $p = 0.035$), the blood radioactivity measured three days after ^{131}I intake was significantly lower in the DTC/+T2DM patients than in those with DTC/−T2DM (0.7 mCi vs. 1.5 mCi, $p < 0.001$).

3.3. Dynamics of Hematological Parameters after the ^{131}I Intake

Figure 1 illustrates the dynamics of absolute lymphocyte counts and the ratios (NLR, PLR) after ^{131}I intake in the DTC/−T2DM group of patients. Lymphocyte count exhibited a decreasing trend of 20% ($p = 0.015$), while neutrophil count, platelet count, and NLR and PLR displayed an opposite trend, with increases of 9%, 11.1%, 19.6%, and 39.1%, respectively ($p = 0.532$, $p = 0.034$, $p = 0.009$ and $p = 0.002$, respectively), in the DTC/−T2DM patients following the administration of the recommended dose of ^{131}I.

Table 2. Clinical data in the two study groups.

Variables	DTC/−T2DM $n = 56$	DTC/+T2DM $n = 24$	p-Value
Age (years) [a]	57.3 ± 9.1	62.7 ± 6.5	0.153
Height (m) [b]	1.64 (1.60–1.65)	1.63 (1.60–1.65)	0.754
Weight (kg) [b]	81.8 (69.05–90.74)	91.48 (80.12–101.44)	0.032
BMI (kg/m^2) [b]	29.6 (26.2–33.9)	33.3 (30.8–37.9)	<0.001
Blood Volume (mL) [b]	4364.1 (3976.3–4825.1)	4880.1 (4613.8–5112.3)	0.018
Administered Activity of ^{131}I (mCi) [b]	88.7 (60.7–129.4)	107.9 (88.9–137)	0.035
Whole-blood radioactivity (mCi) [b]	1.5 (0.7–2.3)	0.7 (0.4–0.9)	<0.001

BMI, body mass index; DTC/−T2DM, differentiated thyroid cancer without type 2 diabetes mellitus; DTC/+T2DM, differentiated thyroid cancer associated with type 2 diabetes mellitus; ^{131}I, radioiodine; [a] mean ± standard deviation; [b] Data are expressed as median and interquartile ranges (25–75%).

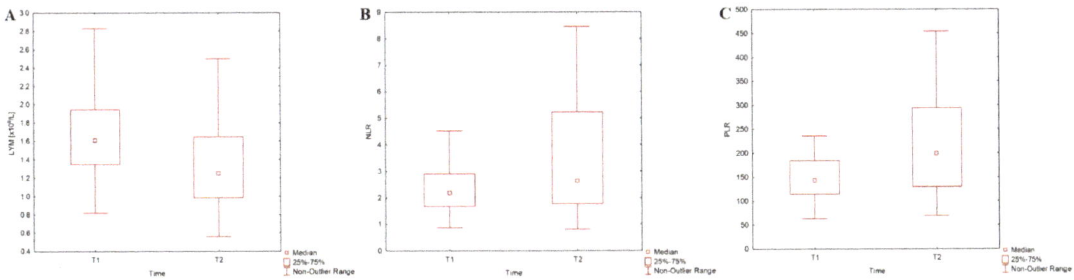

Figure 1. Dynamics of absolute lymphocyte counts (LYM) (**A**), neutrophil-to-lymphocyte ratio (NLR) (**B**), and platelet-to-lymphocyte ratio (PLR) (**C**) three days after ^{131}I administration in differentiated thyroid cancer patients without type 2 diabetes mellitus.

In contrast, in the DTC/+T2DM group, the time course of lymphocytes, neutrophils, and platelets did not show statistically significant changes (8% increase—Figure 2A, 1.7% increase, and 1% decrease, respectively; $p > 0.05$). However, NLR and PLR exhibited a statistically significant decrease of 10% ($p = 0.032$) and 13.4% ($p = 0.021$) three days after ^{131}I administration, as depicted in Figure 2B,C.

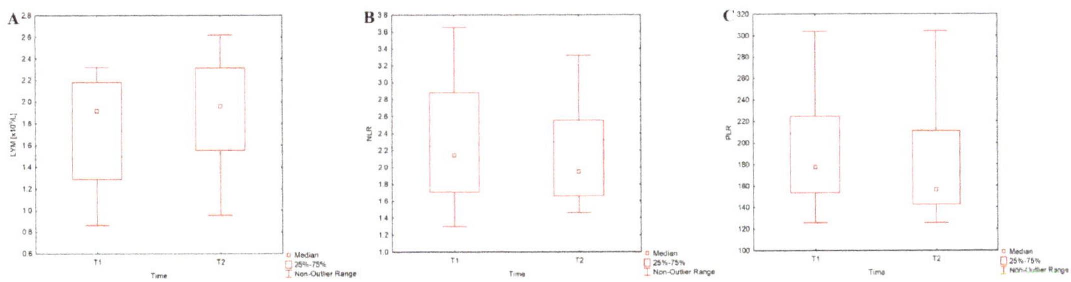

Figure 2. Dynamics of absolute lymphocyte counts (LYM) (**A**), neutrophil-to-lymphocyte ratio (NLR) (**B**), and platelet-to-lymphocyte ratio (PLR) (**C**) three days after ^{131}I administration in differentiated thyroid cancer patients with type 2 diabetes mellitus.

3.4. Correlations in the DTC/−T2DM Group

In the DTC/−T2DM group, there was a positive relationship between the administered ^{131}I dose and whole-blood radioactivity measured three days after ^{131}I intake ($r = 0.64$, $p < 0.001$), as we previously showed [21]. It should be mentioned that the BMI of the patients enrolled in this group was not correlated with whole-blood radioactivity. Furthermore, both administered ^{131}I activity and whole-blood radioactivity were correlated with absolute lymphocyte count (r = −0.51 and r = −0.56, $p < 0.001$), absolute neutrophil count (r = 0.49 and r = 0.54, $p < 0.001$), and absolute platelet count (r = 0.46 and r = 0.51, $p < 0.001$) and strongly correlated with NLR (r = 0.69 and r = 0.74, $p < 0.001$) and PLR (r = 0.69 and r = 0.75, $p < 0.001$). The relationship between whole-blood radioactivity and absolute lymphocyte count, absolute neutrophile count, NLR, and PLR is presented in Figure 3.

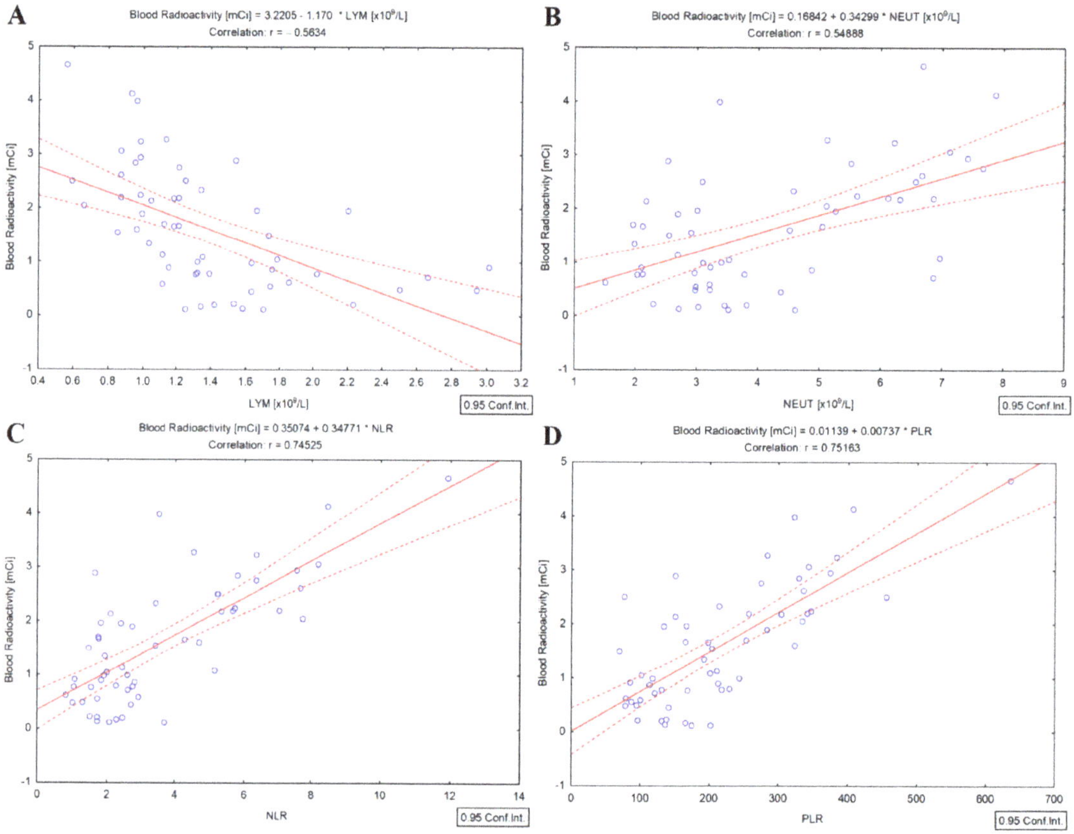

Figure 3. Correlation between the whole-blood radioactivity and absolute lymphocyte count (**A**), absolute neutrophile count (**B**), NLR (**C**), and PLR (**D**) in differentiated thyroid cancer patients without type 2 diabetes mellitus (measured three days after ^{131}I intake); ("—" fitted linear regression curve, "- - -" equality line).

3.5. Correlations in the DTC/+T2DM Group

Unlike the DTC/−T2DM group, the presence of T2DM led to a different kind of portrait of the relationships between the investigated parameters. An overview of the results presented in Figure 4 shows that whole-blood radioactivity was positively correlated with BMI (r = 0.83, $p < 0.001$). However, unexpectedly, whole-blood radioactivity was not correlated with the administered dose of ^{131}I.

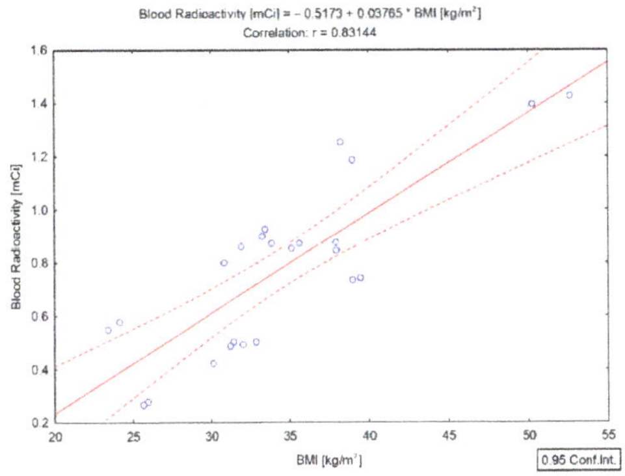

Figure 4. Correlation between whole-blood radioactivity and BMI in differentiated thyroid cancer patients with type 2 diabetes mellitus (measured at three days after ^{131}I intake); (— fitted linear regression curve, - - - equality line).

Likewise, the ^{131}I activity administered to the patients was not correlated with any investigated hematological parameter. A significant statistical relationship was measured only between whole-blood radioactivity and absolute lymphocyte count ($r = 0.42$, $p = 0.039$) (Figure 5A), absolute neutrophil count ($r = 0.69$, $p < 0.001$) (Figure 5B), NLR ($r = 0.58$, $p = 0.003$) (Figure 5C), and PLR ($r = -0.50$, $p = 0.11$) (Figure 5D).

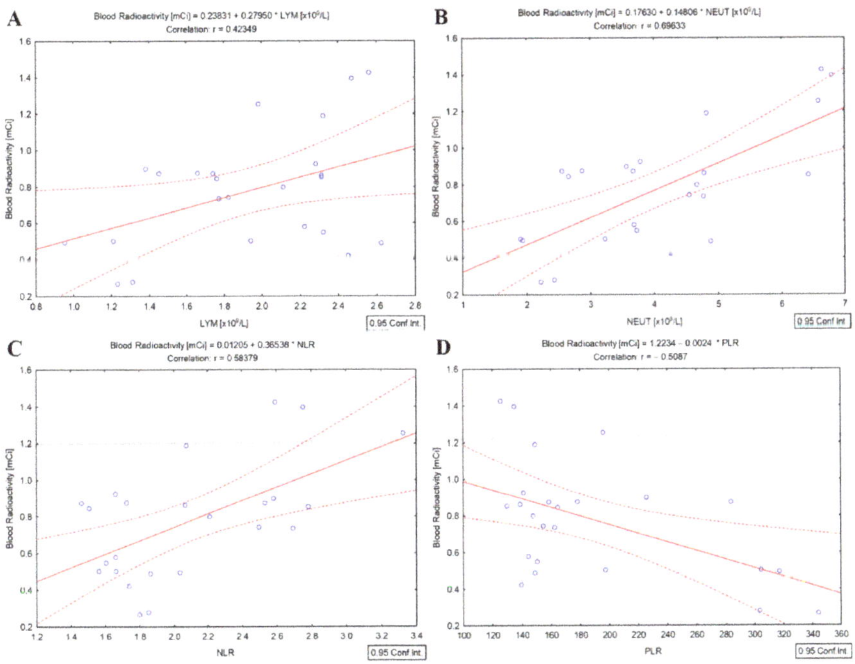

Figure 5. Correlation between whole-blood radioactivity and absolute lymphocyte count (**A**), absolute neutrophile count (**B**), NLR (**C**), and PLR (**D**) in differentiated thyroid cancer patients with type 2 diabetes mellitus (measured three days after ^{131}I intake); ("—" fitted linear regression curve, "- - -" equality line).

BMI was only correlated with neutrophils and NLR both before (r = 0.57, $p = 0.004$ and r = 0.54, $p = 0.008$, respectively) and after ^{131}I administration (r = 0.58, $p = 0.003$ and r = 0.53, $p = 0.008$, respectively) (Figure 6A,B).

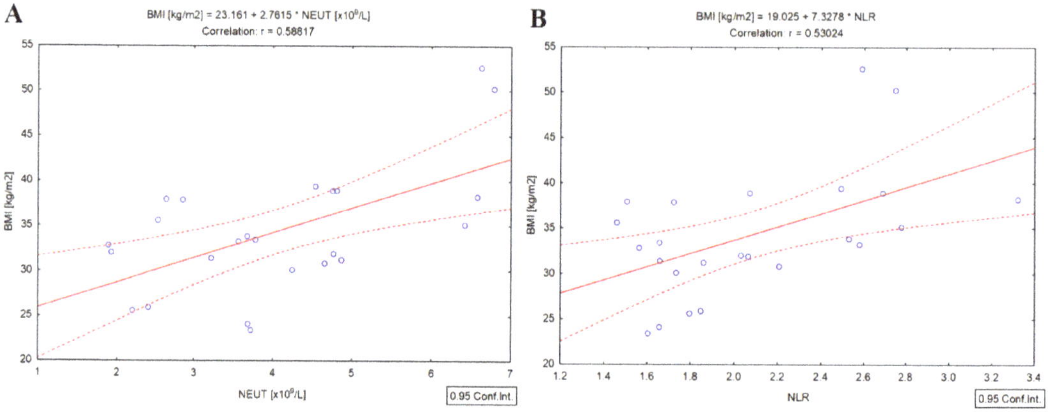

Figure 6. Correlation between the BMI and absolute neutrophile count (**A**) and NLR (**B**) in differentiated thyroid cancer patients with type 2 diabetes mellitus (measured three days after ^{131}I intake); ("—" fitted linear regression curve, "- - -" equality line).

4. Discussion

The present study reveals several key findings: Firstly, the blood radioactivity measured three days after ^{131}I intake was significantly lower in the DTC/+T2DM patients compared to the DTC/−T2DM patients, despite higher administered doses and BMI values. Secondly, there was a strong positive correlation between blood radioactivity and BMI (r = 0.83, $p < 0.001$) in the DTC/+T2DM patients, but no correlation was observed with the administered dose of ^{131}I. Thirdly, ^{131}I therapy demonstrated immune-suppressive effects, resulting in increased NLR and PLR in the DTC/−T2DM patients. Lastly, in the context of chronic inflammation in T2DM, ^{131}I therapy amplified immune metabolism, leading to a decrease in NLR and PLR.

Our study found that the whole-blood radioactivity measured three days after the ^{131}I intake was significantly lower in the DTC/+T2DM patients than in the DTC/−T2DM patients ($p < 0.001$), despite higher administered doses and BMI ($p = 0.035$ and $p = 0.012$). These results align with our previous publication [21], which demonstrated a biphasic course of ^{131}I blood concentration in DTC/−T2DM patients. The initial rapid decrease in whole-blood radioactivity was attributed to fast clearance by the kidneys, followed by a slight increase due to the release of ^{131}I in the blood by residual thyroid tissue. Further investigations are needed to determine if DTC/+T2DM patients exhibit a similar biphasic course of ^{131}I blood concentration. Nevertheless, our results confirm the theory proposed in other studies that the iodine uptake in the blood of T2DM patients is lower compared to healthy individuals. Several explanations could account for this difference:

(i) Expression of NIS: NIS expression has been detected in various tissues, including the pancreas, where ductal cells, exocrine parenchymal cells, and islets of Langerhans show positive staining [13,14]). It is possible that, in the presence of T2DM, iodine uptake is relatively high in pancreatic tissues, especially in the islets of Langerhans, which are known to exhibit dysfunction in T2DM [10,14]. It is well known that the thyroid gland concentrates iodine by a factor of 20–40 times compared to plasma [12]. Cumulatively, these factors may contribute to decreased ^{131}I uptake in the bloodstream.

(ii) Changes in biomolecule conformation: The uptake of ^{131}I in the blood is dependent on the iodination of proteins, carbohydrates, and lipids [28]. In the presence of T2DM, structural conformational changes in biomolecules from the blood, resulting from the disease itself, could reduce the number of binding sites and consequently decrease ^{131}I uptake in this group [28].

(iii) Increased urination: Obesity, often associated with T2DM, can lead to increased intra-abdominal pressure, resulting in increased urine production or frequency [29]. This, coupled with the common symptom of increased urination in T2DM [30], could lead to a higher excretion of ^{131}I in T2DM patients compared to those without T2DM.

The correlation between BMI and the administered radiation dose has been extensively studied in various settings, starting from diagnosis (mammography or computed tomography) to conventional radiotherapy. However, studies examining the correlation between BMI, administered dose, and external dose rates specifically for patients treated with ^{131}I have produced contradictory results. Our findings are consistent with those obtained by Lahfi et al. [31] and Pickering et al. [32], who reported higher external dose rate values, with 11% and 10%, respectively, in the normal BMI group compared to the obese group for administered ^{131}I doses exceeding 150 mCi. Lahfi et al. [31] attributed these results to increased gamma ray attenuation in obese patients. However, this explanation does not apply when analyzing whole-blood radioactivity. In our study, whole-blood radioactivity was 53% higher in the group without T2DM than in the obese group with T2DM. Notably, a statistically significant correlation between whole-blood radioactivity and BMI was found only in the presence of T2DM ($r = 0.83$, $p < 0.001$), as shown in Figure 4. Moreover, contrary to expectations, in the DTC/+T2DM patients, whole-blood radioactivity was not correlated with the administrated dose of ^{131}I.

The strong correlation measured between the low whole-blood radioactivity and high BMI (Figure 4) implies the existence of a possible connection between the ^{131}I uptake in the bloodstream and the specific systemic chronic inflammation of T2DM (chronic low-grade inflammation of the adipose tissue along with chronic physiological stimulation of the innate immune system). One of the concepts explaining the association between obesity and T2DM in our study, obesity class I (BMI = 33.3 kg/m^2) in DTC/+T2DM patients, is the theory of chronic, low-grade systemic inflammation orchestrated by the metabolic cells in response to excess nutrients and energy, called metaflammation. As additional evidence of this connection between the ^{131}I uptake in the bloodstream and chronic low-grade inflammation of the adipose tissue, both BMI and whole-blood radioactivity were positively correlated with absolute neutrophil count ($r = 0.58$, $p = 0.003$ and $r = 0.69$, $p < 0.001$) (Figures 6A and 5B) and NLR ($r = 0.53$, $p = 0.008$ and $r = 0.58$, $p = 0.003$) (Figures 6B and 5C). It seems that the administration of the therapeutic dose of ^{131}I led to the activation of immune metabolism. Immune metabolism refers to the interaction between metabolism and immune response to the action of targeted radionuclide therapy. It is well known that, during obesity-induced chronic inflammation, the number of neutrophils increases in the first phase in the peripheral circulation, and from there, neutrophils begin to infiltrate the adipose tissue [33] and the endothelium of blood vessels [34]. Consequently, in obesity-induced chronic inflammation, neutrophils are the first immune cells recruited in adipose tissue [35], and NLR is the expression of the relationship between innate (neutrophils) and adaptive (lymphocytes) immune responses. It seems that, in the presence of T2DM, the bidirectional crosstalk between neutrophils and obesity (statistically significant correlation between high BMI and neutrophils) leads to the limitation of ^{131}I uptake in the bloodstream (statistically significant correlation between high BMI, neutrophils, and whole-blood radioactivity).

The most severe side effect of radiotherapy in cancer patients is the suppression of hematopoiesis. Its curative effect is mainly based on modulating the immune response in the chronic inflammatory tissue. Therefore, systemic inflammation and their immune status are essential parameters influencing the response to radiotherapy. Although the overall mechanisms are not entirely understood, targeted radionuclide therapy (in our study, therapy with high doses of ^{131}I) exerts both anti-tumor immunogenic and immune-suppressive effects. Practically, radionuclide therapy assumes that cells are not only irradiated for minutes as in conventional radiotherapy but are continuously irradiated over a much more extended period (with the intensity of the dose decreasing over time) depending on the effective half-life of the radionuclide. This continuous exposure of the peripheral blood cells to ^{131}I with a median whole-body effective half-life of 13 h results in cell renewal, apoptosis, and the redistribution of hematopoietic cells, with hematological toxicity being the most common adverse effect of ^{131}I therapy [18,22]. In our study, ^{131}I intake led to a 22.4% drop in lymphocyte count and an increase of 15.4% in NLR and 28.1% in PLR in the DTC/−T2DM patients (Figure 1). These results align with studies by Yi et al. [22] and Rui et al. [18], which reported a 37% and 11.5% reduction in lymphocyte count following ^{131}I therapy. Because peripheral blood lymphocytes are the most radiosensitive mammalian cells, they are constantly regenerating, and their drop after irradiation confirms this. Moreover, the whole-blood radioactivity measured three days after the ^{131}I intake was negatively correlated with the absolute lymphocyte count ($r = -0.56$, $p < 0.001$), as shown in Figure 3A. If, in the DTC/−T2DM group, the lymphocyte count decreased, in the presence of T2DM, the count increased by 2.6%; however, this increase was without statistical significance. This slight increase was marked by the positive correlation between the whole-blood radioactivity measured three days after ^{131}I intake and the absolute lymphocyte count at this time (Figure 5A). An explanation for this could lie in the different radiosensitivity of T and B lymphocytes [36], T lymphocytes predominating in patients with DTC/−T2DM and, most likely, B lymphocytes in T2DM. Even if macrophages are the most abundant type of immune cell in adipose tissue, other immune cells, such as B cells, are also present and play an essential role in regulating adipose tissue inflammation in T2DM, with even a higher ratio of B-cell subsets than bone marrow [37].

Because lymphocytes are a mainstay of anticancer immunity, NLR and PLR reflect immune status after radiotherapy. The overall picture in which targeted radionuclide therapy exerts immune-suppressive effects leading to the increase in NLR and PLR in DTC/−T2DM patients was also shown by Chew et al. [17] after ^{90}Y radioembolization in hepatocellular carcinoma. In our study, whole-blood radioactivity was strongly positively correlated with NLR ($r = 0.74$, $p < 0.001$) and PLR ($r = 0.75$, $p < 0.001$) in the DTC/−T2DM group (Figure 3C,D). In these patients, the local and systemic immune systems were activated differently by ^{131}I therapy than by conventional radiotherapy, leading to sustained tumor response. If conventional radiotherapy induces apoptosis, targeted radionuclide therapy can predominantly induce necrosis, which is considered inflammatory cell death [38]. Therefore, the increased production of cytokines and chemokines leads to the activation of immune cells. Further, the enhanced immune system leads to increased NLR and PLR, demonstrating the immune-modulatory effects of ^{131}I in a clinical setting. This picture is changed in the presence of T2DM because, after ^{131}I irradiation, NLR dropped by 10%, and PLR dropped by 13.4%. Moreover, whole-blood radioactivity measured three days after the ^{131}I intake was positively correlated with NLR ($r = 0.58$, $p = 0.003$) (Figure 5C) and negatively correlated with PLR ($r = -0.50$, $p = 0.11$) (Figure 5D). Because our patients did not receive any additional treatment apart from ^{131}I, the changes in NLR and PLR are considered to be solely attributed to ^{131}I. These observations suggest that the immunomodulatory effects of ^{131}I therapy differ between patients with and without T2DM.

The limitations of our study include its single-center cross-sectional design and relatively small sample size. Despite these limitations, the study included patients referred from across the country to our Department of Radionuclide Therapy. Additionally, the sample size, although small, was sufficient for statistical calculations with a 95% confidence interval and a Z-score of 1.96. Furthermore, the sample size reflects the rarity of the association between DTC and T2DM. On the other hand, all blood samples collected three days after ^{131}I intake were radioactive. The risk of healthcare professionals' radioactive contamination must be considered. Moreover, the study population consisted solely of women due to sex-related differences in clinical outcomes and result interpretation, as sex hormones significantly influence the regulation of thyroid and immune functions. Between estradiol, progesterone, androgens, thyroid hormones, and the immune system is a complex crosstalk [39]. Sex hormones can modulate the immune response to ^{131}I therapy. If, in women, progesterone has extensive anti-inflammatory effects and estradiol improves cellular and humoral mediated immune responses, in men, androgens (dihydrotestosterone and testosterone) suppress the activity of immune cells, leading to low immune responses [40]. The immune system functions in a sexually dimorphic manner, with females exhibiting more robust immune responses than males [41].

5. Conclusions

In conclusion, our study reveals correlations between whole-blood radioactivity, BMI, and NLR, indicating a possible connection between ^{131}I uptake in the bloodstream and the chronic inflammation characteristic of T2DM. The bidirectional crosstalk between neutrophils and obesity appears to limit ^{131}I uptake in the bloodstream in the presence of T2DM. Moreover, ^{131}I therapy demonstrated immunosuppressive effects in the DTC/−T2DM patients, leading to increased NLR and PLR. In contrast, in the context of chronic inflammation in T2DM, ^{131}I therapy amplified immune metabolism, resulting in decreased NLR and PLR. These findings suggest that reducing B lymphocytes could be a potential treatment direction for DTC/+T2DM patients. Further research is needed to elucidate the underlying mechanisms and explore the relationship between prescribed ^{131}I activity, whole-blood radioactivity, and peripheral blood cells at multiple time points in DTC/+T2DM patients.

Author Contributions: Conceptualization, A.E.S.; methodology, A.E.S. and A.H.; formal analysis, M.M.S.; investigation, A.E.S. and A.H.; data curation, M.M.S. and A.E.S.; writing—original draft preparation, A.E.S.; writing—review and editing, A.E.S., A.H., M.M.S., M.G., D.C.G., V.M.P. and A.Z.-C.-A.; visualization, A.E.S., A.H., M.M.S., M.G., D.C.G., V.M.P. and A.Z.-C.-A.; supervision, A.E.S., A.H. and A.Z.-C.-A. All authors have read and agreed to the published version of the manuscript.

Funding: This research received no external funding.

Institutional Review Board Statement: The study was conducted according to the guidelines of the Declaration of Helsinki and approved by the Institute of Oncology Bucharest Medical Ethics Committee (No.15140/10 September 2019).

Informed Consent Statement: Informed consent was obtained from all subjects involved in the study.

Data Availability Statement: The data presented in this study are available upon request from the corresponding author.

Conflicts of Interest: The authors declare no conflict of interest.

References

1. International Diabetes Federation. *IDF Atlas*, 10th ed. Available online: https://diabetesatlas.org/atlas/tenth-edition/ (accessed on 14 February 2023).
2. The American Diabetes Association. Classification and Diagnosis of Diabetes: Standards of Medical Care in Diabetes—2021. *Diabetes Care* **2021**, *44*, S15–S33. [CrossRef]
3. Zhu, B.; Qu, S. The Relationship Between Diabetes Mellitus and Cancers and Its Underlying Mechanisms. *Front. Endocrinol.* **2022**, *13*, 800995. [CrossRef] [PubMed]
4. Kalra, S.; Aggarwal, S.; Khandelwal, D. Thyroid Dysfunction and Type 2 Diabetes Mellitus: Screening Strategies and Implications for Management. *Diabetes Ther.* **2019**, *10*, 2035–2044. [CrossRef] [PubMed]
5. Tuttle, R.M.; Ahuja, S.; Avram, A.M.; Bernet, V.J.; Bourguet, P.; Daniels, G.H.; Dillehay, G.; Draganescu, C.; Flux, G.; Führer, D.; et al. Controversies, Consensus, and Collaboration in the Use of ^{131}I Therapy in Differentiated Thyroid Cancer: A Joint Statement from the American Thyroid Association, the European Association of Nuclear Medicine, the Society of Nuclear Medicine and Molecular Imaging, and the European Thyroid Association. *Thyroid* **2019**, *29*, 461–470. [CrossRef] [PubMed]
6. Gulec, S.A.; Ahuja, S.; Avram, A.M.; Bernet, V.J.; Bourguet, P.; Draganescu, C.; Elisei, R.; Giovanella, L.; Grant, F.D.; Greenspan, B.; et al. A Joint Statement from the American Thyroid Association, the European Association of Nuclear Medicine, the European Thyroid Association, the Society of Nuclear Medicine and Molecular Imaging on Current Diagnostic and Theranostic Approaches in the Management of Thyroid Cancer. *Thyroid* **2021**, *31*, 1009–1019. [CrossRef]

7. Gherghe, M.; Lazar, A.M.; Mutuleanu, M.D.; Stanciu, A.E.; Martin, S. Radiomics Analysis of [^{18}F]FDG PET/CT Thyroid Incidentalomas: How Can It Improve Patients' Clinical Management? A Systematic Review from the Literature. *Diagnostics* **2022**, *12*, 471. [CrossRef]
8. Avram, A.M.; Giovanella, L.; Greenspan, B.; Lawson, S.A.; Luster, M.; Van Nostrand, D.; Peacock, J.G.; Ovčariček, P.P.; Silberstein, E.; Tulchinsky, M.; et al. SNMMI Procedure Standard/EANM Practice Guideline for Nuclear Medicine Evaluation and Therapy of Differentiated Thyroid Cancer: Abbreviated Version. *J. Nucl. Med.* **2022**, *63*, 15N–35N. [PubMed]
9. Pacini, F.; Fuhrer, D.; Elisei, R.; Handkiewicz-Junak, D.; Leboulleux, S.; Luster, M.; Schlumberger, M.; Smit, J.W. 2022 ETA Consensus Statement: What are the indications for post-surgical radioiodine therapy in differentiated thyroid cancer? *Eur. Thyroid. J.* **2022**, *11*, e210046. [CrossRef]
10. Roh, E.; Noh, E.; Hwang, S.Y.; Kim, J.A.; Song, E.; Park, M.; Choi, K.M.; Baik, S.H.; Cho, G.J.; Yoo, H.J. Increased Risk of Type 2 Diabetes in Patients with Thyroid Cancer After Thyroidectomy: A Nationwide Cohort Study. *J. Clin. Endocrinol. Metab.* **2021**, *107*, e1047–e1056. [CrossRef]
11. Riedel, C.; Levy, O.; Carrasco, N. Post-transcriptional regulation of the sodium/iodide symporter by thyrotropin. *J. Biol. Chem.* **2001**, *276*, 21458–21463. [CrossRef]
12. Salvatore, D.; Davies, T.F.; Schlumberger, M.J.; Hay, I.D.; Larsen, P.R. Thyroid physiology and diagnostic evaluation of patients with thyroid disorders. In *Williams Textbook of Endocrinology*, 12th ed.; Melmed, S., Polonsky, K.S., Larsen, P.R., Kronenberg, H.M., Eds.; Elsevier: Philadelphia, PA, USA, 2011; pp. 327–475.
13. Spitzweg, C.; Joba, W.; Schriever, K.; Goellner, J.R.; Morris, J.C.; Heufelder, A.E. Analysis of human sodium iodide symporter immunoreactivity in human exocrine glands. *J. Clin. Endocrinol. Metab.* **1999**, *84*, 4178–4184. [CrossRef]
14. Samadi, R.; Shafiei, B.; Azizi, F.; Ghasemi, A. Radioactive Iodine Therapy and Glucose Tolerance. *Cell J.* **2017**, *19*, 184–193. [CrossRef] [PubMed]
15. Prattichizzo, F.; De Nigris, V.; Spiga, R.; Mancuso, E.; La Sala, L.; Antonicelli, R.; Testa, R.; Procopio, A.D.; Olivieri, F.; Ceriello, A. Inflammageing and metaflammation: The yin and yang of type 2 diabetes. *Ageing Res. Rev.* **2018**, *41*, 1–17. [CrossRef] [PubMed]
16. Kuryłowicz, A.; Koźniewski, K. Anti-Inflammatory Strategies Targeting Metaflammation in Type 2 Diabetes. *Molecules* **2020**, *25*, 2224. [CrossRef] [PubMed]
17. Chew, V.; Lee, Y.H.; Pan, L.; Nasir, N.J.M.; Lim, C.J.; Chua, C.; Lai, L.; Hazirah, S.N.; Lim, T.K.H.; Goh, B.K.P.; et al. Immune activation underlies a sustained clinical response to Yttrium-90 radioembolisation in hepatocellular carcinoma. *Gut* **2019**, *68*, 335–346. [CrossRef]
18. Rui, Z.; Wu, R.; Zheng, W.; Wang, X.; Meng, Z.; Tan, J. Effect of ^{131}I Therapy on Complete Blood Count in Patients with Differentiated Thyroid Cancer. *Med. Sci. Monit.* **2021**, *27*, e929590. [CrossRef]
19. Du, W.; Dong, Q.; Lu, X.; Liu, X.; Wang, Y.; Li, W.; Pan, Z.; Gong, Q.; Liang, C.; Gao, G. Iodine-131 therapy alters the immune/inflammatory responses in the thyroids of patients with Graves' disease. *Exp. Ther. Med.* **2017**, *13*, 1155–1159. [CrossRef]
20. Sabri, O.; Zimny, M.; Schulz, G.; Schreckenberger, M.; Reinartz, P.; Willmes, K.; Buell, U. Success Rate of Radioiodine Therapy in Graves' Disease: The Influence of Thyrostatic Medication. *J. Clin. Endocrinol. Metab.* **1999**, *84*, 1229–1233. [CrossRef]
21. Stanciu, A.E.; Verzia, A.; Stanciu, M.M.; Zamfirescu, A.; Gheorghe, D.C. Analysis of the Correlation between the Radioactive Iodine Activity and Neutrophil-to-Lymphocyte Ratio in Patients with Differentiated Thyroid Cancer. *Cancers* **2022**, *14*, 1899. [CrossRef]
22. Yi, W.; Kim, B.H.; Kim, M.; Ryang, S.R.; Jang, M.H.; Kim, J.M.; Kim, E.H.; Jeon, Y.K.; Kim, S.S.; Kim, I.J. Short-term bone marrow suppression in differentiated thyroid cancer patients after radioactive iodine treatment. *Endocr. J.* **2020**, *67*, 1193–1198. [CrossRef]
23. Stanciu, A.E.; Stanciu, M.M.; Zamfirescu, A.; Gheorghe, D.C. Cardiovascular Effects of Cumulative Doses of Radioiodine in Differentiated Thyroid Cancer Patients with Type 2 Diabetes Mellitus. *Cancers* **2022**, *14*, 2359. [CrossRef]
24. The American Thyroid Association Taskforce on Radioiodine Safety; Sisson, J.C.; Freitas, J.; McDougall, I.R.; Dauer, L.T.; Hurley, J.R.; Brierley, J.D.; Edinboro, C.H.; Rosenthal, D.; Thomas, M.J.; et al. Radiation safety in the treatment of patients with thyroid diseases by radioiodine ^{131}I: Practice recommendations of the American Thyroid Association. *Thyroid* **2011**, *21*, 335–346. [CrossRef]
25. Bedel, C.; Korkut, M.; Armağan, H.H. NLR, d-NLR and PLR can be affected by many factors. *Int. Immunopharmacol.* **2021**, *90*, 107154. [CrossRef]
26. Weir, C.B.; Jan, A. BMI Classification Percentile and Cut off Points. In *StatPearls*; [Updated 29 June 2021]; StatPearls Publishing: Treasure Island, FL, USA, 2022. Available online: https://www.ncbi.nlm.nih.gov/books/NBK541070/ (accessed on 10 March 2023).
27. Lassmann, M.; Hanscheid, H.; Chiesa, C.; Hindorf, C.; Flux, G.; Luster, M.; EANM Dosimetry Committee. EANM Dosimetry Committee series on standard operational procedures for pretherapeutic dosimetry I: Blood and bone marrow dosimetry in differentiated thyroid cancer therapy. *Eur. J. Nucl. Med. Mol. Imaging* **2008**, *35*, 1405–1412. [CrossRef]
28. Ravindra, M.; Vivek, R.J.; Ayaz, K.M.; Gouda, B.K.M.; Jeevan, K.S.; Prakash, M.; Revathi, P.S.; Shivaraj, B. A comparative study on iodination of normal and diabetic serum. *Int. J. Appl. Biol. Pharm. Technol.* **2011**, *2*, 328–333.
29. Hagovska, M.; Švihra, J.; Buková, A.; Horbacz, A.; Dračková, D.; Lupták, J.; Švihra, J., Jr. The Relationship between Overweight and Overactive Bladder Symptoms. *Obes. Facts.* **2020**, *13*, 297–306. [CrossRef]
30. Ali, J.; Haider, S.M.S.; Ali, S.M.; Haider, T.; Anwar, A.; Hashmi, A.A. Overall Clinical Features of Type 2 Diabetes Mellitus with Respect to Gender. *Cureus* **2023**, *15*, e35771. [CrossRef]

31. Lahfi, Y.; Anjak, O. The impact of body mass index on the external dose rate from patients treated with radioiodine-131: A preliminary study. *Iran. J. Nucl. Med.* **2015**, *23*, 89–95.
32. Pickering, C.A.; Mas, J.; Dykes, J.N.; Domingo, M.T.; Yamauchi, D.M.; Lopatin, G. Williams LE. Exposure levels associated with Na(131)I thyroid cancer patients: Correlation with initial activity and clinical physical parameters. *Health Phys.* **2014**, *107*, S163–S165. [CrossRef] [PubMed]
33. Elgazar-Carmon, V.; Rudich, A.; Hadad, N.; Levy, R. Neutrophils transiently infiltrate intra-abdominal fat early in the course of high-fat feeding. *J. Lipid Res.* **2008**, *49*, 1894–1903. [CrossRef]
34. Zernecke, A.; Bot, I.; Djalali-Talab, Y.; Shagdarsuren, E.; Bidzhekov, K.; Meiler, S.; Krohn, R.; Schober, A.; Sperandio, M.; Soehnlein, O.; et al. Protective role of CXC receptor 4/CXC ligand 12 unveils the importance of neutrophils in atherosclerosis. *Circ. Res.* **2008**, *102*, 209–217. [CrossRef]
35. Watanabe, Y.; Nagai, Y.; Honda, H.; Okamoto, N.; Yanagibashi, T.; Ogasawara, M.; Yamamoto, S.; Imamura, R.; Takasaki, I.; Hara, H.; et al. Bidirectional crosstalk between neutrophils and adipocytes promotes adipose tissue inflammation. *FASEB J.* **2019**, *33*, 11821–11835. [CrossRef] [PubMed]
36. Heylmann, D.; Ponath, V.; Kindler, T.; Kaina, B. Comparison of DNA repair and radiosensitivity of different blood cell populations. *Sci. Rep.* **2021**, *11*, 2478. [CrossRef] [PubMed]
37. Srikakulapu, P.; McNamara, C.A.B. Lymphocytes and Adipose Tissue Inflammation. *Arter. Thromb. Vasc. Biol.* **2020**, *40*, 1110–1122. [CrossRef] [PubMed]
38. Park, Y.; Chang, A.R. Neutrophil to Lymphocyte Ratio and Platelet to Lymphocyte Ratio in Hepatocellular Carcinoma Treated with Stereotactic Body Radiotherapy. *Korean J. Gastroenterol.* **2022**, *79*, 252–259. [CrossRef]
39. Ren, B.; Zhu, Y. A New Perspective on Thyroid Hormones: Crosstalk with Reproductive Hormones in Females. *Int. J. Mol. Sci.* **2022**, *23*, 2708. [CrossRef] [PubMed]
40. Irelli, A.; Sirufo, M.M.; D'Ugo, C.; Ginaldi, L.; De Martinis, M. Sex and Gender Influences on Cancer Immunotherapy Response. *Biomedicines* **2020**, *8*, 232. [CrossRef]
41. Chakraborty, B.; Byemerwa, J.; Krebs, T.; Lim, F.; Chang, C.Y.; McDonnell, D.P. Estrogen Receptor Signaling in the Immune System. *Endocr. Rev.* **2023**, *44*, 117–141. [CrossRef]

cancers

MDPI

Article

Clinical Implication of Bilateral and Unilateral Multifocality in Papillary Thyroid Carcinoma: A Propensity Score-Matched Study

Youngmin Kim, Solji An, Joonseon Park, Ja Seong Bae, Jeong Soo Kim and Kwangsoon Kim *

Department of Surgery, College of Medicine, The Catholic University of Korea, Seoul 06591, Republic of Korea; ym.e.kim@gmail.com (Y.K.); solji1130@hanmail.net (S.A.); joonsunny@naver.com (J.P.); jaseong@gmail.com (J.S.B.); btskim@catholic.ac.kr (J.S.K.)

* Correspondence: noar99@naver.com; Tel.: +82-2-2258-6784; Fax: +82-2-2258-2138

Simple Summary: Multifocality is often found in PTC. There are contradicting evidences regarding clinical implications of cancer laterality in multifocal PTC. The current study compared the clinicopathological characteristics and the long-term oncological outcomes of bilateral and unilateral multifocal PTC. Patients with bilateral PTC were more likely to present with aggressive features, including high tumor stage, cervical LN metastasis, gross ETE, and lymphatic and perineural invasion. On the multivariate analysis using Cox regression, gross ETE, perineural invasion, LN metastasis, N1b stage, and RAI therapy were significant risk factors of recurrence. However, bilaterality was not associated with an increased risk of recurrence. In order to reduce selection bias, a subgroup analysis of patients who underwent total thyroidectomy was conducted using propensity score matching. After matching, unilateral multifocality, vascular invasion, and RAI therapy were significant risk factors of recurrence. Patients with unilateral multifocal PTC showed significantly poorer DFS than those with bilateral PTC on the Kaplan-Meier analysis.

Abstract: Papillary thyroid cancer (PTC) is commonly characterized by multifocality, which is associated with aggressive features and a less favorable prognosis. The current study aimed to compare the clinicopathologic characteristics and long-term oncological outcomes of bilateral and unilateral multifocal PTC. The medical records of 1745 patients with multifocal PTC who underwent thyroid surgery at Seoul St. Mary's Hospital were retrospectively reviewed. The clinicopathological characteristics and recurrence rates were compared based on cancer laterality. Further, 357 patients who underwent total thyroidectomy were matched to investigate the recurrence risk and disease-free survival (DFS). Before propensity score matching (PSM), there was no significant difference in the recurrence rate between the bilateral and unilateral multifocal PTC groups. Cancer laterality was not a predictor of DFS based on the Cox regression analyses. However, after PSM, unilateral multifocality was associated with a significantly high risk of recurrence. Similarly, unilateral multifocality was associated with a significantly poor DFS based on the Kaplan–Meier analysis. Compared with bilateral PTC, unilateral multifocal PTC was associated with a poor DFS. A comprehensive preoperative examination should be performed to detect multifocality before the initial surgical intervention for optimal treatment. Postoperative short-term follow-up is recommended for unilateral multifocal PTC for recurrence surveillance.

Keywords: bilaterality; unilateral multifocality; papillary thyroid carcinoma; disease-free survival; propensity score matching

1. Introduction

Over the years, the incidence of thyroid cancer has been continuously increasing particularly in developed countries, partly due to advancements in imaging technology and increasing accuracy of pathologic evaluation [1,2]. Papillary thyroid cancer (PTC) is the most prevalent subtype of thyroid carcinoma, accounting for up to 89.1% of all diagnosed cases [3].

The incidence of multifocal PTC ranges from 18% to 87% [4–6]. It is not uncommon for PTC to present as a multifocal disease at diagnosis. Moreover, multifocal PTC is often incidentally diagnosed during postoperative pathologic evaluation. Multifocality is defined as the presence of two or more distinct malignant foci in the thyroid gland. According to the location of the malignant foci, multifocality can be divided into either unilateral—if multiple foci are limited to a single lobe—or bilateral—if malignant foci are found in two lobes. However, there is still a debate whether to consider multiple foci as a characteristic of independent synchronous malignancies or intraglandular metastases from a single focus [4,7].

Several studies have shown that bilaterality is an independent predictor of lymph node metastasis in PTC. Further, it is related to a more aggressive disease, with an increased risk of gross extrathyroidal extension (ETE), positive resection margin, locoregional recurrence, and distant metastasis [7–9]. According to the National Comprehensive Cancer Network (NCCN) guidelines, total thyroidectomy (TT) is the recommended surgical extent for bilateral PTC. If macroscopic multifocality is diagnosed postoperatively upon pathologic examination, a complete thyroidectomy should be performed [10].

On the contrary, some studies have revealed that although bilateral PTC is associated with more aggressive features, patients with this condition do not necessarily have a poor clinical outcome [11,12]. Further, compared with TT, unilateral lobectomy may be sufficient for treating low-risk unilateral multifocal PTC without cervical LN metastasis, with no negative impact on recurrence-free survival [13]. Thus, the negative effect of multifocality on clinical course remains unclear.

The current study aimed to compare the clinicopathological characteristics and long-term oncological outcomes of unilateral multifocal and bilateral PTC via a propensity score-matched analysis to reduce selection bias.

2. Materials and Methods

2.1. Patients

Between March 2008 and June 2014, 4591 patients diagnosed with PTC underwent a thyroidectomy at Seoul St. Mary's Hospital. In total, 139 patients were excluded due to insufficient data (n = 84) and loss to follow-up (n = 55). The medical records of the remaining 4452 patients were reviewed retrospectively. Then, 1745 patients with multifocal PTC were included in the analysis. Moreover, 1002 and 743 patients had bilateral and unilateral multifocal PTC. All patients with bilateral disease underwent total thyroidectomy (TT), and 371 (49.9%) of 743 patients with unilateral multifocal disease underwent TT. TNM classification was based on the eighth edition of the AJCC TNM staging system [14]. Testing for $BRAF^{V600E}$ mutation was carried out via real-time PCR of tumor specimen acquired by either fine-needle biopsy or surgical resection, as well as $BRAF^{V600E}$-specific staining of tumors. A positive result was considered as positive for BRAF mutation. The average follow-up duration was 105.4 ± 22.2 (range: 55–139) months.

This study was conducted in accordance with the Declaration of Helsinki (revised in 2013). It was approved by the Institutional Review Board of Seoul St. Mary's Hospital, Catholic University of Korea (no.: KC22RISI0682). The need for informed consent was waived due to the retrospective nature of this study.

2.2. Follow-Up Assessment

Postoperative care and follow-up evaluation were conducted according to the American Thyroid Association (ATA) management guidelines for differentiated thyroid cancer [15]. During regular follow-up evaluations, all patients underwent a physical examination, blood tests, including serum thyroid function, thyroglobulin and anti-thyroglobulin antibody assessment, and neck ultrasonography at 3, 6, and 12 months after surgery and annually after the first year. Radioactive iodine (RAI) ablation was performed 6–8 weeks after the surgery in patients who underwent TT and those who are at intermediate or high risk according to the risk stratification system of the ATA management guidelines. A whole-body scan was performed 5–7 days after RAI ablation. To determine the location and extent of recurrence, patients suspected with recurrence underwent additional diagnostic imaging tests, including a computed tomography scan, positron emission tomography/computed tomography scan, and/or whole-body RAI scan. If a structural recurrence appeared on imaging studies, either ultrasound-guided fine-needle aspiration/core needle biopsy or surgical excision was performed for pathologic confirmation.

2.3. Primary and Secondary Endpoint

The primary endpoint was disease-free survival (DFS) between the unilateral multifocal and bilateral PTC groups after propensity score matching (PSM). The secondary endpoint was clinicopathological characteristics between the two groups before and after PSM.

2.4. Statistical Analysis

Continuous variables were analyzed with the Student's *t*-test and were presented as means and standard deviations. Categorical variables were assessed with the Fisher's exact test and were expressed as numbers and percentages. Univariate and multivariate Cox regression analyses were performed to validate the predictors of DFS, and hazard ratios (HRs) with 95% confidence intervals (CIs) were calculated. The Kaplan–Meier method with the log-rank test was used to compare the DFS.

To control potential confounding factors, the individual patient propensity scores were calculated via logistic regression analysis. Next, patients with unilateral multifocal PTC were matched to those with bilateral PTC at a 1:1 ratio using the propensity scores. Then, the DFS and long-term oncological outcomes were compared between the matched unilateral multifocal and bilateral PTC groups. After PSM, the DFS predictors were validated using univariate and multivariate Cox regression analyses, similar to the approach before matching. A p value of <0.05 was considered statistically significant. All statistical analyses were performed using the Statistical Package for the Social Sciences software (version 24.0; IBM Corp., Armonk, NY, USA).

3. Results

3.1. Comparison of Bilateral and Unilateral Multifocal PTC

Table 1 shows the baseline clinicopathological characteristics of bilateral and unilateral multifocal PTC. The mean age of the bilateral PTC group was significantly higher than that of the unilateral multifocal PTC group, while the two groups did not show a difference in sex. All patients with bilateral PTC underwent TT with central lymph node dissection and/or modified radical neck dissection. Meanwhile, 50.1% of patients with unilateral multifocal disease underwent thyroid lobectomy with central lymph node dissection only. On pathological examination, patients with bilateral PTC had significantly larger tumors than those with unilateral multifocal PTC (1.2 ± 0.9 cm vs. 0.9 ± 0.6 cm, $p < 0.001$). Moreover, the bilateral PTC group more commonly presented with gross ETE (9.5% vs. 3.9%, $p < 0.001$), lymphatic invasion (36.6% vs. 26.1%, $p < 0.001$), and perineural invasion (3.9% vs. 1.3%, $p = 0.001$) than the unilateral multifocal PTC group. Patients with bilateral PTC had a higher number of harvested lymph nodes and metastatic lymph nodes than those with unilateral multifocal PTC (19.1 ± 21.4 vs. 13.2 ± 16.0, $p < 0.001$ and 3.9 ± 6.3 vs. 2.4 ± 4.5, $p < 0.001$, respectively). Accordingly, the bilateral PTC group had a higher proportion of patients with more advanced T and N stages than the unilateral multifocal PTC group ($p < 0.001$, both). Although not statistically significant, the bilateral PTC group had a higher proportion of patients with M1 disease than the unilateral multifocal group (0.4% vs. 0.1%, $p = 0.402$). Approximately 72.5% of patients in the bilateral PTC group and 36.2% in the unilateral multifocal group received RAI therapy after surgical treatment

($p < 0.001$). However, the two groups did not significantly differ in terms of recurrence (4.3% vs. 4.4%, $p = 0.906$).

Table 1. Comparison of baseline clinicopathological characteristics between bilateral and unilateral-multifocal PTC.

	Bilateral (n = 1002)	Unilateral Multifocal (n = 743)	p-Value
Age (years)	48.9 ± 12.1 (range, 15–83)	47.5 ± 11.7 (range, 16–82)	0.018
Male gender	199 (19.9%)	168 (22.6%)	0.172
Extent of surgery			<0.001
Less than TT	0	372 (50.1%)	
TT and/or mRND	1002 (100%)	371 (49.9%)	
Subtype of PTC			0.111
Non-aggressive	848 (84.6%)	649 (87.3%)	
Aggressive	154 (15.4%)	94 (12.7%)	
Tumor size (cm)	1.2 ± 0.9 (range, 0.2–6.7)	0.9 ± 0.6 (range, 0.2–6.5)	<0.001
Gross ETE	95 (9.5%)	29 (3.9%)	<0.001
Lymphatic invasion	367 (36.6%)	194 (26.1%)	<0.001
Vascular invasion	34 (3.4%)	24 (3.2%)	0.893
Perineural invasion	39 (3.9%)	10 (1.3%)	0.001
BRAFV600E positivity	712/853 (83.5%)	489/596 (82.0%)	0.479
Harvested LNs	19.1 ± 21.4	13.2 ± 16.0	<0.001
Positive LNs	3.9 ± 6.3	2.4 ± 4.5	<0.001
T stage			<0.001
T1	826 (82.4%)	689 (92.7%)	
T2	68 (6.8%)	23 (3.1%)	
T3a	13 (1.3%)	2 (0.3%)	
T3b	93 (9.3%)	27 (3.6%)	
T4a	2 (0.2%)	2 (0.3%)	
N stage			<0.001
N0	387 (38.6%)	359 (48.3%)	
N1a	455 (45.4%)	310 (41.7%)	
N1b	160 (16.0%)	74 (10.0%)	
M stage			0.402
M1	4 (0.4%)	1 (0.1%)	
TNM stage			0.002
Stage I	802 (80.0%)	643 (86.5%)	
Stage II	196 (19.6%)	100 (13.5%)	
Stage III	2 (0.2%)	0	
Stage IVb	2 (0.2%)	0	
RAI therapy	726 (72.5%)	269 (36.2%)	<0.001
Recurrence	43 (4.3%)	33 (4.4%)	0.906

Data are expressed as patient's number (%) or mean ± standard deviation. The aggressive subtypes of PTC include tall cell, columnar, hobnail, diffuse sclerosing, and solid variant. A statistically significant difference was defined as $p < 0.05$. Abbreviation: PTC, papillary thyroid carcinoma; TT, total thyroidectomy; mRND, modified radical neck dissection; ETE, extrathyroidal extension; LN, lymph node; T, tumor; N, node; M, metastasis; RAI, radioactive iodine.

3.2. Univariate and Multivariate Analyses of the Risk Factors of Recurrence before PSM

In the univariate analysis, male sex, tumor size > 1 cm, gross ETE, lymphatic, vascular invasion, and perineural invasion, LN metastasis, T stage of $\geq$2, N1 stage, M1 disease, and RAI therapy were considered the risk factors of recurrence (Table 2). Based on the multivariate analysis, only gross ETE, perineural invasion, LN metastasis, N1b stage, and RAI therapy were significantly associated with recurrence. However, bilaterality was not a significant risk factor of recurrence.

Table 2. Univariate and multivariate analyses of recurrence risk factors.

	Univariate		Multivariate	
	HR (95% CI)	***p*-Value**	**HR (95% CI)**	***p*-Value**
Gender				
Female	ref.			
Male	1.770 (1.091–2.870)	0.021		
Extent of surgery				
Less than TT	ref.			
TT and/or mRND	1.408 (0.760–2.610)	0.277		
Subtype of PTC				
Non-aggressive	ref.			
Aggressive	1.523 (0.866–2.681)	0.144		
Tumor size				
≤1 cm	ref.			
>1 cm	2.877 (1.821–4.547)	<0.001		
Gross ETE	3.376 (1.919–5.940)	<0.001	12.674 (1.6119–99.713)	0.016
Multifocality				
Unilateral	ref.			
Bilateral	0.953 (0.605–1.500)	0.835		
Lymphatic invasion	3.738 (2.345–5.957)	<0.001		
Vascular invasion	3.581 (1.721–7.451)	0.001		
Perineural invasion	5.011 (2.499–10.050)	<0.001	2.273 (1.005–5.139)	0.049
Harvested LNs	1.017 (1.010–1.024)	<0.001		
Positive LNs	1.078 (1.060–1.096)	<0.001	1.102 (1.053–1.154)	<0.001
T stage				
T1	ref.			
T2	2.741 (1.301–5.776)	0.008		
T3a	4.257 (1.036–17.488)	0.044		
T3b	3.635 (2.012–6.568)	<0.001		
T4b	9.142 (1.261–66.257)	0.029		
N stage				
N0	ref.		ref.	
N1a	7.535 (3.215–17.662)	<0.001	2.303 (0.912–5.819)	0.078
N1b	14.065 (5.770–34.286)	<0.001	3.565 (1.086–11.710)	0.036
M stage	10.883 (2.668–44.389)	0.001		
RAI therapy	18.685 (5.880–59.289)	<0.001	7.760 (2.275–26.470)	0.001

Data are expressed as hazard ratio (HR) and 95% confidence interval (CI). The aggressive subtypes of PTC include tall cell, columnar, hobnail, diffuse sclerosing, and solid variant. A statistically significant difference was defined as $p < 0.05$. Abbreviations: TT, total thyroidectomy; mRND, modified radical neck dissection; PTC, papillary thyroid carcinoma; ETE, extrathyroidal extension; LN, lymph node; T, tumor; N, node; M, metastasis; RAI, radioactive iodine.

3.3. Comparison of Patients with Bilateral and Unilateral Multifocal PTC Who Underwent TT

Table 3 shows the baseline clinicopathological characteristics of bilateral and unilateral multifocal PTC in patients who underwent TT before and after PSM. All patients with bilateral PTC underwent TT. Meanwhile, 371 of 743 patients with unilateral multifocal PTC underwent TT. Before matching, the bilateral PTC group had a significantly higher proportion of patients with gross ETE than the unilateral multifocal PTC group (9.5% vs. 5.7%, $p = 0.028$). Similarly, the bilateral PTC group had a higher proportion of patients with T2 and T3 disease than the unilateral multifocal group (6.8% vs. 4.3% and 10.6% vs. 5.7%, respectively, $p = 0.015$). After PSM, the unilateral multifocal PTC group had a higher recurrence rate than the bilateral PTC group (2.2% vs. 5.9%, $p = 0.021$).

Table 3. Comparison of baseline clinicopathological characteristics between bilateral and unilateral multifocal PTC in patients who underwent total thyroidectomy before and after propensity score matching.

	Before Matching			After Matching		
	Bilateral (n = 1002)	Unilateral Multifocal (n = 371)	p-Value	Bilateral (n = 357)	Unilateral Multifocal (n = 357)	p-Value
Age (years)	48.9 ± 12.1 (range, 15–83)	48.1 ± 12.2 (range, 20–82)	0.305	46.5 ± 12.4 (range, 14–79)	46.2 ± 11.8 (range, 11–81)	0.793
Male gender	199 (19.9%)	89 (24.0%)	0.101	83 (23.2%)	83 (23.2%)	1.000
Subtype of PTC			0.933			0.336
Non-aggressive	848 (84.6%)	315 (84.9%)		311 (87.1%)	301 (84.3%)	
Aggressive	154 (15.4%)	56 (15.1%)		46 (12.9%)	56 (15.7%)	
Tumor size (cm)	1.2 ± 0.9 (range, 0.2–6.7)	1.0 ± 0.7 (range, 0.2–6.5)	<0.001	1.0 ± 0.6 (range, 0.2–4.5)	1.0 ± 0.7 (range, 0.2–6.5)	0.893
Gross ETE	95 (9.5%)	21 (5.7%)	0.028	22 (6.2%)	21 (5.9%)	1.000
Lymphatic invasion	367 (36.6%)	135 (36.4%)	0.950	128 (35.9%)	126 (35.3%)	0.938
Vascular invasion	34 (3.4%)	11 (3.0%)	0.865	10 (2.8%)	11 (3.1%)	1.000
Perineural invasion	39 (3.9%)	8 (2.2%)	0.134	14 (3.9%)	8 (2.2%)	0.279
$BRAF^{V600E}$ positivity	712/853 (83.5%)	254/307 (82.7%)	0.789	255/298 (85.6%)	248/298 (83.2%)	0.498
Harvested LNs	19.1 ± 21.4	19.2 ± 20.5	0.986	19.1 ± 21.4	19.2 ± 20.5	0.463
Positive LNs	3.9 ± 6.3	3.9 ± 5.7	0.824	3.9 ± 6.3	3.9 ± 5.7	0.781
T stage			0.015			0.987
T1	826 (82.4%)	333 (89.7%)		318 (89.1%)	319 (89.4%)	
T2	68 (6.8%)	16 (4.3%)		16 (4.5%)	16 (4.5%)	
T3a	13 (1.3%)	1 (0.3%)		1 (0.3%)	1 (0.3%)	
T3b	93 (9.3%)	20 (5.4%)		20 (5.6%)	20 (5.6%)	
T4a	2 (0.2%)	1 (0.3%)		2 (0.6%)	1 (0.3%)	
N stage			0.189			0.842
N0	387 (38.6%)	131 (35.3%)		128 (35.9%)	129 (36.1%)	
N1a	455 (45.4%)	166 (44.8%)		157 (44.0%)	162 (45.4%)	
N1b	160 (16.0%)	74 (19.9%)		72 (20.2%)	66 (18.5%)	
M stage			0.579			N/A
M1	4 (0.4%)	0		0	0	
TNM stage			0.391			0.303
Stage I	802 (80.0%)	309 (83.3%)		288 (80.7%)	296 (82.9%)	
Stage II	196 (19.6%)	62 (16.7%)		67 (18.8%)	61 (17.1%)	
Stage III	2 (0.2%)	0		2 (0.6%)	0	
Stage IVb	2 (0.2%)	0		0	0	
RAI therapy	726 (72.5%)	251 (67.7%)	0.093	246 (68.9%)	242 (67.8%)	0.809
Recurrence	43 (4.3%)	21 (5.7%)	0.313	8 (2.2%)	21 (5.9%)	0.021

Data are expressed as patient's number (%) or mean ± standard deviation. The aggressive subtypes of PTC include tall cell, columnar, hobnail, diffuse sclerosing, and solid variant. A statistically significant difference was defined as $p < 0.05$. The p-value for M stage is unavailable since none of the patients had M1 disease after matching. Abbreviation: PTC, papillary thyroid carcinoma; ETE, extrathyroidal extension; LN, lymph node; T, tumor; N, node; M, metastasis; RAI, radioactive iodine.

3.4. Univariate and Multivariate Analyses of Recurrence Risk Factors after PSM

Table 4 depicts the risk factors of recurrence after PSM based on the univariate and multivariate analyses. Based on the univariate analysis, tumor size > 1 cm, gross ETE, unilateral multifocality, lymphatic/vascular/perineural invasion, lymph node positivity, T3b and T4b stages, N1a and N1b stages, and RAI therapy were significant risk factors of recurrence. Based on the multivariate analysis, only unilateral multifocality (hazard ratio (HR): 2.664, 95% CI: 1.180–6.017; p = 0.018), vascular invasion (HR: 3.839, 95% CI: 1.331–11.073; p = 0.013), and RAI therapy (HR: 12.124, 95% CI: 1.640–89.630; p = 0.014) were significant predictors of recurrence. In the Kaplan–Meier analysis, patients with unilateral multifocal disease had a significantly lower DFS than those with bilateral disease (p = 0.014, Figure 1).

Table 4. Univariate and multivariate analyses of recurrence risk factors after propensity score matching.

	Univariate		Multivariate	
	HR (95% CI)	***p*-Value**	**HR (95% CI)**	***p*-Value**
Tumor size				
≤1 cm	ref.			
>1 cm	2.102 (1.014–4.358)	0.046		
gross ETE	3.458 (1.318–9.070)	0.012		
Multifocality				
Bilateral	ref.		ref.	
Unilateral	2.660 (1.178–6.004)	0.019	2.664 (1.180–6.017)	0.018
Lymphatic invasion	3.586 (1.667–7.712)	0.001		
Vascular invasion	5.768 (2.006–16.582)	0.001	3.839 (1.331–11.073)	0.013
Perineural invasion	3.882 (1.175–12.833)	0.026		
Positive LNs	1.057 (1.023–1.093)	0.001		
T stage				
T1	ref.			
T3b	3.041 (1.047–8.830)	0.041		
T4b	12.909 (1.727–96.474)	0.013		
N stage				
N0	ref.			
N1a	4.437 (1.293–15.228)	0.018		
N1b	6.678 (1.836–24.288)	0.004		
RAI therapy	13.334 (1.814–98.005)	0.011	12.124 (1.640–89.630)	0.014

Data are expressed as hazard ratio (HR) and 95% confidence interval (CI); a statistically significant difference was defined as $p < 0.05$. Abbreviations: ETE, extrathyroidal extension; LN, lymph node; T, tumor; N, node; RAI, radioactive iodine.

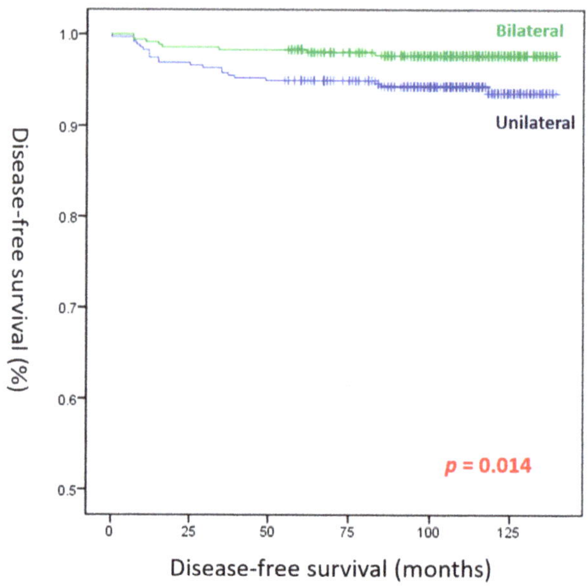

Figure 1. Disease-free survival curves of the bilateral and unilateral multifocal groups (log-rank test, $p = 0.014$).

4. Discussion

Previous studies have reported that bilateral PTC is a predictor of aggressive disease and an independent risk factor of recurrence [8,9,16]. However, in the current study, unilateral multifocality, rather than bilaterality, was associated with a high risk of recurrence.

PTC is the most prevalent subtype of thyroid malignancies [3]. Generally, PTC is a relatively indolent tumor with an excellent long-term prognosis. Its overall survival rate is 90–95% [17]. Multifocal PTC is common, with an incidence rate of 18–87%, based on the diagnostic approach [4–6]. According to the ATA guidelines, multifocal PTC is associated with a low risk for structural disease recurrence unless it is accompanied by other high-risk features such as ETE, LN metastasis, and vascular invasion [15]. Nonetheless, several studies have reported that multifocality is associated with a high risk of contralateral disease and that bilateral multifocality is a predictor of LN metastasis and poorer clinical outcome, including locoregional recurrence and distant metastasis [18–23]. Feng et al. showed that both multifocality and bilaterality were associated with aggressive features. However, multifocality was the only predictor of recurrence [24]. Similarly, Yan et al. found that bilateral multifocality is associated with aggressive features such as large tumor size, ETE, and lymph node metastasis, but not with prognosis [25]. Therefore, whether multifocality or bilaterality can be a prognostic factor remains controversial.

Results showed that patients with bilateral PTC had significantly larger tumors and more extensive lymph node involvement and advanced T and N stages compared with those with unilateral multifocal PTC. Moreover, bilateral disease was more likely characterized by aggressive features, including gross ETE and lymphatic and perineural invasion. These findings are in accordance with those of previous reports showing that bilateral PTC is associated with more aggressive clinicopathological features compared with unilateral multifocal disease [11,24,25]. Interestingly, the incidence of $BRAF^{V600E}$ mutation and the recurrence rate did not significantly differ between the bilateral and the unilateral multifocal PTC groups, which was in contrast to previously reported outcomes [26,27].

Patients with bilateral PTC are routinely treated with TT. Meanwhile, patients with unilateral multifocal PTC undergo either TT or lobectomy. The surgical extent may have an effect on locoregional disease control and may subsequently affect long-term outcomes. Hence, patients who underwent TT were analyzed. Approximately 49.9% of patients with unilateral multifocal disease who underwent TT were included in the research. Results showed that the bilateral PTC group had a significantly larger tumor size and higher frequency of gross ETE, thereby leading to a greater proportion of patients with a more advanced T stage. Otherwise, the two groups did not significantly differ in terms of other aggressive features, such as aggressive PTC subtypes, cervical LN metastasis, $BRAF^{V600E}$ positivity, and lymphatic, vascular, and perineural invasion.

We conducted PSM to further reduce selection bias. After matching, unilateral multifocality, vascular invasion, and RAI therapy were the only significant risk factors of recurrence. Interestingly, unilateral multifocality was a predictor of recurrence based on the multivariate analysis, with an HR of 2.664. This result is in contrast to that of previous studies showing that bilateral PTC is a risk factor of recurrence [8,9,16].

PSM yielded rather an unexpected outcome. Before matching, the bilateral and the unilateral multifocal PTC groups did not show a significant difference in recurrence, which became significant once PSM was conducted. It suggests that the clinicopathologic characteristics, such as tumor size and gross extrathyroidal extension, play an important role in determining the oncological outcome. Therefore, it is important to correct for the possibly confounding factors in order to make an accurate comparison of cancer laterality regarding prognosis. Our findings showed that the surgical extent for unilateral multifocal PTC should be planned cautiously. Postoperatively, patients with unilateral multifocal PTC must be closely monitored with short-term follow-up for the early detection of recurrent disease.

A molecular analysis of multifocal PTCs by Bansal and colleagues revealed that PTCs arising from different molecular origins, representing multiple synchronous primary tumors (MSPTs), frequently appear in different lobes, while the majority of tumors that share the same mutation status were located in the same lobe [28]. Similarly, Cai et al. have shown that unilateral multifocality and bilateral multifocality should be considered as two molecularly separate entities. They found that unilateral multifocal disease is associated with an increased risk of central neck metastasis compared with bilateral disease (single lesion in each lobe) [29]. Together, these findings suggest that unilateral multifocal PTC may be more aggressive in nature because it arises through intraglandular tumor dissemination rather than synchronous development of independent primary tumors.

Further, vascular invasion was a strong predictor of recurrence in our study, with an HR of 3.839. Reilly et al. showed that vascular invasion is associated with aggressive tumor factors, such as lymphatic and capsular invasion, ETE, and lymph node metastasis, in papillary cancer [30]. Our findings are in accordance with those of previous studies showing that vascular invasion is associated with a high risk of recurrence and poor prognosis in PTC [30,31].

RAI therapy is recommended for intermediate- and high-risk patients who underwent TT or near TT, according to the current ATA guidelines [15]. However, the effect of RAI therapy in improving prognosis remains controversial, with a RAI-refractory PTC rate of 20–30% [32]. Tang J. et al. performed a retrospective study using the SEER program. Results showed that RAI therapy improved disease-specific survival in patients with a tumor measuring <2 cm and distant metastasis or those with a tumor measuring >2 cm accompanied by one of the following risk factors: gross ETE, age >45 years, lymph node metastasis, and distant metastasis. Otherwise, there was no significant improvement in disease-specific survival even after RAI therapy [33]. In the current study, RAI therapy was a significant risk factor of recurrence based on the multivariate analysis.

RAI therapy was conducted in patients who underwent TT and had intermediate to high risk disease according to the ATA 2015 risk stratification system for structural disease control. In other words, patients who underwent RAI therapy generally had a more advanced disease than those who did not, with larger primary tumors, more positive lymph nodes, and/or aggressive pathologic features such as vascular invasion and extrathyroidal extension. It is unlikely that RAI therapy itself increases risk for recurrence. Rather, RAI therapy may have been ineffective in reducing recurrence in patients with multifocal PTC. We surmise that this is partially due to high rate of RAI-refractory PTC. Further study should explore the efficacy of RAI therapy as adjuvant therapy for differentiated thyroid malignancies. Because RAI therapy may cause several complications such as xerostomia, sialoadenitis, and pulmonary fibrosis, cautious patient selection for RAI therapy candidates is required.

The current study had several limitations. Although the subgroup analysis aimed to eliminate the effect of surgical extent on long-term outcomes, we might have inadvertently introduced selection bias in the process of including patients with unilateral multifocal PTC who underwent TT. Large tumor size, clinical LN positivity, and other aggressive features are considered when performing TT for unilateral disease, thereby selectively including patients at a higher risk of recurrence. Further, this study was retrospective in nature and was conducted at a single center, and it included a relatively small sample size. However, all patients were treated and followed-up uniformly according to a single protocol, which is considered a strength of this research. Nevertheless, the molecular profile of the tumors, which may have important implications for clinical course and prognosis, was not investigated. Correlating the findings of our study with the standard immunohistochemical markers for aggressiveness of PTC, such as Gal-3, CK-19, and HBME-1, would provide further insight into cancer laterality as a prognostic factor for multifocal PTC.

5. Conclusions

Compared with bilateral PTC, unilateral multifocal PTC is significantly associated with a higher recurrence risk and poorer DFS. Our findings could affect decision making regarding surgical extent in patients with unilateral multifocal PTC. For postoperative care, patients should undergo short-term follow-up to screen for recurrence. A subsequent investigation with a larger study cohort and additional information on molecular characteristics may provide further insight about the clinical course of multifocal PTC and may help in establishing optimal treatment and follow-up strategies.

Author Contributions: Conceptualization: K.K.; methodology: K.K., J.S.B. and J.S.K.; software: K.K.; validation: K.K. and Y.K.; formal analysis: K.K., J.P. and Y.K.; investigation: K.K., J.P. and Y.K.; resources: K.K., J.S.B. and J.S.K.; data curation: K.K., S.A. and Y.K.; writing—original draft preparation: K.K. and Y.K.; writing—review and editing: all authors; visualization: K.K. and Y.K.; supervision: J.S.K. and J.S.B.; project administration: K.K. All authors have read and agreed to the published version of the manuscript.

Funding: This research received no external funding.

Institutional Review Board Statement: This study was conducted in accordance with the Declaration of Helsinki and was approved by the Institutional Review Board of Seoul St. Mary's Hospital, The Catholic University of Korea (registration no: KC22RISI0682 and approval date: 2023/9/26).

Informed Consent Statement: The need for patient consent was waived due to the retrospective nature of this study.

Data Availability Statement: The data supporting the findings of this study are available upon request from the corresponding author and are not publicly available due to privacy or ethical restrictions.

Acknowledgments: The authors wish to acknowledge the financial support of the Catholic Medical Center Research Foundation made in the program year of 2022.

Conflicts of Interest: The authors declare no conflict of interest.

References

1. Xu, S.; Han, Y. The overdiagnosis of thyroid micropapillary carcinoma: The rising incidence, inert biological behavior, and countermeasures. *J. Oncol.* **2021**, *2021*, 5544232. [CrossRef] [PubMed]
2. Davies, L.; Welch, H. Increasing incidence of thyroid cancer in United States. *JAMA* **2006**, *295*, 2164–2167. [CrossRef] [PubMed]
3. Megwalu, U.; Moon, P. Thyroid cancer incidence and mortality trends in the United States: 2000–2018. *Thyroid* **2022**, *32*, 560–570. [CrossRef] [PubMed]
4. Iida, F.; Yonekura, M.; Miyakawa, M. Study of intraglandular dissemination of thyroid cancer. *Cancer* **1969**, *24*, 764–771. [CrossRef]
5. Katoh, R.; Sasaki, J.; Kurihara, H.; Suzuki, K.; Iida, Y.; Kawaoi, A. Multiple thyroid involvement (intraglandular metastasis) in papillary thyroid carcinoma: A clinicopathologic study of 105 consecutive patients. *Cancer* **1992**, *70*, 1585–1590. [CrossRef]
6. Tam, A.A.; Ozdemir, D.; Cuhaci, N.; Baser, H.; Aydin, C.; Yazgan, A.K.; Ersoy, R.; Cakir, B. Association of multifocality, tumor number, and total tumor diameter with clnicopathological features in papillary thyroid cancer. *Endocrine* **2016**, *53*, 774–783. [CrossRef] [PubMed]
7. Shattuck, T.M.; Westra, W.H.; Ladenson, P.W.; Arnold, A. Independent clonal origins of distinct tumor foci in multifocal papillary thyroid carcinoma. *N. Engl. J. Med.* **2005**, *352*, 2406–2412. [CrossRef]
8. Kim, S.K.; Park, I.; Woo, J.-W.; Lee, J.H.; Choe, J.-H.; Kim, J.-H.; Kim, J.S. Predictive factors for lymph node metastasis in papillary thyroid microcarcinoma. *Ann. Surg. Oncol.* **2016**, *23*, 2866–2873. [CrossRef]
9. Genpeng, L.; Jianyong, L.; Jiaying, Y.; Ke, J.; Zhihui, L.; Rixiang, G.; Lihan, Z.; Jingqiang, Z. Independent predictors and lymph node metastasis characteristics of multifocal papillary thyroid cancer. *Medicine* **2018**, *97*, e9619. [CrossRef]
10. Haddad, R.I.; Bischoff, L.; Ball, D.; Bernet, V.; Blomain, E.; Busaidy, N.L.; Campbell, M.; Dickson, P.; Duh, Q.-Y.; Ehya, H.; et al. Thyroid carcinoma, version 2.2022, NCCN clinical practice guidelines in oncology. *J. Natl. Compr. Canc. Netw.* **2022**, *20*, 925–951. [CrossRef]
11. Kim, H.J.; Sohn, S.Y.; Jang, H.W.; Kim, S.W.; Chung, J.H. Multifocality, but not bilaterality, is a predictor of disease recurrence/persistence of papillary thyroid carcinoma. *World J. Surg.* **2013**, *37*, 376–384. [CrossRef] [PubMed]
12. Polat, S.B.; Cakir, B.; Evranos, B.; Baser, H.; Cuhaci, N.; Aydin, C.; Ersoy, R. Preoperative predictors and prognosis of bilateral multifocal papillary thyroid carcinomas. *Surg. Oncol.* **2019**, *28*, 145–149. [CrossRef] [PubMed]
13. Jeon, Y.W.; Gwak, H.G.; Lim, S.T.; Schneider, J.; Suh, Y.J. Long-term prognosis of unilateral and multifocal papillary thyroid microcarcinoma after unilateral lobectomy versus total thyroidectomy. *Ann. Surg. Oncol.* **2019**, *26*, 2952–2958. [CrossRef]
14. Tuttle, M.; Morris, L.F.; Haugen, B.; Shah, J.; Sosa, J.A.; Rohren, E.; Subramaniam, R.M.; Hunt, J.L.; Perrier, N.D. 2017 Thyroid differentiated and anaplastic carcinoma. In *AJCC Cancer Staging Manual*, 8th ed.; Amin, M.B., Edge, S.B., Eds.; Springer International Publishing: New York, NY, USA, 2017; ISBN 978-3319406176.

15. Haugen, B.R.; Alexander, E.K.; Bible, K.C.; Doherty, G.M.; Mandel, S.J.; Nikiforov, Y.E.; Pacini, F.; Randolph, G.W.; Sawka, A.M.; Schlumberger, M.; et al. 2015 American Thyroid Association management guidelines for adult patients with thyroid nodules and differentiated thyroid cancer: The American Thyroid Association Guidelines Task Force on Thyroid Nodules and Differentiated Thyroid Cancer. *Thyroid* **2016**, *26*, 1–133. [CrossRef] [PubMed]
16. Wada, N.; Duh, Q.Y.; Sugino, K.; Iwasaki, H.; Kameyama, K.; Mimura, T.; Ito, K.; Takami, H.; Takanashi, Y. Lymph node metastasis from 259 papillary thyroid carcinomas: Frequency, pattern of occurrence and recurrence and optimal strategy for neck dissection. *Ann. Surg.* **2003**, *237*, 399–407. [CrossRef] [PubMed]
17. Cramer, J.D.; Fu, P.; Harth, K.C.; Margevicius, S.; Wilhelm, S.M. Analysis of the rising incidence of thyroid cancer using the Surveillance, Epidemiology and End Results national cancer data registry. *Surgery* **2010**, *148*, 1147–1153. [CrossRef]
18. Karatzas, T.; Vasileiadis, I.; Charitoudis, G.; Karakostas, E.; Tseleni-Balafouta, S.; Kouraklis, G. Bilateral versus unilateral papillary thyroid microcarcinoma: Predictive factors and associated histopathological findings following total thyroidectomy. *Hormones* **2013**, *12*, 529–536. [CrossRef]
19. Kim, K.; Zheng, X.; Kim, J.K.; Lee, C.R.; Kang, S.-W.; Lee, J.; Jeong, J.J.; Nam, K.-H.; Chung, W.Y. The contributing factors for lateral neck lymph node metastasis in papillary thyroid microcarcinoma (PTMC). *Endocrine* **2020**, *69*, 149–156. [CrossRef]
20. Kim, S.K.; Park, I.; Woo, J.-W.; Lee, J.H.; Choe, J.-H.; Kim, J.-H.; Kim, J.S. Predicting factors for bilaterality in papillary thyroid carcinoma with tumor size < 4cm. *Thyroid* **2017**, *27*, 207–214. [CrossRef]
21. Wang, N.; Qian, L.-X. Predictive factors for occult bilateral papillary thyroid carcinoma. *Acad. Rad.* **2021**, *28*, 328–332. [CrossRef]
22. Zhou, Y.-L.; Gao, E.-L.; Zhang, W.; Yang, H.; Guo, G.-L.; Zhang, X.-H.; Wang, O.-C. Factors predictive of papillary thyroid microcarcinoma with bilateral involvement and central lymph node metastasis: A retrospective study. *World J. Surg. Oncol.* **2012**, *10*, 67. [CrossRef] [PubMed]
23. Qu, N.; Zhang, L.; Wu, W.-L.; Ji, Q.-H.; Lu, Z.-W.; Zhu, Y.-X.; Lin, D.-Z. Bilaterality weighs more than unilateral multifocallity in predicting prognosis in papillary thyroid cancer. *Tumour. Biol.* **2016**, *37*, 8783–8789. [CrossRef]
24. Feng, J.-W.; Qu, Z.; Qin, A.-C.; Pan, H.; Ye, J.; Jiang, Y. Significance of multifocality in papillary thyroid carcinoma. *Eur. J. Surg. Oncol.* **2020**, *46*, 1820–1828. [CrossRef] [PubMed]
25. Yan, T.; Qiu, W.; Song, J.; Ying, T.; Fan, Y.; Yang, Z. Bilateral multifocality, a marker for aggressive disease, is not an independent prognostic factor for papillary thyroid microcarcinoma: A propensity score matching analysis. *Clin. Endocrinol.* **2021**, *95*, 209–216. [CrossRef] [PubMed]
26. Liu, Z.; Lv, T.; Xie, C.; Di, Z. BRAF V600E gene mutation is associated with bilateral malignancy of papillary thyroid cancer. *Am. J. Med. Sci.* **2018**, *356*, 130–134. [CrossRef] [PubMed]
27. Wang, W.; Zhao, W.; Wang, H.; Teng, X.; Wang, H.; Chen, X.; Li, Z.; Yu, X.; Fahey, T.J.; Teng, L. Poorer prognosis and higher prevalence of BRAFV600E mutation in synchronous bilateral papillary thyroid carcinoma. *Ann. Surg. Oncol.* **2012**, *19*, 31–36. [CrossRef]
28. Bansal, M.; Gandhi, M.; Ferris, R.L.; Nikiforova, M.N.; Yip, L.; Carty, S.E.; Nikiforov, Y.E. Molecular and histopathologic characteristics of multifocal papillary thyroid carcinoma. *Am. J. Surg. Pathol.* **2013**, *37*, 158–1591. [CrossRef]
29. Cai, J.; Fang, F.; Chen, J.; Xiang, D. Unilateral multifocality and bilaterality could be two different multifocal entities in patients with papillary thyroid microcarcinoma. *BioMed Res. Int.* **2020**, *2020*, 9854964. [CrossRef]
30. Reilly, J.; Faridmoayer, E.; Lapkus, M.; Pastewski, J.; Sun, F.; Elassar, H.; Studzinski, D.M.; Callahan, R.E.; Czako, P.; Nagar, S. Vascular invasion predicts advanced tumor characteristics in papillary thyroid carcinoma. *Am. J. Surg.* **2022**, *223*, 487–491. [CrossRef]
31. Kim, J.W.; Roh, J.-L.; Gong, G.; Cho, K.-J.; Choi, S.-H.; Nam, S.Y.; Kim, S.Y. Recurrence in patients with clinically early-stage papillary thyroid carcinoma according to tumor size and surgical extent. *Am. J. Surg.* **2016**, *212*, 419–425. [CrossRef]
32. Shobab, L.; Gomes-Lima, C.; Zeymo, A.; Feldman, R.; Jonklaas, J.; Wartofsky, L.; Burman, K.D. Clinical, pathological, and molecular profiling for radioactive iodine refractory differentiated thyroid cancer. *Thyroid* **2019**, *29*, 1262–1268. [CrossRef] [PubMed]
33. Tang, J.; Kong, D.; Cui, Q.; Wang, K.; Zhang, D.; Liao, X.; Gong, Y.; Wu, G. The role of radioactive iodine therapy in papillary thyroid cancer: An observation study based on SEER. *Onco. Targets Ther.* **2018**, *11*, 3551–3560. [CrossRef] [PubMed]

cancers

MDPI

Article

Radioiodine-131 Therapy Used for Differentiated Thyroid Cancer Can Impair Titanium Dental Implants: An In Vitro Analysis

Doina Piciu [1,2], Simion Bran [3], Marioara Moldovan [4], Simona Varvara [5], Andra Piciu [6,*], Stanca Cuc [4], Cristina Moisescu-Goia [1], Elena Barbus [1], Alexandru Mester [7] and Florin Onisor [3]

1 Department of Endocrine Tumors and Nuclear Medicine, Institute of Oncology "Ion Chiricuta", 400015 Cluj-Napoca, Romania
2 Doctoral School, University of Medicine and Pharmacy "Iuliu Hatieganu", 400012 Cluj-Napoca, Romania
3 Department of Maxillofacial Surgery and Implantology, University of Medicine and Pharmacy "Iuliu Hatieganu", 400012 Cluj-Napoca, Romania
4 Institute of Chemistry "Raluca Ripan", University Babes-Bolyai, 400294 Cluj-Napoca, Romania
5 Faculty of Exact Sciences and Engineering, "1 Decembrie 1918" Alba Iulia University, 510009 Alba Iulia, Romania
6 Department of Medical Oncology, University of Medicine and Pharmacy "Iuliu Hatieganu", 400012 Cluj-Napoca, Romania
7 Department of Oral Health, University of Medicine and Pharmacy "Iuliu Hatieganu", 400012 Cluj-Napoca, Romania
* Correspondence: andra.piciu@umfcluj.ro

Simple Summary: The alterations on dental implants seen after therapeutic radioiodine-131 exposure have important clinical impact. Several microstructural alterations start to appear at 24 h up to 2 weeks after exposure; this affects the pores walls which tend to be eroded.

Abstract: Background: The aim was to assess, in vitro, the effects of radioiodine-131 (I-131) on the structure of titanium implants. Material and Methods: A total of 28 titanium implants were divided into 7 groups ($n = 4$) and irradiated at 0, 6, 12, 24, 48, 192 and 384 hours. At the end of the experiment, each sample was investigated via scanning electron microscopy (SEM) and electrochemical measures. Results: The control sample revealed a smooth and compact surface. The small micro-sized porosity is slightly visible at the macroscopic level, but the precise details cannot be observed. A mild exposure to the radioactive solution for 6 to 24 h showed a good preservation of the macro-structural aspects such as thread details and surface quality. Significant changes occurred after 48 h of exposure. It was noticed that the open-circuit potential (OCP) value of the non-irradiated implants move toward more noble potentials during the first 40 min of exposure to the artificial saliva and then stabilizes at a constant value of −143 mV. A displacement of the OCP values toward more negative values was observed for all irradiated implants; these potential shifts are decreasing, as the irradiation period of the tested implants increased. Conclusion: After exposure to I-131, the structure of titanium implants is well preserved up to 12 h. The eroded particles start to appear in the microstructural details after 24 h of exposure and their numbers progressively increase up to 384 h after exposure.

Keywords: titanium implant; osseointegration; radioiodine-131; differentiated thyroid cancer

1. Introduction

Thyroid cancer is the most frequent endocrine tumor, even if it is considered to be a rare cancer; however, incidences of thyroid cancer are a maximum of 6 cases in 100,000 inhabitants—and this is continuously increasing [1]. According to the 2022 WHO (World Health Organization) classification of thyroid neoplasm, thyroid cancer is classified by its histology in malignant follicular cell-derived neoplasms, stratified based on molecular profiles and aggressiveness, medullary thyroid cancer, anaplastic thyroid cancer and some other rare forms [2]. From the total of thyroid cancers, more than 80% are represented by the malignant follicular cell-derived neoplasms, mostly papillary thyroid cancers [2].

The treatment of the malignant follicular cell-derived neoplasms is established in multidisciplinary committee and is made according to the stage of the disease [3,4]. The first intention procedure in the treatment of the thyroid cancer is the thyroidectomy or the lobectomy, with or without lymphadenectomy [5]. Radioiodine-131 (I-131) therapy is the procedure used for the irradiation of the remnant iodine avid tissue and/or iodine avid metastases using radioiodine (I-131), orally administered [3,5]. Further, hormone therapy for the thyroid function should be administered, using TSH substitutive/suppressing doses of Levothyroxine (LT4), according to the risk of recurrence classification [6].

In the multidisciplinary context of thyroid malignancy, dentistry has a clear role in defining the patients' quality of life. Oral complications can compromise the protocols of radioiodine I-131 therapy, possibly making it necessary to adjust the administered activities, to change the treatment protocol, or even to avoid the therapy [7,8]. The role of the dental practitioner is to prevent and to erase the oral acute and late side effects of the radioiodine therapy [9]. The effect of radioiodine on salivary glands and its potential inflammatory effect, leading to chronic sialadenitis [9–11], is well known; moreover, many publications focus on this side effect and on strategies for preventing its occurrence. Other complications that may arise could be candidiasis, stomatitis, xerostomia, carious lesions, periodontal disease, nerve damage (e.g., facial nerve) or neoplasia [12–15].

Therapeutic approaches to reduce the infectious risk by treating the carious lesions and removing deficient tooth restorations are essential for preventing periodontal disease [15]. The characteristic of radioiodine to penetrate tooth structure is an important aspect that should be taken into account [15]. Salivary side effects correlate with cumulative radioiodine activity, and thus, dentists managing oral health thyroid patients need to intervene with measures that reduce oral complications. When it comes to oral rehabilitation of thyroid cancer patients with dental implants, the current scientific literature is scarce. Patients with differentiated thyroid cancer during radioiodine therapy are instructed to follow comprehensive rules after taking I-131 for a specific period, as I-131 has a physical half-life of 8 days. The effective half-life in DTC with thyroidectomy is controversial, but many researchers estimate for an activity of 3.7 GBq I-131—the effective half-life in final phase—at 38.6 h [16]. It is rational to consider the complete absence of any radioiodine trace and any direct salivary effect at 10 half-life, approximatively 2 weeks (384 h); this interval could be safe. Therefore, the aim of our study was to characterize the effects of I-131 on the structure on titanium implants up to 384 h after I-131 exposure.

2. Materials and Methods

2.1. Radioiodine-131 Irradiation Protocol and Sample Preparation

For this study, ethics committee approval was not necessary. Our in vitro model analogue with the in vivo conditions of thyroid cancer patients treated with radioiodine-131 consisted in a solution of 592 MBq (16 mCi) I-131 dissolved in 50 mL of artificial saliva [14,17]. This experimental model was already tested in other in vitro publications by the authors [14,17]. In the prepared solution, titanium implants (n = 24) were introduced and were then taken out at 6, 12, 24, 48, 192 and 384 hours post-irradiation [16]. The control dental implants (n = 4) were submerged in 20 mL of artificial saliva. Every implant was separately soaked in exactly the same quantity of saliva and I-131 activity. A calibrator (Curiementor 3, Freiburg, Germany) was used to measure the radioactivity of the implants after different exposure times.

2.2. Electrochemical Measurements

Electrochemical measurements were conducted in a conventional three-electrode cell using the implant specimens as working electrodes, while a saturated calomel electrode (SCE) and a large Pt foil served as reference and counter electrodes, respectively

For the corrosion testing, the tip of each miniscrew up to a standardized 5 mm level was exposed to the electrolyte solution (artificial saliva), while the remaining part of the implant was carefully coated with Parafilm and insulated from solution by a home-made plastic tube. The electrical connection was established using a copper rod. The surface area of samples exposed to the electrolyte was estimated at 1 cm^2. A volume of 30 mL of artificial saliva was used for the electrochemical experiments.

Prior to the electrochemical measurement, the dental sample was cleaned with ultrapure water, pure ethanol and dried at room temperature. Then, the implant was left for 2 h in the electrolyte solution to attain the steady-state condition, while measuring the value of open-circuit potential (OCP) as a function of time. Electrochemical impedance spectroscopy (EIS) measurements were acquired at the open-circuit potential using a PARSTAT 2273 potentiostat/galvanostat in the frequency range between 10 kHz and 10 mHz, with 5 points per Hz decade and an AC voltage amplitude of $\pm$10 mV. The fitting of experimental EIS data was performed with ZSimpWin 3.21 software (Ametek, Berwyn, PA, USA). Potentiodynamic polarization measurements were carried out using a Gill AC potentiostat (ACM Instruments, Cartmel, United Kingdom), in the potential range from $-$300 mV to +3000 mV vs. OCP, with a scan rate of 1 mV/s. The analysis of the polarization results was performed by means of the Gill AC potentiostat software (version 5).

2.3. Scanning Electron Microscopy Assessment

Titanium screw samples were rinsed very well with deionized water to remove all traces of radioactive solution exposure and perfectly dried and stored in sterile vials. Their surface was investigated by scanning electron microscopy (SEM) using a Hitachi SU8230 microscope, Hitachi Hi-Tec Corporation, Tokyo, Japan, using an acceleration voltage of 30 kV in high vacuum mode. The macroscopic aspect of the samples was observed at a magnification of $\times$30, overall microstructure aspect was investigated at $\times$1000 magnification and microstructural details were observed at a magnification of $\times$5000.

3. Results

3.1. Scanning Electron Microscopy Analysis

The control sample macrostructure (Figure 1A(a)) reveals a smooth and compact surface of the thread helix and the constant pitch; moreover, the thread end is observed on the right side of the observation field. The thread root is very smooth and compact; crests are well contoured with a right profile. The small micro-sized porosity is slightly visible at the macroscopic level, but the precise details cannot be observed. A mild exposure to the radioactive solution for 6 to 24 h (Figure 1B(a),C(a),D(a)) shows a good preservation of the macro-structural aspects such as thread details and surface quality.

Significant changes occur after 48 h of exposure (Figure 1E(a)). The thread crest presents some local dimensional alteration prone observed on the right side of the observation field, but the root seems to be well preserved along with the surface porosity which seems to be slightly affected. The thread helix with both crest and root is significantly damaged after 192 and 384 h of exposure to the radioactive solution (Figure 1F(a),G(a)). Surface quality depreciation is also noticed after long-time exposure to the radioactive environment. A more detailed microscopic investigation is required to evidence the specific alterations.

Surface microstructure is very complex due to an interlocked porous structure formed by large alveolus of about 10–20 μm in diameter with smaller pores on their walls of about 2.5 μm diameter (Figure 1A(b)). The pore structure is sustained by a complex network of well sintered titanium particles (e.g., pores walls represent the sintering necks between titanium particles). The microstructural aspects are well preserved at moderate exposure times such as 6 to 12 h (Figure 1B(b),C(b)), with no visible alterations.

Several microstructural alterations start to appear after 24–48 h of exposure that affects the pore walls, which tend to be eroded such as evidenced by the flattened and enlarged pore wall observed in Figure 1D(b),E(b). The prolonged exposure to the I-131 substance at

192 and 384 h facilitated the erosive pattern proliferation (Figure 1F(b),G(b)). The eroded material is dismantled from the pore walls and precipitates inside the pores as boulder particles; their shape and size are well observed at the microstructural details.

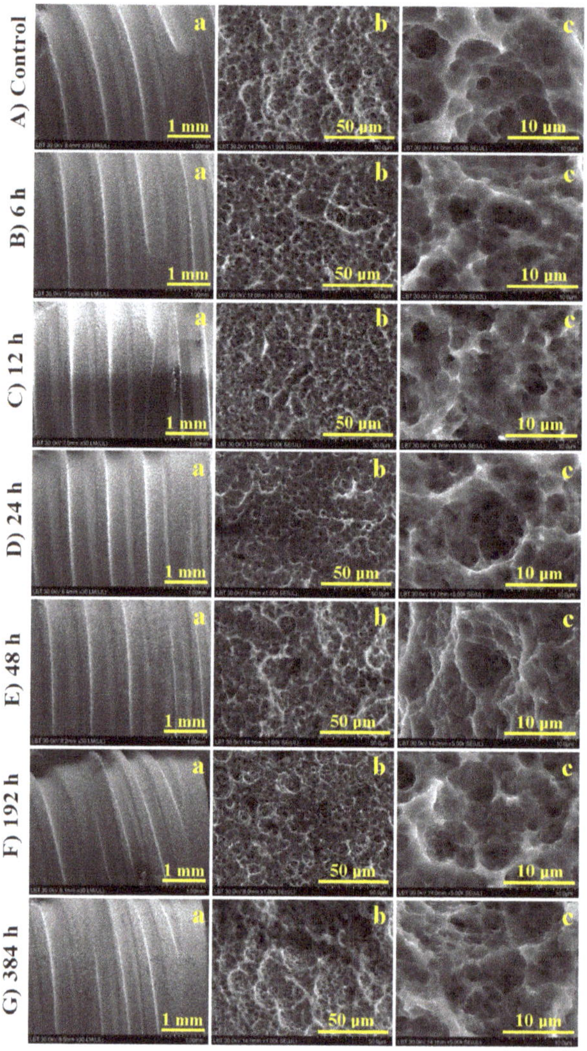

Figure 1. SEM images for Ti screws: macroscopic view (**a**), microstructure (**b**) and fine microstructural details (**c**) exposed to radioactive environment for: (**A**) control, (**B**) 6 h, (**C**) 12 h, (**D**) 24 h, (**E**) 48 h, (**F**) 192 h and (**G**) 384 h.

3.2. Open-Circuit Potential Measurements

The evolution of the open-circuit potential (OCP) values for the non-irradiated and irradiated implants during the immersion is shown in Figure 2. In this figure, it can be noticed that the OCP value of the non-irradiated Ti-6Al-4V implant moves toward more noble potentials during the first 40 min of exposure to the artificial saliva and then stabilizes at a constant value of −142 mV vs. SCE. A displacement of the OCP values toward more negative values was observed for all irradiated implants during the immersion in the I-131.

These potential shifts are more negative, as the irradiation period of the tested implants increased. For instance, in case of the sample irradiated for 6 h, the OCP value stabilizes at about −172 mV vs. SCE, after 120 min of immersion in artificial saliva. Instead, the open-potential values of the implant irradiated for 384 h drop sharply to a very negative potentials within the first 15 min of immersion and then stabilizes at about −298 V vs. SCE by the end of the exposure period.

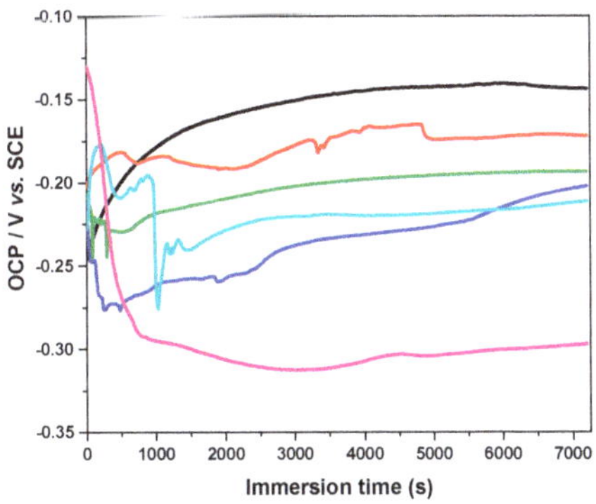

Figure 2. Variation of the open circuit potential of the non-irradiated and irradiated implants exposed for 2 h in artificial saliva solution. Irradiation period (hours): 0 (—); 6 (—); 12 (—); 48 (—); 192 (—); 384 (—).

3.3. *Electrochemical Impedance Spectroscopy*

The EIS tests were further performed after 2 h exposure of the non-irradiated and irradiated implants in artificial saliva solution and the obtained impedance spectra are presented in Figure 2. The data are displayed in complex impedance (Nyquist diagram) and in Bode amplitude and phase angle plots. As depicted in Figure 2, a single broad capacitive loop is visible in the impedance spectra corresponding to all tested implant specimens exposed for 2 h in the artificial saliva, disregarding their initial condition (non-irradiated or irradiated for different periods). A decrease of the diameter of the capacitive semicircle could be noticed for the irradiated Ti-6Al-4V samples as compared to the untreated one. Likewise, the impedance modulus determined at low frequency (0.01 Hz), $|Z|_{0.01Hz}$ presents smaller values in the case of the treated Ti-6Al-4V implants, with the lowest $|Z|_{0.01Hz}$ values of 214 kΩ cm^2 and 189 kΩ cm^2 being attained for the specimens irradiated for 192 h and 384 h, respectively. Moreover, the phase angle maximum in artificial saliva was found to lie in the range of −78° to −70°.

As the impedance spectra from Figure 3 consisted of one-time relaxation constant, the equivalent electrical circuit depicted in Figure 4 was further used to reproduce the experimental data and to extract the corresponding R-Q parameters. As depicted in Table 1, the values of the resistance of the passive film are lower in the case of all irradiated samples as compared to the non-irradiated samples. The smallest R_p values were calculated for the samples which were irradiated for the longest periods (192 h and 384 h). The Q values for the irradiated samples were lower than those corresponding to the untreated one, while the values of n were found within the range of 0.797–0.893, indicating the surface heterogeneity of Ti-6Al-4V samples.

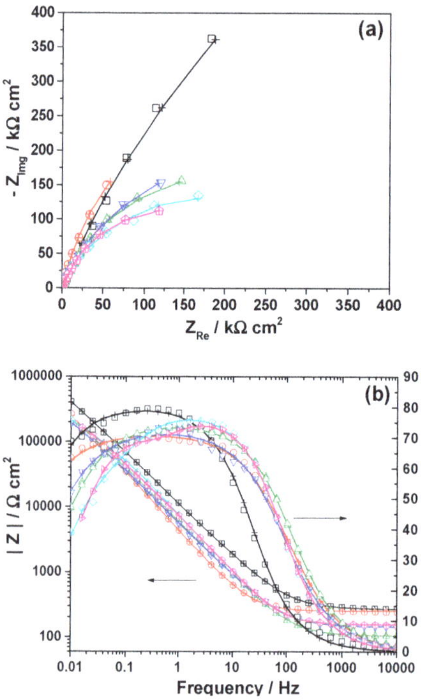

Figure 3. Nyquist (**a**) and Bode (**b**) diagrams corresponding to the non-irradiated (□) and irradiated Ti-6Al-4V implant specimens for 6 h (○); 12 h (△); 48 h (∇); 192 ( ) and 384 h (⬠) after their exposure for 2 h in the artificial saliva. Symbols correspond to the experimental data and the line with cross (—+—) to the calculated data.

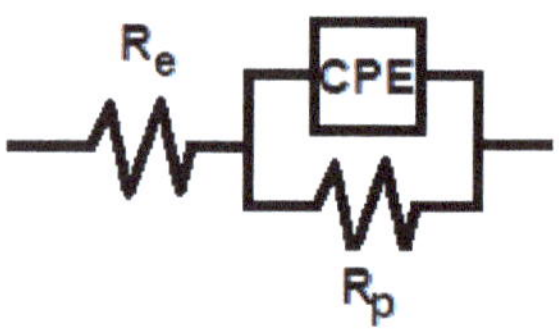

Figure 4. Electrical equivalent circuit used for the computer fitting of experimental data.

Table 1. EIS parameters for non-irradiated and irradiated implants after 2 h immersion in artificial saliva solution.

Irradiation Period (Hours)	R_e (Ω cm^2)	Rp (kΩ cm^2)	Q (μF s^{n-1} cm^{-2})	n	C (μF cm^{-2})
0	255	1100	44.9	0.893	71.7
6	301	1090	19.5	0.797	57.2
12	105	436.7	36.2	0.833	63.1
48	144	532.7	40.6	0.809	84.1
192	153	295.3	28.7	0.861	37.6
384	152	285.5	30.6	0.848	45.1

4. Discussion

Thyroid cancer is the most frequent endocrine tumor, with specific therapies that succeed in offering complete remission in more than 90% of patients [18]. One of the early side effects of radioiodine used to treat malignant differentiated thyroid disease is acute sialadenitis; the prevalence of salivary dysfunction varies among studies between 16 and 54% [19]. In the majority of cases, sialadenitis resolves within days; however, in some circumstances (high doses, recurrent doses, etc.), there is damage to acinar cells and the inflammatory effect of salivary ducts lead to fluid reduction and chronic sialadenitis, finally ending with xerostomia [19]. The standard protocol to reduce the salivary gland damage is to stimulate the salivary fluid before and after the therapy with lemon juice, and drops for several hours for 2–3 days [9,10].

The quality of life of thyroid cancer patients is an essential issue considering the high rates of curability. Among many other aspects, oral health is an important topic that should be considered in the evaluation of life quality. A previous study performed by our team has evaluated, in vitro, the alteration of enamel and dentin after I-131 exposure using histopathological assessment, scanning electron microscopy (SEM) and atomic force microscopy (AFM) [14]. The results of our research demonstrated that the alterations are extended into the enamel depth after 6 h; furthermore, this is more important after 12 h and the microstructure is modified after 8 days. The next focus was to study if there are any alterations of different types of dental implants in cases of patients with thyroid cancer who underwent radioiodine therapies. The investigated titanium dental implant is produced by powder metallurgy techniques assuring a well-defined surface quality and a precise thread detail, as well as a very well-controlled micro-sized porosity. The microstructural porosity is necessary for the penetration of body fluid, which promotes the hard tissue adhesion onto the implant. According to our latest search in the scientific English language publications database, this is the first study considering the I-131 effects on dental implants.

Complex pore structure nanostructure details within the control sample are observed in Figure 1A(c), with larger alveolus observed and the fine pores observed on their walls. This structure is well preserved after I-131 exposure up to 12 h (Figure 1B(c),C(c)). Eroded particles start to appear in the microstructural details after 24 h of exposure (Figure 1D(c)) as small boulders of about 2 μm which are sank on the pore bottoms. Their diameter strongly increases at about 3–6 μm after 48 h of exposure, as observed in Figure 1E(c), and their number progressively increases up to 192 h of exposure as observed in Figure 1F(c). The longest exposure time of 384 h conducts larger eroded bolder particles of about 8 μm diameter as observed in Figure 1G(c).

The presence of titanium implants in irradiated areas can create a deleterious effect on bone tissue. While studies on external irradiation were previously done, they are completely missing for internal I-131 irradiation. High-energy beta-emitters from I-131—the gamma rays and electrons at the tissue–metal interface—may compromise bone repair. In addition, ionizing radiation induces persistent hypoxia in small blood vessels and decreases the activity and quantity of osteoblasts and osteocytes, which can increase the occurrence of necrosis [20,21]. Implant morphology has a crucial role in bone-implant contact and can enhance the osseointegration process [20,21].

The microscopic alterations on dental implants seen after therapeutic radioiodine exposure have important clinical impact. Firstly, in order to prevent any damage and further dental complication, the patients with thyroid cancer that are candidates for radioiodine therapies will be advised to have their dental implants of titanium after the radioiodine therapy, with a safe period of a minimum of 2 weeks. Secondly, for patients who already have dental implants—and before our clinical evaluation of radioiodine therapy—we need to include data about the type of implants and the clear recommendation to extend the standard salivary stimulation protocol at minimum 2 weeks after irradiation.

5. Conclusions

This is the first study considering the effects of the therapeutic I-131 on titanium dental implants. After exposure to radioiodine, the structure of dental implants are well preserved up to 12 h; the eroded particles start to appear in the microstructural details after 24 h of exposure and their number progressively increases up to 384 h after exposure at about 8 μm diameter.

According to our results, there are two major clinical impacts of microscopic alterations on dental implants after radioiodine exposure: (1) in order to prevent any damage and further dental complication, the patients with thyroid cancer that are candidates for radioiodine therapies will be advised to have their dental implants after the radioiodine therapy, with a safe period of a minimum of 2 weeks; and (2) for patients who already have dental implants, we recommend registering their information about the type of dental implants in our clinical files and extending the standard salivary stimulation protocol at minimum 2 weeks after irradiation. Studies on larger cohorts are necessary in order to establish a safe appropriate time.

Author Contributions: Conceptualization, D.P. and A.M.; methodology, D.P., A.M., M.M. and S.C.; validation, A.M. and F.O.; formal analysis, D.P., S.B., M.M., S.V. and F.O.; investigation, D.P., M.M., S.V., S.C., C.M.-G. and E.B.; writing—original draft preparation, D.P., M.M., S.V., A.P., A.M. and S.C.; writing—review and editing, D.P., A.P. and A.M.; supervision, D.P. and A.M. All authors have read and agreed to the published version of the manuscript.

Funding: This research received no external funding.

Institutional Review Board Statement: Not applicable.

Informed Consent Statement: Not applicable.

Data Availability Statement: The data presented in this study are available on request from the corresponding author.

Acknowledgments: The authors acknowledge the support of TAV Dental Implant for providing titanium implant for this research.

Conflicts of Interest: The authors declare no conflict of interest.

References

1. Sung, H.; Ferlay, J.; Siegel, R.L.; Laversanne, M.; Soerjomataram, I.; Jemal, A.; Bray, F. Global Cancer Statistics 2020: GLOBOCAN Estimates of Incidence and Mortality Worldwide for 36 Cancers in 185 Countries. *CA Cancer J. Clin.* **2021**, *71*, 209–249. [CrossRef] [PubMed]
2. Baloch, Z.W.; Asa, S.L.; Barletta, J.A.; Ghossein, R.A.; Juhlin, C.C.; Jung, C.K.; LiVolsi, V.A.; Papotti, M.G.; Sobrinho-Simões, M.; Tallini, G.; et al. *Overview of the 2022 WHO Classification of Thyroid Neoplasms*; Springer: New York, NY, USA, 2022; Volume 33, ISBN 1202202209.
3. Filetti, S.; Durante, C.; Hartl, D.; Leboulleux, S.; Locati, L.D.; Newbold, K.; Papotti, M.G.; Berruti, A. Thyroid cancer: ESMO Clinical Practice Guidelines for diagnosis, treatment and follow-up. *Ann. Oncol. Off. J. Eur. Soc. Med. Oncol.* **2019**, *30*, 1856–1883. [CrossRef] [PubMed]
4. Borda, A.; Zahan, A.-E.; Piciu, D.; Barbuș, E.; Berger, N.; Nechifor-Boilă, A. A 15 year institutional experience of well-differentiated follicular cell-derived thyroid carcinomas; impact of the new 2017 TNM and WHO Classifications of Tumors of Endocrine Organs on the epidemiological trends and pathological characteristics. *Endocrine* **2020**, *67*, 630–642. [CrossRef] [PubMed]
5. Haugen, B.R.; Alexander, E.K.; Bible, K.C.; Doherty, G.; Mandel, S.J.; Nikiforov, Y.E.; Pacini, F.; Randolph, G.; Sawka, A.; Schlumberger, M.; et al. American Thyroid Association Management Guidelines for Adult Patients with Thyroid Nodules and Differentiated Thyroid Cancer: The American Thyroid Association Guidelines Task Force on Thyroid Nodules and Differentiated Thyroid Cancer. *Thyroid* **2015**, *26*, 1–133. [CrossRef]
6. Sugitani, I.; Ito, Y.; Takeuchi, D.; Nakayama, H.; Masaki, C.; Shindo, H.; Teshima, M.; Horiguchi, K.; Yoshida, Y.; Kanai, T.; et al. Indications and Strategy for Active Surveillance of Adult Low-Risk Papillary Thyroid Microcarcinoma: Consensus Statements from the Japan Association of Endocrine Surgery Task Force on Management for Papillary Thyroid Microcarcinoma. *Thyroid* **2021**, *31*, 183–192. [CrossRef] [PubMed]
7. Baudin, C.; Lussey-Lepoutre, C.; Bressand, A.; Buffet, C.; Menegaux, F.; Soret, M.; Broggio, D.; Bassinet, C.; Huet, C.; Armengol, G.; et al. Salivary Dysfunctions and Consequences After Radioiodine Treatment for Thyroid Cancer: Protocol for a Self-Controlled Study (START Study). *JMIR Res. Protoc.* **2022**, *11*, e35565. [CrossRef] [PubMed]

8. Walshaw, E.G.; Smith, M.; Kim, D.; Wadsley, J.; Kanatas, A.; Rogers, S.N. Systematic review of health-related quality of life following thyroid cancer. *Tumori J.* **2022**, *108*, 291–314. [CrossRef]
9. Auttara-Atthakorn, A.; Sungmala, J.; Anothaisintawee, T.; Reutrakul, S.; Sriphrapradang, C. Prevention of salivary gland dysfunction in patients treated with radioiodine for differentiated thyroid cancer: A systematic review of randomized controlled trials. *Front. Endocrinol.* **2022**, *13*, 960265. [CrossRef] [PubMed]
10. Liu, Y.; Wang, Y.; Zhang, W. Optimal administration time of vitamin C after (131)I therapy in differentiated thyroid cancer based on propensity score matching. *Front. Surg.* **2022**, *9*, 993712. [CrossRef] [PubMed]
11. Le Roux, M.-K.; Graillon, N.; Guyot, L.; Taieb, D.; Galli, P.; Godio-Raboutet, Y.; Chossegros, C.; Foletti, J.-M. Salivary side effects after radioiodine treatment for differentiated papillary thyroid carcinoma: Long-term study. *Head Neck* **2020**, *42*, 3133–3140. [CrossRef] [PubMed]
12. Lee, S.L. Complications of radioactive iodine treatment of thyroid carcinoma. *J. Natl. Compr. Cancer Netw.* **2010**, *8*, 1277–1286, quiz 1287. [CrossRef] [PubMed]
13. Badam, R.K.; Suram, J.; Babu, D.B.G.; Waghray, S.; Marshal, R.; Bontha, S.C.; Lavanya, R.; Kanth, S. Assessment of Salivary Gland Function Using Salivary Scintigraphy in Pre and Post Radioactive Iodine Therapy in Diagnosed Thyroid Carcinoma Patients. *J. Clin. Diagn. Res.* **2016**, *10*, ZC60-2. [CrossRef] [PubMed]
14. Mester, A.; Moldovan, M.; Taulescu, M.; Sarosi, C.; Petean, I.; Vulpoi, A.; Piciu, A.; Voina-Tonea, A.; Moisescu-Goia, C.; Barbus, E.; et al. The Side Effects of Therapeutic Radioiodine-131 on the Structure of Enamel and Dentin in Permanent Human Teeth. *Biology* **2021**, *10*, 284. [CrossRef] [PubMed]
15. Mester, A.; Piciu, A.; Lucaciu, O.; Apostu, D.; Piciu, D.; Voina-Tonea, A. Assessment and Care of Oral Lesions for Patients Who Undergo Radioiodine Treatment for Thyroid Cancer. *Am. J. Med. Sci.* **2021**, *361*, 8–13. [CrossRef] [PubMed]
16. Tabei, F.; Asli, I.N.; Azizmohammadi, Z.; Javadi, H.; Assadi, M. Assessment of radioiodine clearance in patients with differentiated thyroid cancer. *Radiat. Prot. Dosim.* **2012**, *152*, 323–327. [CrossRef] [PubMed]
17. Mester, A.; Piciu, A.; Piciu, D.; Petean, I.; Lucaciu, P.O.; Apostu, D.; Moisescu-Goia, C.; Voina-Tonea, A.; Moldovan, M. Disorders of Dental Hard Tissues Induced by Radioiodine-131 (I-131) Therapy Used in Differentiated Thyroid Cancer: An In Vitro Study. *Biomedicines* **2020**, *8*, 475. [CrossRef] [PubMed]
18. Tuttle, R.M.; Ahuja, S.; Avram, A.M.; Bernet, V.J.; Bourguet, P.; Daniels, G.H.; Dillehay, G.; Draganescu, C.; Flux, G.; Führer, D.; et al. Controversies, Consensus, and Collaboration in the Use of (131)I Therapy in Differentiated Thyroid Cancer: A Joint Statement from the American Thyroid Association, the European Association of Nuclear Medicine, the Society of Nuclear Medicine and Molecula. *Thyroid* **2019**, *29*, 461–470. [CrossRef] [PubMed]
19. Sunavala-Dossabhoy, G. Radioactive iodine: An unappreciated threat to salivary gland function. *Oral Dis.* **2018**, *24*, 198–201. [CrossRef] [PubMed]
20. Chrcanovic, B.R.; Albrektsson, T.; Wennerberg, A. Dental implants in irradiated versus nonirradiated patients: A meta-analysis. *Head Neck* **2016**, *38*, 448–481. [CrossRef] [PubMed]
21. Soares, P.B.F.; Soares, C.J.; Limirio, P.H.J.O.; Lara, V.C.; Moura, C.C.G.; Zanetta-Barbosa, D. Biomechanical and morphological changes produced by ionizing radiation on bone tissue surrounding dental implant. *J. Appl. Oral Sci.* **2020**, *28*, e20200191. [CrossRef] [PubMed]

cancers

MDPI

Article

Thyroglobulin Value Predict Iodine-123 Imaging Result in Differentiated Thyroid Cancer Patients

Alfredo Campennì [1,*], Rosaria Maddalena Ruggeri [2], Massimiliano Siracusa [1], Davide Romano [1], Giulia Giacoppo [1], Ludovica Crocè [1], Helena Rosarno [1], Simona Russo [1], Davide Cardile [1], Francesca Capoccetti [3], Angela Alibrandi [4], Sergio Baldari [1] and Luca Giovanella [5,6]

[1] Unit of Nuclear Medicine, Department of Biomedical and Dental Sciences and Morpho-Functional Imaging, University of Messina, 98124 Messina, Italy
[2] Unit of Endocrinology, Department of Clinical and Experimental Medicine, University of Messina, 98125 Messina, Italy
[3] Nuclear Medicine Unit, Service Department Macerata Hospital, ASUR Marche AV3, 62100 Macerata, Italy
[4] Unit of Statistical and Mathematical Sciences, Department of Economics, University of Messina, 98125 Messina, Italy
[5] Clinic for Nuclear Medicine and Competence Centre for Thyroid Diseases, Imaging Institute of Southern Switzerland, Ente Ospedaliero Cantonale, 6500 Bellinzona, Switzerland
[6] Clinic for Nuclear Medicine, University Hospital and University of Zurich, 8006 Zurich, Switzerland
* Correspondence: acampenni@unime.it; Tel.: +39-090-2217367; Fax: +39-090-2212842

Simple Summary: This study was prompted to assess the diagnostic performance of ^{123}I-Dx-WBS-SPECT/CT in the identification of incomplete structural response in the early follow-up of DTC patients and derived optimized basal-Tg thresholds as a yardstick for scintigraphic imaging. In this light, we reviewed the records of 124 low or intermediate-risk DTC patients who underwent thyroid surgery followed by radioiodine therapy. The response to initial treatments was evaluated 6–12 months after radioiodine therapy. According to 2015 ATA criteria, 87, 19 and 18 patients were classified to have excellent response (ER), indeterminate/incomplete biochemical response (BIndR/BIR) or structural incomplete response (SIR), respectively. Among 37 patients with less than ER, 18 had a positive ^{123}I-Dx-WBS-SPECT/CT. Interestingly, metastatic disease noted at ^{123}I-Dx-WBS-SPECT/CT mainly involved lymph nodes of the central compartment with a corresponding negative ultrasound of the neck. The optimized basal-Tg cut-off was settled at 0.39 ng/mL by ROC curve analysis (AUC = 0.852) aiming to discriminate patients with positive or negative ^{123}I-Dx-WBS-SPECT/CT, respectively. Basal-Tg exceeding this cutoff level independently predicts a positive ^{123}I-Dx-WBS-SPECT/CT. In conclusion, ^{123}I-WBS-SPECT/CT identified lymph node metastases in 14/37 patients with less than ER and negative neck ultrasound, thus modifying the management of such patients. The diagnostic performance of ^{123}I-Dx-WBS-SPECT/CT imaging significantly increases in patients with basal-Tg levels $\geq$ 0.39 ng/mL.

Abstract: Background: In differentiated thyroid cancer (DTC) patients, the response to initial treatments is evaluated 6–12 months after radioiodine therapy (RIT) according to the 2015 American Thyroid Association (2015 ATA) criteria. In selected patients, diagnostic 131-radioiodine whole-body scintigraphy (Dx-WBS) is recommended. We evaluated the diagnostic performance of ^{123}I-Dx-WBS-SPECT/CT imaging in detecting incomplete structural responses in the early follow-up of DTC patients and, additionally, derived optimized basal-Tg value as a yardstick for scintigraphic imaging. **Methods:** We reviewed the records of 124 low or intermediate-risk DTC patients with negative anti-thyroglobulin antibody. All patients had undergone (near)-total-thyroidectomy followed by RIT. The response to initial treatments was evaluated 6–12 months after RIT. **Results:** According to the 2015 ATA criteria, 87, 19 and 18 DTC patients were classified to have excellent response (ER), indeterminate/incomplete biochemical response (BIndR/BIR) or structural incomplete response (SIR), respectively. Among patients with less than ER, 18 had a positive ^{123}I-Dx-WBS-SPECT/CT. Metastatic disease at ^{123}I-Dx-WBS-SPECT/CT mainly involved lymph nodes within the central compartment, and corresponding neck ultrasound examinations were negative. The ROC curve analysis was performed to define the best basal-Tg cut-off (i.e., 0.39 ng/mL; AUC = 0.852) able to discriminate patients with and without positive ^{123}I-Dx-WBS-SPECT/CT, respectively. The overall sensitivity, specificity, accuracy, PPV and NPV were 77.8%, 89.6%, 87.9%, 56.0% and 95.9%, respectively. Basal-Tg cut-off was an independent risk factor for having a positive ^{123}I-Dx-WBS-SPECT/CT. **Conclusion:** ^{123}I-Dx-WBS-SPECT/CT identified lymph node metastases in 14/37 patients with less than ER and a negative neck ultrasound, thus modifying the management of such patients. The diagnostic performance of ^{123}I-Dx-WBS-SPECT/CT significantly increased in patients with basal Tg values $\geq$ 0.39 ng/mL.

Keywords: iodine-123 imaging; SPECT/CT; radioiodine diagnostic scintigraphy; differentiated thyroid cancer; thyroglobulin

1. Introduction

Thyroid cancer represents the most frequent endocrine malignancy [1–4], with differentiated thyroid cancer (DTC) being the most common subtype (80% and more of all thyroid cancers). The incidence of DTC has been increasing in the last decades with an overall increased annual incidence of about 3%, mainly represented by papillary histotype, small tumors and female patients [5–10]. Thyroidectomy followed by risk-adapted ^{131}I therapy (RIT) and levothyroxine (LT4) therapy are the standard of care leading to excellent response in more than 80% of patients. Notwithstanding, long-term follow-up is recommended after primary treatment since the risk of persistent or recurrent disease is not negligible, especially among intermediate to high-risk patients [5,11–14]. According to the 2015 ATA guidelines [15], the response to initial treatments is evaluated at 6–12 months by using basal and/or stimulated serum thyroglobulin (Tg) and neck-ultrasound (nUS). The use of diagnostic whole-body scintigraphy (Dx-WBS) with iodine radioisotopes (^{123}I or ^{131}I) is suggested in selected DTC patients [5,15,16]. Additional single photon emission computed tomography/computed tomography (SPECT/CT) is recommended in addition to planar imaging whenever possible [16]. Indeed, SPECT/CT is able to: (i) detect a higher number of radioiodine-avid foci than planar imaging; (ii) improve anatomic/topographic localization of radioiodine-avid foci; and (iii) distinguish pathological from aspecific uptakes, respectively. As per consequence, the diagnostic performance of radioiodine imaging significantly increased after the introduction of SPECT/CT in clinical practice, especially in detecting small metastatic lymph nodes within the central compartment [5,15–18]. The diagnostic performance of radioiodine imaging improves in patients with higher Tg levels (either basal and/or stimulated). Thus, the present study was prompted to assess the diagnostic performance of ^{123}I-Dx-WBS-SPECT/CT in detecting structural incomplete response (SIR) at early DTC follow-up. In addition, we assessed the relationship between basal/stimulated Tg levels and ^{123}I-Dx-WBS-SPECT/CT results to derive optimized Tg cut-off(s) to select patients for ^{123}I-Dx-WBS-SPECT/CT, thus reducing the number of useless studies.

2. Patients and Methods

2.1. Patients

We retrospectively reviewed the records of 124 consecutive DTC patients [F = 94, M = 30; female to male ratio (F/M) = 3.1:1; mean age ± SD = 47.1 ± 14.1, median age = 46, range = 18–81 years] affected by low [n = 61; F = 49, M = 12; female to male ratio (F/M) = 4.1:1; mean age ± SD = 47.5 ± 13.7, median age= 46, range = 27–78 years] or intermediate [n = 63; F = 45, M = 18; female to male ratio (F/M): 2.5:1; mean age ± SD = 46.7 ± 14.3, median age = 44, range = 18–81 years] risk DTC [pT1-T3, Nx (0/1), Mx] referred to the Nuclear Medicine Unit at "G. Martino" University Hospital in Messina (Italy) from 1 January 2018 to 31 December 2021.

The study was conducted in accordance with the Declaration of Helsinki. In addition, the protocol was approved by the Ethics Committee of the "G. Martino" University Hospital

(Project identification code 19/17). All subjects gave informed consent for their inclusion prior to enrollment in the study.

From the present study, patients with (i) positive (i.e., >40 IU/mL, see response assessment section) anti-thyroglobulin antibody (TgAb); (ii) age <18 years; and (iii) poorly-DTC were excluded. Most patients carried papillary thyroid carcinoma (PTC) (n = 112 out of 124, 90.3%; F = 85, M = 27; F/M = 3.1:1; mean age ± SD 46.3 ± 13.6, median = 44.5, range 18–81) while 7 and 5 patients only had a follicular thyroid carcinoma (FTC) (F = 5, M = 2; F/M = 2.5:1; mean age ± SD 57.0 ± 12.2, median = 56, range = 39–74) or a Hurthle cell carcinoma (HC), respectively (F = 4, M = 1; F/M = 4:1; mean age ± SD 52.0 ± 19.7, median = 54, range = 28–75). Among PTC patients, 71 (63.4%) had no aggressive variant (e.g., classic variant) while in 41 (36.6%), an aggressive variant was diagnosed (e.g., sclerosing variant, Tall-cell variant and hob-nail variant).

2.2. Methods

All patients had undergone (near)-total-thyroidectomy [(n)-TT] followed by RIT within 3 months. Before RIT (i.e., postoperative period), all patients were assessed by a neck ultrasound (nUS) and laboratory test [1 month after surgery] before performing RIT. Afterward, patients underwent RIT after rhTSH administration according to standard protocol (i.e., intra-muscle injection of 0.9 mg rhTSH daily for 2 consecutive days). Administered ^{131}I activities ranged from 2220 to 3700 MBq for ablative purpose and 3700 to 5550 MBq for adjuvant purpose, respectively. A post-therapy whole-body scan with single photon emission tomography-computed tomography (PT-WBS-SPECT/CT) was obtained in all patients (5 to 7 days after RIT), as already described [19,20]. Then, all patients were revaluated 3 months after ^{131}I therapy by a clinical examination and laboratory test (TSH, FT4, Tg and TgAb), while a laboratory test and additional nUS and ^{123}I-Dx-WBS-SPECT/CT were obtained about 9–12 months later (i.e., response to initial treatments, see specific paragraph). ^{123}I-Dx-WBS-SPECT/CT examinations were performed to assess the response to initial treatment in patients fulfilling the 2015 ATA criteria for scintigraphic reassessment, including those with positive PT-WBS-SPECT/CT and/or isthmus topography of malignancy, as already reported [16,21]. Additional diagnostic [e.g., fine needle cytology (FNC) and Tg measurement in the aspirate washout] or therapeutic approaches (e.g., lymph node dissection or ^{131}I therapy) were performed according to the patient's response to initial treatment and the judgement of the attending physician.

The response to initial treatments was assessed 8–12 months after ^{131}I therapy by:

(i) Neck-ultrasonography carried out by expert ultrasonographers using high-resolution ultrasound systems (Logiq3 Expert, GE Healthcare, Little Chalfont, United Kingdom or ACUSON 3000 Siemens, Erlangen, Germany) equipped with a high energy linear probe (14 MHz or more);

(ii) Laboratory test. Basal Tg and TgAb values were measured on day 1 (basal), before the first rhTSH administration. Stimulated Tg values were measured on day 3 (early stimulated Tg) and 5 (late stimulated Tg) after the last rhTSH-administration. Serum TSH and TgAb were measured at Core Laboratory "G. Martino" University Hospital in Messina (Italy) by fully automated Access® TSH immunochemiluminescent assay (Beckman Coulter, US; reference range 0.4–4.2 mUI/L) and Elecsys® TgAb chemiluminescence immunoassay (Roche, Switzerland; functional sensitivity 40 IU/mL), respectively. For the purpose of the present study, patients' sera were frozen at −80 °C and centralized at the Laboratory of Clinical Chemistry and Immunology, Department of Laboratory Medicine, Ente Ospedaliero Cantonale, Bellinzona (Switzerland), and serum Tg was measured on the Kryptor® Compact Plus instrument (BRAHMS Thermo Fisher Scientific, Waltham, MA, USA). The Kryptor® hTg-sensitive assay is calibrated against the BCR® 457 international reference standard and the FS (corresponding to inter-assay imprecision of 20%) has been specified as 0.15 μg/L by the manufacturer (Instructions for Use, ThermoFisher). To conform to the 2015 ATA response criteria, Tg values below 0.20 were transformed in 0.20 ng/mL for statistical analysis.

(iii) ^{123}I-Dx-WBS-SPECT/CT was obtained using a double-headed gamma camera (Xeleris, GE Medical System. Chicago, IL, USA; Symens Symbia T-series, Erlangen, Germany) equipped with low-energy high-resolution parallel-hole collimators (HEHRPAR). Whole-body images were obtained from head to proximal thighs (anterior and posterior views, matrix 1024 · 256, magnification: 1, acquisition time: 10 cm/min). The study was integrated by static images of the neck and thorax (anterior and posterior views, magnification: 1; matrix: 256 · 256; frame time: 900 s). SPECT/CT images were obtained in step-and-shoot acquisition mode (40 s/step, 6° angle, 30 steps/detector) while CT images were acquired under the following conditions: tube voltage of 120 kVp, tube current of 80–210 mA, helical thickness of 2.5 mm, table speed of 37 mm/s, table feed per rotation of 18.75 mm/rot, tube rotation time of 0.8 s and pitch of 0.938:1. Using the aforementioned parameters, the overall efficacy doses released to the body linked to the use of ^{123}I and CT imaging were 3.145 and <3 mSv, respectively. Finally, all patients were required to drink at least 1.5 L of water and take laxative drugs 1 day before the examination in order to achieve a better target/background ratio.

According to the 2015 ATA guidelines (15), responses to treatment were classified in three categories: (I) excellent response (ER) [i.e., stimulated Tg < 1 ng/mL, and no loco-regional and/or distant metastases at morphological and/or functional imaging; (II) biochemical indeterminate (BIndR) or incomplete (BIR) response [i.e., negative imaging and stimulated Tg between 1 and 10 ng/mL or >10 ng/mL, respectively]; and (III) structural incomplete response (SIR) [evidence of structural disease independently from Tg and TgAb results].

3. Statistical Analysis

Continuous data were expressed as mean and standard deviation and categorical variables as numbers ratio and relative percentage. The non-parametric approach was used since most of the numerical variables were not normally distributed, as verified by the Kolmogorov—Smirnov test. In order to assess the existence of significant differences between groups of patients (ER vs. less than ER), the Mann—Whitney test was applied with references to numerical parameters [basal Tg (day 1), early and late stimulated Tg (day 3 and day 5, respectively) and the Chi-Square test for categorical variables. The Spearman correlation test was applied in order to assess the possible correlation between the Tg values (day 1, day 3 and day 5) and ^{123}I-Dx-WBS-SPECT/CT results, respectively. The Receiver Operating Characteristic (ROC) curve was plotted in order to set the optimal Tg cut-off for day 1, day 3 and day 5 to predict a positive ^{123}I-Dx-WBS-SPECT/CT result; the area under the curve (AUC) was calculated with a relative 95% Confidence Interval and the significance. Sensitivity, specificity, negative predictive value (NPV), positive predictive value (PPV) and diagnostic accuracy (DA) were evaluated according to cut-offs resulting through ROC analysis (0.39, 0.38 and 0.71 for day 1, day 3 and day 5, respectively). Finally, univariate and multivariate logistic regression models were estimated in order to identify significantly independent predictive factors for positive ^{123}I-Dx-WBS-SPECT/CT. The covariates were gender, age, histotype, histological variant, size, malignant nodule topography and basal Tg (day 1) cut-off. Statistical analyses were performed using SPSS 27.0 for Window package. A p-value lower than 0.05 was considered to be statistically significant.

4. Results

Demographic, clinical and pathological data of the enrolled patients are reported in Table 1.

Table 1. Demographic, clinical and pathological data of the enrolled DTC patients.

	Patients Number (%)	Female (%)	Male (%)	Median Age (Range)	Median Tumor Size (mm) [Range]	Histological Variant (No Aggressive Variant) [e.g.: * CV; § Minimally Invasive] (%)	Histological Variant (Aggressive Variant) [e.g.: ** FV, # TC, ∞ HV, §§ SV, ¶ HC] (%)	Low-Risk Class (2015 ATA) (%)	Intermediate Risk Class (2015 ATA) (%)
PTC	112 (90.3)	85 (75.9)	27 (24.1)	44.5 (19–81)	18.1 (3–39)	71 (63.4)	41 (36.6)	52 (46.4)	60 (53.6)
FTC	7 (5.6)	5 (71.4)	2 (28.6)	56 (39–74)	26 (10–38)	7 (100)	0 (0.0)	6 (85.7)	1 (14.3)
HC	5 (4.1)	4 (80)	1 (20)	54 (28–75)	33 (25–40)	0 (0.0)	5 (100)	3 (60)	2 (40)
TOTAL	124	94 (75.8)	30 (24.2)	46 (19–81)	19.2 (3–40)	78 (62.9)	46 (37.1)	61 (49.2)	63 (50.8)

* Classic variant, § Minimally invasive, ** Follicular variant, # Tall cell, ∞ Hobnail variant, §§ Sclerosing variant, ¶ Hurthle cell.

Overall, 87 (70.2%) patients showed an ER (Group A) while the remaining patients (n = 37, 29.8%) had a less than ER. In particular, 19 out of 124 patients (15.3%) were classified to have BIndR [17 (89.5%); median basal Tg (day1) = 0.35 ng/mL, median stimulated Tg (day 5) = 2.9 ng/mL] or BIR [2 (10.5%); median basal Tg (day 1): 1.95 ng/mL, median stimulated Tg (day 5) = 15.9 ng/mL] (Group B), while SIR was diagnosed in 18 patients (14.5%) (Group C). Among these latter patients, seven had shown metastatic disease (lymph node metastases and lymph node and lung metastases in six and one cases, respectively) at ^{131}I-PT-WBS-SPECT/CT.

Demographic, clinical and pathological data of the patients with ER, BIndR/BIR and SIR are reported in Tables 2–5.

Table 2. Demographic, clinical, pathological and imaging data of the patients with excellent response (ER) to initial treatments (Group A).

	Patients Number (%)	Female (%)	Male (%)	Median Age (Range)	Median Tumor Size (mm) [Range]	Histological Variant: (No Aggressive Variant) [e.g.: * CV; § Minimally Invasive] (%)	Histological Variant (Aggressive Variant) [e.g.: ** FV, # TC, ∞ HV, §§ SV, ¶ HC] (%)	Low-Risk Class (2015 ATA) (%)	Intermediate Risk Class (2015 ATA) (%)	nUS n = Performed Studies [n = Positive studies]	^{123}I-Dx-Imaging n = Performed Studies [n = Positive Studies]
PTC	77 (88.6)	58 (75.3)	19 (24.7)	48.9 (23–81)	20.5 (3–39)	49 (63.6)	28 (36.4)	36 (46.8)	41 (53.2)	n = 77 [n = 0]	n = 77 [n = 0]
FTC	5 (5.7)	4 (80)	1 (20)	49 (39–61)	26 (18–38)	5 (100)	0 (0.0)	4 (80)	1 (20)	n = 5 [n = 0]	n = 5 [n = 0]
HC	5 (5.7)	4 (20)	1 (20)	54 (28–75)	33 (25–40)	0 (0.0)	5 (100)	3 (60)	2 (40)	n = 5 [n = 0]	n = 5 [n = 0]
TOTAL	87	66 (75.9)	21 (24.1)	49.1 (23–81)	22 (3–40)	54 (62.1)	33 (42.9)	43 (49.4)	44 (50.6)	n = 87 [n = 0]	n = 87 [n = 0]

* Classic variant, § Minimally invasive, ** Follicular variant, # Tall cell, ∞ Hobnail variant, §§ Sclerosing variant, ¶ Hurthle cell.

Table 3. Demographic, clinical, pathological and imaging data of the patients with biochemical incomplete/indeterminate response (BIndR/BIR) to initial treatments (Group B).

	Patients Number (%)	Female (%)	Male (%)	Median Age (Range)	Median Tumor Size (mm) [Range]	Histological Variant: (No Aggressive Variant) [e.g.: * CV; § Minimally Invasive] (%)	Histological Variant: (Aggressive Variant) [e.g.: ** FV, # TC, ∞ HV, §§ SV, ¶ HC] (%)	Low-Risk Class (2015 ATA) (%)	Intermediate Risk Class (2015 ATA) (%)	nUS n = Performed Studies [n = Positive Studies]	^{123}I-Dx-Imaging n = Performed Studies [n = Positive Studies]
PTC	18 (94.7)	15 (83.3)	3 (16.7)	38 (18–50)	15 (5–38)	10 (55.6)	8 (44.4)	6	12	n = 18 [n = 0]	n = 18 [n = 0]
FTC	1 (5.3)	0 (0)	1 (100)			1 (100)	0 (0)	1 (100)	0 (0)	n = 1 [n = 0]	n = 1 [n = 0]
TOTAL	19	15 (78.9)	4 (21.1)	38 (18–50)	15 (5–38)	11 (57.9)	8 (42.1)	7 (36.8)	12 (63.2)	n = 19 [n = 0]	n = 19 [n = 0]

* Classic variant, § Minimally invasive, ** Follicular variant, # Tall cell, ∞ Hobnail variant, §§ Sclerosing variant, ¶ Hurthle cell.

Table 4. Demographic, clinical, pathological and imaging data of the patients with structural incomplete response (SIR) to initial treatments (Group C).

	Patients Number (%)	Female (%)	Male (%)	Median Age (Range)	Median Tumor Size (mm) [Range]	Histological Variant: (No Aggressive Variant) [e.g.: * CV; § Minimally Invasive] (%)	Histological Variant (Aggressive Variant) [e.g.: ** FV, # TC, ∞ HV, §§ SV, ¶ HC] (%)	Low-Risk Class (2015 ATA) (%)	Intermediate Risk Class (2015 ATA) (%)	nUS n = Performed Studies [n = Positive Studies]	^{123}I-Dx-Imaging n = Performed Studies [n = Positive Studies]
PTC	17 (94.4)	12 (70.6)	5 (29.4)	42 (24–72)	12 (6–24)	11 (64.7)	6 (35.3)	10 (58.8)	7 (41.2)	n = 17 [n = 4]	n = 17 [n = 17]
FTC	1 (5.6)	1 (100)	0 (0)			1 (100)	0 (0)	1 (100)	0 (0)	n = 1 [n = 0]	n = 1 [n = 1]
TOTAL	18	13 (72.2)	5 (27.8)	42 (24–72)	12 (6–24)	12 (66.7)	6 (33.3)	11 (61.1)	7 (38.9)	n = 18 [n = 4]	n = 18 [n = 18]

* Classic variant, § Minimally invasive, ** Follicular variant, # Tall cell, ∞ Hobnail variant, §§ Sclerosing variant, ¶ Hurthle Cell.

Table 5. Comparison of clinical characteristics of the patients included in different groups.

	Patients Number (%)	Female (%)	Male (%)	Median Age (year)	PTC (%)	FTC (%)	Median Tumor Size (mm)	Histological Variant: (No Aggressive Variant) [e.g.: * CV; § Minimally Invasive] (%)	Histological Variant (Aggressive Variant) [e.g.: ** FV, # TC, ∞ HV, §§ SV, ¶ HC] (%)	Low-Risk Class (2015 ATA) (%)	Intermediate Risk Class (2015 ATA) (%)
Group A	87 (70.2)	66 (75.9)	21 (24.1)	49.1	77 (88.5)	10 (11.5)	22	54 (62.1)	33 (42.9)	43 (49.4)	44 (50.6)
Group B	19 (15.3)	15 (78.9)	4 (21.1)	38	18 (94.7)	1 (5.3)	15	11 (57.9)	8 (42.1)	7 (36.8)	12 (63.2)
Group C	18 (14.5)	13 (72.2)	5 (27.8)	42	17 (94.4)	1 (5.6)	12	12 (66.7)	6 (33.3)	11 (61.1)	7 (38.9)

* Classic variant, § Minimally invasive, ** Follicular variant, # Tall cell, ∞ Hobnail variant, §§ Sclerosing variant, ¶ Hurthle cell.

Interestingly, among patients of the Group B, no one developed structural disease during the subsequent follow-up. Patients with BIndR did not undergo any treatment (i.e., wait and see strategy) and basal Tg decreased and became undetectable over time with corresponding negative nUS examinations. Conversely, as per local protocols, BIR patients underwent an additional ^{131}I therapy course, and relative PT-WBS-SPECT/CT examinations showed radioiodine-avid lymph nodes located in the central compartment.

At follow-up evaluation, one of these patients showed an excellent response after retreatment while the remaining one was down-staged from BIR to BIndR status, respectively. It is noteworthy that 123I-Dx-WBS-SPECT/CT was positive (i.e., abnormal foci) in all SIR patients with sensitivity, specificity, positive predictive value (PPV), NPV and accuracy of 48.6%, 100%, 100%, 82.1% and 84.6%, respectively. Metastatic disease detected at 123I-Dx-WBS-SPECT/CT involved local (i.e., VI, VII Robbins' level), regional (i.e., II–V Robbins' level) and loco-regional (i.e., VI, IV Robbins' level) lymph nodes in 13, four and one patients, respectively. Interestingly, lymph node metastases were located within the tracheo-esophageal space in 9 out of 14 patients with local metastatic disease. The overall mean size of the metastatic lymph nodes was 11.1 ± 3.7 mm (median = 11, range = 6–18 mm). Notably, ^{123}I-planar imaging detected functional disease in 6 out of 18 patients (sensitivity 33%), confirming the significantly higher sensitivity of SPECT/CT imaging (p = 0.006). Notably, nUS was negative in 14 out of 18 patients. In particular, nUS did not detect any local lymph node metastases while pathological lymph nodes were detected in four out of five patients with regional (n = 3) or loco-regional (n = 1) metastatic disease. Accordingly, overall nUS sensitivity, specificity, PPV, NPV and accuracy were 10.8%, 100%, 100%, 72.5% and 73.4%, respectively. However, excluding patients with local lymph node metastases (n = 14), nUS diagnostic performance in detecting regional or loco-regional lymph node metastasis dramatically increased [sensitivity, specificity, positive predictive value (PPV), NPV, accuracy 80%, 100%, 100%, 98.9% and 73.4%, respectively). Regional or loco-regional lymph node metastasis was confirmed in four out of five patients by FNC with Tg washout measurement, and all SIR patients underwent functional lymphadenectomy according to local standard of care (also taking into account that in 9 out of 18 patients, the size of the metastatic lymph node was >10 mm), while no patients accepted a "wait and see" approach. No patients suffered by early or late side effects/complications due to surgical approach while lymph node metastases were confirmed at histopathological analysis in all SIR patients.

Notably, serum Tg values at day 1 (basal measurement), day 3 (early stimulated measurement) and day 5 (late stimulated measurement) were significantly higher in patients with less than ER and positive ^{123}I-Dx-WBS-SPECT/CT (median value day 1, day 3 and day 5: 0.97, 3.5 and 7.6 ng/mL, respectively) than those with negative imaging, respectively (median value day 1, day 3 and day 5: 0.7, 2.15 and 3.6 ng/mL, respectively) (p = 0.036, p = 0.038 and p = 0.047, respectively) (Table 6).

Table 6. Basal, Early and late-stimulated-Tg values of all DTC patients.

	Basal-Tg (Day 1)		Early-Stimulated-Tg (Day 3)		Late-Stimulated-Tg (Day 5)	
	Median (ng/mL)	**Range (ng/mL)**	**Median (ng/mL)**	**Range (ng/mL)**	**Median (ng/mL)**	**Range (ng/mL)**
Group A (n = 87)	0.15	0.15–0.51	0.15	0.15–0.83	0.15	0.15–0.67
Group B (n = 19)	0.70	0.15–2.1	2.15	0.15–16.9	3.6	0.9–19.8
Group C (n = 18)	0.97	0.15–11.4	3.50	0.42–47.3	7.6	0.76–41
All patients (n = 124)	0.15	0.15–11.4	0.15	0.15–47.3	0.15	0.15–41

The optimized serum Tg cut-off points derived by ROC curves to discriminate patients with and without positive 123I-Dx-WBS-SPECT/CT were settled at 0.39 ng/mL (AUC = 0.852), 0.38 ng/mL (AUC = 0.932) and 0.71 ng/mL (AUC = 0.944) for basal (i.e., day 1), early stimulated (i.e., day 3) and late (i.e., day 5) stimulated-Tg values, respectively (Figure 1a–c).

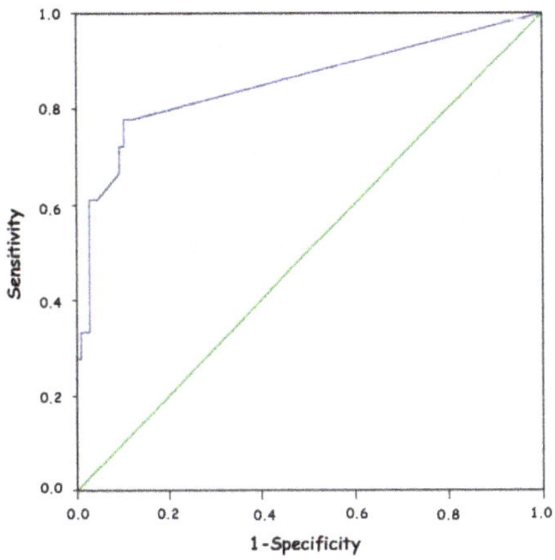

(**a**)

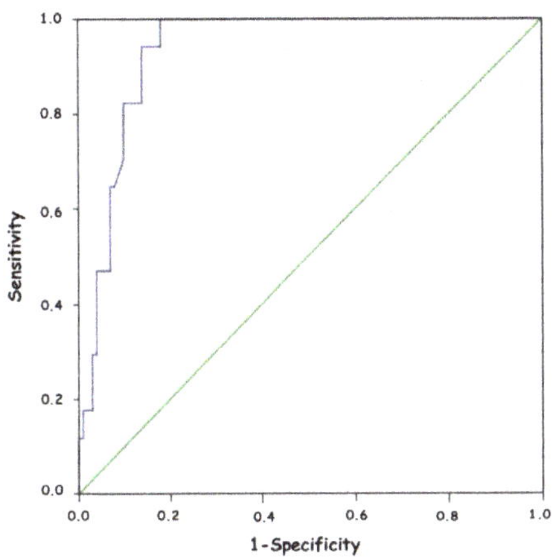

(**b**)

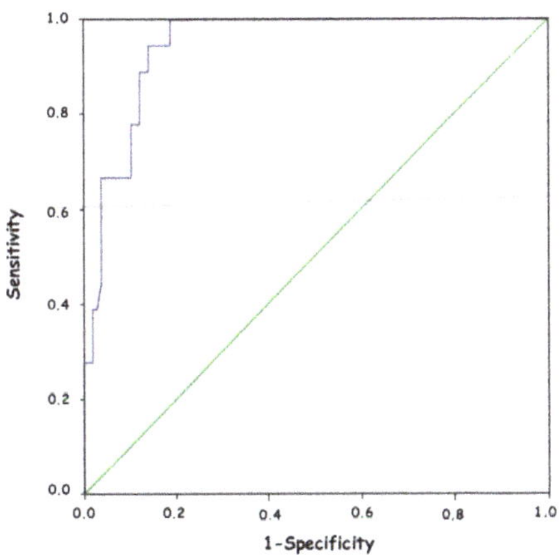

(**c**)

Figure 1. Receiver operating characteristic (ROC) analysis. (**a**) Basal Tg, optimal cutoff = 0.39 ng/mL. Area under the ROC curve (AUC)= 0.852. Sensitivity, specificity, accuracy, positive predictive value

(PPV), and negative predictive value (NPV): 77.8%, 89.6%, 87.9%, 56.0% and 95.9%, respectively. (**b**) Early-stimulated Tg, optimal cutoff = 0.38 ng/mL. Area under the ROC curve (AUC) = 0.932. Sensitivity, specificity, accuracy, positive predictive value (PPV), and negative predictive value (NPV): 100%, 82.0%, 84.6%, 48.6% and 100%, respectively. (**c**) Late-stimulated Tg, optimal cutoff = 0.71 ng/mL. Area under the ROC curve (AUC) = 0.944. Sen-sitivity, specificity, accuracy, positive predictive value (PPV), and negative predictive value (NPV): 100%, 81.1%, 83.9%, 47.4% and 100%, respectively.

The overall sensitivity, specificity, accuracy, PPV and NPV for basal (i.e., day 1), early (i.e., day 3) and late (i.e., day 5) stimulated Tg were 77.8%, 89.6%, 87.9%, 56.0% and 95.9%; 100%, 82.0%, 84.6%, 48.6% and 100%; and 100%, 81.1%, 83.9%, 47.4% and 100%, respectively. In particular, 14 out of 18 SIR patients (Group C) had basal-Tg value > 0.39 ng/mL, while only 24 out of 106 patients (Group A + B patients) had basal Tg > 0.39 ng/mL (p = <0.001).

Positive (+LR) and negative (−LR) likelihood ratios for basal (i.e., day 1), early (i.e., day 3) and late (i.e., day 5) stimulated Tg were 7.49 and 0.25, 5.56 and 0.00 and 5.30 and 0.00, respectively.

Finally, in univariate and multivariate logistic regression analysis, the basal Tg cut-off emerged as the only independent predictor of positive ^{123}I-Dx-WBS-SPECT/CT results regardless of age, gender, histotype, histological variant, tumor size, malignant nodule topography or risk classification, according to 2015 ATA (Table 7).

Table 7. Univariate and multivariate logistic regression analysis for positive ^{123}I-Dx-imaging after initial treatments: basal-Tg $\geq$ 0.39 ng/mL.

Independent Variables	Univariate Models			Multivariate Model		
	OR	95% CI	p-Value	OR	95% CI	p-Value
Age	0.997	0.962–1.033	0.866	1.000	0.953–1.049	0.994
Gender	0.802	0.261–2.471	0.701	1.045	0.223–4.902	0.955
Histotype	0.508	0.062–4.195	0.530	0.212	0.008–5.338	0.346
Histological variant *	0.830	0.299–2.308	0.721	1.594	0.362–7.019	0.538
Basal-Tg (≥0.39 ng/mL)	30.227	8.450–108.123	**<0.001**	34.625	8.359–143.421	**<0.001**
Tumor size	0.964	0.917–1.012	0.142	0.979	0.925–1.036	0.460
Risk classification # (2015 ATA)	0.568	0.205–1.578	0.278	0.406	0.105–1.570	0.192
Malignant nodule topography	0.980	0.111–8.660	0.986	0.634	0.035–11.401	0.757

Abbreviations: OR, Odds Ratio; CI, Confidence Interval; * No aggressive variant: Classic variant, Minimally invasive tumor; Aggressive variant: Follicular variant, Tall-cell variant, Hobnail variant, Sclerosing variant, Hurthle cell. # Low-risk cancer; Intermediate risk cancer.

Interestingly, the risk of having a positive ^{123}I-Dx-WBS-SPECT/CT result was 36% higher in DTC patients with basal Tg $\geq$ 0.39 ng/mL than others (Odds ratio = 3.60) (Figure 2).

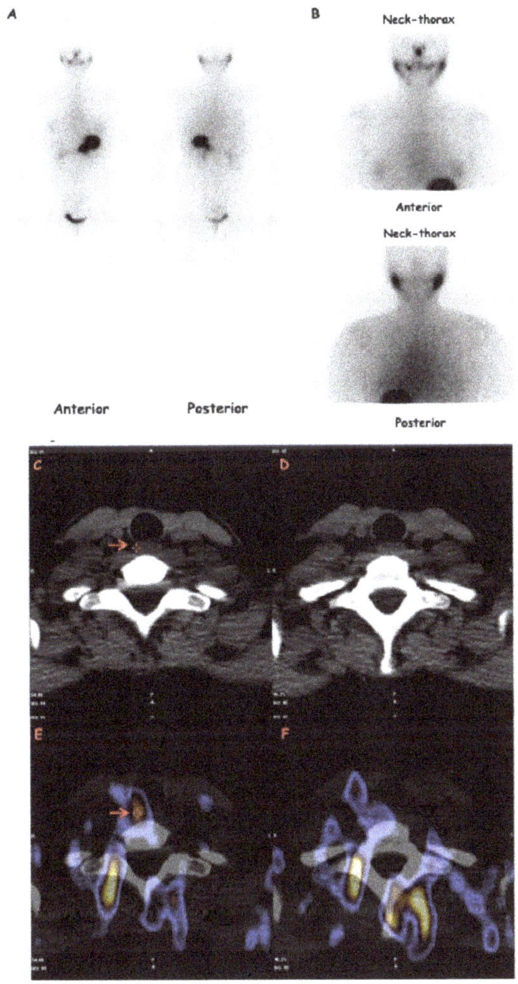

Figure 2. Forty year old woman, pT1b, Nx, Mx-PTC (classic variant), multifocal and bilateral. The largest malignant nodule (14 mm in size) was located in the lower part of the right lobe. (**A**) Dx-WBS (anterior and posterior views) and (**B**) static images (anterior and posterior views) of the neck-thoracic region were obtained 3 h after iodine-123 administration (259 MBq after rhTSH stim-ulation). No pathological radioiodine uptake was noted. On the contrary, axial SPECT-CT images (**C**–**F**) showed abnormal radioiodine uptake in a small para-tracheal lymph-node (red arrows) of the right central compartment (VI Robbins' level). At the time of 123I-Dx-WBS-SPECT/CT study, nUs did not show any lymph-node with suspected/pathological features. Basal-Tg was 0.9 ng/mL while early and late-stimulated-Tg levels were <10 ng/mL (2.7 and 7.7 ng/mL, respectively). The patient underwent functional lymphadenectomy of the right central compartment and histophatological analysis confirmed the presence of micrometastasis in 4 out of 13 removed lymph-nodes.

5. Discussion

Thyroid surgery followed by postoperative risk-adapted RIT therapy is the standard of care in many DTC patients, leading to an excellent response in more than 80% of patients. The response to initial treatment is commonly assessed 6–12 months after RIT by using a laboratory test (i.e., basal and stimulated Tg measurements) and nUS. In addition, the use of $^{131-123}$I-Dx-WBS is also recommended in selected DTC patients (e.g., high risk cancers, positive TgAb, poorly informative post-therapy whole-body scintigraphy) according to the 2015 ATA guidelines [15]. More recently, its use has also been suggested in lower risk DTC patients having a malignant nodule located in the isthmus [19,21].

All in all, the use of diagnostic whole-body scintigraphy has markedly decreased in DTC management over the last decades, likely due to suboptimal diagnostic performances in terms of both sensitivity and detection rate. In addition, the so-called stunning effect due to diagnostic ^{131}I activity administration further contributed to the reduced use of diagnostic whole-body scintigraphy, since it may reduce the effectiveness of subsequent RIT cycles, as reported by some authors, while others have contradicted this hypothesis [15,22–25]. Notably, the improved sensitivity of both Tg assays and nUS also contributed to the decreased use of diagnostic whole-body scintigraphy in clinical practice [12,13,25]. All in all, a consensus on the use of diagnostic whole-body scintigraphy after initial RIT has not been reached until now [26–28].

However, the aforementioned limits have been overtaken by the availability of both hybrid imaging (i.e., SPECT/CT) and ^{123}I (rather than ^{131}I), that significantly improved diagnostic performances of diagnostic whole-body scintigraphy, as reported in the literature [11,16–18,29–33].

Our present results are well in line with previous ones and showed a significantly better diagnostic performance of hybrid over planar imaging ($p = 0.006$). Indeed, ^{123}I planar images were positive in 6 out of 37 patients with less than ER (15.4%) and in 6 out of 18 patients with SIR (33%), respectively.

Moreover, hybrid imaging overperformed nUS in detecting lymph node metastasis within the central neck compartment. Indeed, this is not surprising due to the well-known anatomical limitations of the ultrasound exploration of such a district. As per consequence, it can be difficult for well-trained ultra sonographers to detect lymph node metastasis (especially small sized metastatic disease).

In our cohort of DTC patients with less than ER to initial treatments, ^{123}I-Dx-WBS-SPECT/CT changed response classification from BIndR (n = 10) or BIR (n = 4) (better prognosis) to SIR (worse prognosis) in 37.8% of patients with increased Tg and negative nUS. Accordingly, a change in patients' management was prompted.

On the other hand, negative ^{123}I-Dx-WBS-SPECT/CT results occurred in 19 out of 37 DTC patients with BIndR (n = 17) or BIR (n = 2). In such patients, nUS was negative as well. It should be noted that many patients in the BIndR range will spontaneously reach and maintain undetectable basal Tg levels during follow-up, thus making a Tg follow-up the most reasonable approach in such cases [15].

Interestingly, serum Tg values at day 1, day 3 and day 5 were all significantly higher in patients with positive ^{123}I-Dx-WBS-SPECT/CT than negative ^{123}I-Dx-WBS-SPECT/CT ($p = 0.036$, $p = 0.038$ and $p = 0.047$, respectively).

The most relevant result of our present study has been to set an optimized basal Tg cutoff at 0.39 ng/mL able to provide high diagnostic performance and retain an independent prognostic role, regardless of other routinely considered risk factors such as age, gender, histotype, histological variant, tumor size, malignant nodule topography and risk classification according to 2015 ATA. In addition, the risk of having a positive 123I-Dx-WBS-SPECT/CT result in DTC patients with basal Tg $\geq$ 0.39 ng/mL was 36% higher than in other ones (Odds ratio = 3.60).

Even if the Tg interpretation criteria are adapted to the methods employed in clinical practice due to the high inter-assay Tg variability, our results are well in line with previous studies where highly sensitive assays were adopted. Interestingly, no structural recurrences were detected over time in patients with basal hsTg values below ~0.3–0.4 µg/L in newly available highly sensitive assays, including the method adopted in our study, and basal hsTg emerged as the only independent predictor of cancer relapse in multivariate analysis, conferring hazard ratios for reduced disease-free survival of 67.94 and 81.61, depending on the assay employed [33,34].

As per consequence, the basal-Tg cut-off value could be useful to address the use of ^{123}I-Dx-WBS-SPECT/CT in DTC patients with basal-Tg values $\geq$ 0.39 ng/mL and rule out such procedure in patients with lower basal-Tg values (NPV 95.9%). Some potential limitations of our study must be also addressed. First, considering the retrospective design, a selection bias cannot be completely excluded. However, the study is not interventional, clinical practice in our centers is homogeneous and strict inclusion criteria were adopted, making a significant effect unlikely. Second, the follow-up length might not be considered sufficient in our patients; nevertheless, some recurrences could turn out positive during lifelong follow-up. Indeed, most relapses occur during early follow-up and significant bias is unlikely. Third, nUS were performed in different services by different operators and this may have reduced the overall accuracy. On the other hand, it should be noted that all ultrasonographers were well trained in DTC patients' management, and used high standing US machines. Moreover, many metastatic lymph nodes were located in anatomical regions difficult to approach by nUS, such as the central neck compartment.

Finally, the differences between different Tg assays in terms of analytical and clinical performance should be carefully accounted for to correctly use Tg assays in clinical practice [13]. Accordingly, cut-off limits reported in our study should be considered with caution, and their transferability to local settings carefully evaluated.

6. Conclusions

^{123}I-Dx-WBS is a useful diagnostic tool to integrate Tg measurement and nUS in assessing the response to initial treatments in DTC patients. Planar imaging should be completed by SPECT/CT imaging whenever possible to improve the diagnostic performance of the method, especially in detecting small sized lymph node metastases within anatomical regions (i.e., the central compartment) difficult to explore by nUS. In our series, ^{123}I-Dx-WBS-SPECT/CT changed the response assessment (from BIndR/BIR to SIR) and, consequently, the clinical management of more than 35% DTC patients with less than ER to initial treatments. The accuracy of ^{123}I-Dx-WBS-SPECT/CT increases when patients are selected based on a basal serum Tg level above 0.39 ng/mL. Thus, the use of basal Tg values is suggested to increase the diagnostic accuracy of ^{123}I-Dx-WBS-SPECT/CT and reduce the number of useless radioiodine imaging.

Author Contributions: A.C.: contributed to conception and design and wrote the manuscript. R.M.R. and M.S.: acquired, analyzed and interpreted the data. D.R., G.G., L.C., H.R., S.R. and D.C.: acquired the data. F.C.: acquired, analyzed and interpreted the data. A.A.: wrote the statistical analysis. S.B.: revised the manuscript. L.G.: contributed to conception and design and revised the manuscript. All authors have read and agreed to the published version of the manuscript.

Funding: This research received no external funding.

Institutional Review Board Statement: The study was conducted in accordance with the Declaration of Helsinki, and approved by the Ethics Committee of the "G. Martino" University Hospital (Project identification code 19/17, 17 July 2017).

Informed Consent Statement: Informed consent was obtained from all subjects involved in the study.

Data Availability Statement: The data that support the findings of this study are available on request from the corresponding author [A.C.].

Acknowledgments: We gratefully acknowledge the work of past and present members of our team.

Conflicts of Interest: The authors declare no conflict of interest.

References

1. Campenni, A.; Giovanella, L. Nuclear medicine therapy of thyroid cancer post-thyroidectomy. In *Biomedical Sciences*; Elsevier: Amsterdam, The Netherlands, 2022.
2. Siegel, R.L.; Miller, K.D.; Fuchs, H.E.; Jemal, A. Cancer Statistics, 2021. *CA Cancer J. Clin.* **2021**, *71*, 7–33. [CrossRef] [PubMed]

3. Howlader, N.; Noone, A.M.; Krapcho, M.; Miller, D.; Bishop, K.; Kosary, C.L.; Yu, M.; Ruhl, J.; Tatalovich, Z.; Mariotto, A.; et al. *SEER Cancer Statistics Review, 1975–2014*; National Cancer Institute: Bethesda, MD, USA, 2017. Available online: https://seer.cancer.gov/archive/csr/1975_2014/ (accessed on 5 April 2017).
4. Campennì, A.; Giovanella, L.; Pignata, S.A.; Violi, M.A.; Siracusa, M.; Alibrandi, A.; Moleti, M.; Amato, E.; Ruggeri, R.M.; Vermiglio, F.; et al. Thyroid remnant ablation in differentiated thyroid cancer: Searching for the most effective radioiodine activity and stimulation strategy in a real-life scenario. *Nucl. Med. Commun.* **2015**, *36*, 1100–1106. [CrossRef] [PubMed]
5. Campennì, A.; Ruggeri, R.M.; Siracusa, M.; Comis, A.D.; Romano, D.; Vento, A.; Lanzafame, H.; Capoccetti, F.; Alibrandi, A.; Baldari, S.; et al. Early preablation rhTSH-stimulated thyroglobulin predicts outcome of differentiated thyroid cancer (DTC) patients. *Eur. J. Nucl. Med. Mol. Imaging* **2021**, *48*, 2466–2475. [CrossRef] [PubMed]
6. Lim, H.; Devesa, S.S.; Sosa, J.A.; Check, D.; Kitahara, C.M. Trends in Thyroid Cancer Incidence and Mortality in the United States, 1974–2013. *JAMA* **2017**, *317*, 1338–1348. [CrossRef]
7. Davies, L.; Welch, H.G. Increasing incidence of thyroid cancer in the United States, 1973–2002. *JAMA* **2006**, *295*, 2164–2167. [CrossRef]
8. Horn-Ross, P.L.; Lichtensztajn, D.Y.; Clarke, C.A.; Dosiou, C.; Oakley-Girvan, I.; Reynolds, P.; Gomez, S.L.; Nelson, D.O. Continued rapid increase in thyroid cancer incidence in california: Trends by patient, tumor, and neighborhood characteristics. *Cancer Epidemiol. Biomark. Prev. Publ. Am. Assoc. Cancer Res. Cosponsored Am. Soc. Prev. Oncol.* **2014**, *23*, 1067–1079. [CrossRef]
9. *Cancer Statistics Review, 1975–2013*; Based on November 2015 SEER Data Submission; National Cancer Institute: Bethesda, MD, USA, 2016. Available online: https://seer.cancer.gov/archive/csr/1975_2013/ (accessed on 5 April 2017).
10. Howlader, N.; Noone, A.M.; Krapcho, M.; Miller, D.; Brest, A.; Yu, M.; Ruhl, J.; Tatalovich, Z.; Mariotto, A.; Lewis, D.R.; et al. *SEER Cancer Statistics Review, 1975–2018*; National Cancer Institute: Bethesda, MD, USA, 2021. Available online: https://seer.cancer.gov/csr/1975_2018/ (accessed on 5 April 2017).
11. Campennì, A.; Barbaro, D.; Guzzo, M.; Capoccetti, F.; Giovanella, L. Personalized management of differentiated thyroid cancer in real life-practical guidance from a multidisciplinary panel of experts. *Endocrine* **2020**, *70*, 280–291. [CrossRef]
12. Tuttle, R.M.; Ahuja, S.; Avram, A.M.; Bernet, V.J.; Bourguet, P.; Daniels, G.H.; Dillehay, G.; Draganescu, C.; Flux, G.; Führer, D.; et al. Controversies, Consensus, and Collaboration in the Use of ^{131}I Therapy in Differentiated Thyroid Cancer: A Joint Statement from the American Thyroid Association, the European Association of Nuclear Medicine, the Society of Nuclear Medicine and Molecular Imaging, and the European Thyroid Association. *Thyroid. Off. J. Am. Thyroid. Assoc.* **2019**, *29*, 461–470. [CrossRef]
13. Giovanella, L.; Duntas, L.H. Management of Endocrine Disease: The role of rhTSH in the management of differentiated thyroid cancer: Pros and cons. *Eur. J. Endocrinol.* **2019**, *181*, R133–R145. [CrossRef]
14. Luster, M.; Clarke, S.E.; Dietlein, M.; Lassmann, M.; Lind, P.; Oyen, W.J.; Tennvall, J.; Bombardieri, E.; European Association of Nuclear Medicine (EANM). Guidelines for radioiodine therapy of differentiated thyroid cancer. *Eur. J. Nucl. Med. Mol. Imaging* **2008**, *35*, 1941–1959. [CrossRef]
15. Haugen, B.R.; Alexander, E.K.; Bible, K.C.; Doherty, G.M.; Mandel, S.J.; Nikiforov, Y.E.; Pacini, F.; Randolph, G.W.; Sawka, A.M.; Schlumberger, M.; et al. 2015 American Thyroid Association Management Guidelines for Adult Patients with Thyroid Nodules and Differentiated Thyroid Cancer: The American Thyroid Association Guidelines Task Force on Thyroid Nodules and Differentiated Thyroid Cancer. *Thyroid. Off. J. Am. Thyroid. Assoc.* **2016**, *26*, 1–133. [CrossRef]
16. Campennì, A.; Vrachimis, A.; Siracusa, M.; Baldari, S.; Giovanella, L. Usefulness of ^{123}I-spect/ct to assess the response to initial therapy in differentiated thyroid cancer patients. *Endocrine* **2021**, *74*, 193–196. [CrossRef]
17. Spanu, A.; Nuvoli, S.; Gelo, I.; Mele, L.; Piras, B.; Madeddu, G. Role of Diagnostic ^{131}I SPECT/CT in Long-Term Follow-up of Patients with Papillary Thyroid Microcarcinoma. *J. Nucl. Med. Off. Publ. Soc. Nucl. Med.* **2018**, *59*, 1510–1515. [CrossRef]
18. Spanu, A.; Nuvoli, S.; Marongiu, A.; Gelo, I.; Mele, L.; Piras, B.; Madeddu, G. Neck lymph node metastasis detection in patients with differentiated thyroid carcinoma (DTC) in long-term follow-up: A ^{131}I-SPECT/CT study. *BMC Cancer* **2020**, *20*, 239. [CrossRef]
19. Campennì, A.; Giovanella, L.; Siracusa, M.; Stipo, M.E.; Alibrandi, A.; Cucinotta, M.; Ruggeri, R.M.; Baldari, S. Is malignant nodule topography an additional risk factor for metastatic disease in low-risk differentiated thyroid cancer? *Thyroid. Off. J. Am. Thyroid. Assoc.* **2014**, *24*, 1607–1611. [CrossRef]
20. Campennì, A.; Giovanella, L.; Pignata, S.A.; Vento, A.; Alibrandi, A.; Sturiale, L.; Laudicella, R.; Comis, A.D.; Filice, R.; Giuffrida, G.; et al. Undetectable or low (<1 ng/ml) postsurgical thyroglobulin values do not rule out metastases in early stage differentiated thyroid cancer patients. *Oncotarget* **2018**, *9*, 17491–17500. [CrossRef]
21. Campennì, A.; Ruggeri, R.M.; Siracusa, M.; Giacoppo, G.; La Torre, F.; Saccomanno, A.; Alibrandi, A.; Dionigi, G.; Tuccari, G.; Baldari, S.; et al. Isthmus topography is a risk factor for persistent disease in patients with differentiated thyroid cancer. *Eur. J. Endocrinol.* **2021**, *185*, 397–404. [CrossRef]
22. Pacini, F.; Schlumberger, M.; Dralle, H.; Elisei, R.; Smit, J.W.; Wiersinga, W.; European Thyroid Cancer Taskforce. European consensus for the management of patients with differentiated thyroid carcinoma of the follicular epithelium. *Eur. J. Endocrinol.* **2006**, *154*, 787–803. [CrossRef]
23. American Thyroid Association (ATA) Guidelines Taskforce on Thyroid Nodules and Differentiated Thyroid Cancer; Cooper, D.S.; Doherty, G.M.; Haugen, B.R.; Kloos, R.T.; Lee, S.L.; Mandel, S.J.; Mazzaferri, E.L.; McIver, B.; Pacini, F.; et al. Revised American Thyroid Association management guidelines for patients with thyroid nodules and differentiated thyroid cancer. *Thyroid. Off. J. Am. Thyroid. Assoc.* **2009**, *19*, 1167–1214. [CrossRef]

24. Sisson, J.C.; Avram, A.M.; Lawson, S.A.; Gauger, P.G.; Doherty, G.M. The so-called stunning of thyroid tissue. *J. Nucl. Med. Off. Publ. Soc. Nucl. Med.* **2006**, *47*, 1406–1412.
25. Lamartina, L.; Deandreis, D.; Durante, C.; Filetti, S. Endocrine Tumours: Imaging in the follow-up of differentiated thyroid cancer: Current evidence and future perspectives for a risk-adapted approach. *Eur. J. Endocrinol.* **2016**, *175*, R185–R202. [CrossRef] [PubMed]
26. Pirich, C.; Schweighofer-Zwink, G. Less is more: Reconsidering the need for regular use of diagnostic whole body radioiodine scintigraphy in the follow-up of differentiated thyroid cancer. *Eur. J. Nucl. Med. Mol. Imaging* **2017**, *44*, 741–743. [CrossRef] [PubMed]
27. Dietlein, M.; Dressler, J.; Eschner, W.; Grünwald, F.; Lassmann, M.; Leisner, B.; Luster, M.; Reiners, C.; Schicha, H.; Schober, O. Procedure guideline for iodine-131 whole-body scintigraphy for differentiated thyroid cancer (version 3). *Nucl. Med.* **2007**, *g46*, 206–212.
28. Gonzalez Carvalho, J.M.; Görlich, D.; Schober, O.; Wenning, C.; Riemann, B.; Verburg, F.A.; Vrachimis, A. Evaluation of ^{131}I scintigraphy and stimulated thyroglobulin levels in the follow up of patients with DTC: A retrospective analysis of 1420 patients. *Eur. J. Nucl. Med. Mol. Imaging* **2017**, *44*, 744–756. [CrossRef] [PubMed]
29. Barwick, T.; Murray, I.; Megadmi, H.; Drake, W.M.; Plowman, P.N.; Akker, S.A.; Chew, S.L.; Grossman, A.B.; Avril, N. Single photon emission computed tomography (SPECT)/computed tomography using Iodine-123 in patients with differentiated thyroid cancer: Additional value over whole body planar imaging and SPECT. *Eur. J. Endocrinol.* **2010**, *162*, 1131–1139. [CrossRef]
30. Spanu, A.; Solinas, M.E.; Chessa, F.; Sanna, D.; Nuvoli, S.; Madeddu, G. 131I SPECT/CT in the follow-up of differentiated thyroid carcinoma: Incremental value versus planar imaging. *J. Nucl. Med Off. Publ. Soc. Nucl. Med.* **2009**, *50*, 184–190. [CrossRef]
31. Alzahrani, A.S.; AlShaikh, O.; Tuli, M.; Al-Sugair, A.; Alamawi, R.; Al-Rasheed, M.M. Diagnostic value of recombinant human thyrotropin-stimulated ^{123}I whole-body scintigraphy in the follow-up of patients with differentiated thyroid cancer. *Clin. Nucl. Med.* **2012**, *37*, 229–234. [CrossRef]
32. Siddiqi, A.; Foley, R.R.; Britton, K.E.; Sibtain, A.; Plowman, P.N.; Grossman, A.B.; Monson, J.P.; Besser, G.M. The role of 123I-diagnostic imaging in the follow-up of patients with differentiated thyroid carcinoma as compared to 131I-scanning: Avoidance of negative therapeutic uptake due to stunning. *Clin. Endocrinol.* **2001**, *55*, 515–521. [CrossRef]
33. Trimboli, P.; Imperiali, M.; Piccardo, A.; Campennì, A.; Giordani, I.; Ruggeri, R.M.; Baldari, S.; Orlandi, F.; Giovanella, L. Multicentre clinical evaluation of the new highly sensitive Elecsys® thyroglobulin II assay in patients with differentiated thyroid carcinoma. *Clin. Endocrinol.* **2018**, *88*, 295–302. [CrossRef]
34. Trimboli, P.; Zilioli, V.; Imperiali, M.; Ceriani, L.; Giovanella, L. High-sensitive basal serum thyroglobulin 6–12 months after thyroid ablation is strongly associated with early response to therapy and event-free survival in patients with low-to-intermediate risk differentiated thyroid carcinomas. *Eur. J. Endocrinol.* **2017**, *176*, 497–504. [CrossRef]

cancers

MDPI

Review

Theranostic Risk Stratification for Thyroid Cancer in the Genomic Paradigm

Seza A. Gulec [1,2,*] and Evander Meneses [1]

1 Miami Cancer Research Center, Miami, FL 33181, USA; evander.meneses@hcahealthcare.com
2 Herbert Wertheim College of Medicine, Florida International University, Miami, FL 33199, USA
* Correspondence: seza.gulec@hcahealthcare.com

Simple Summary: Risk stratification for differentiated thyroid cancer is a well-established tool for prognostication and selection of the appropriate initial therapy for "differentiated thyroid cancers". The current risk stratification systems include a system used in current guidelines, based on surgical pathology features identified postoperatively and a more dynamic model that includes all perioperative clinical, radiologic, and pathologic data as well as the response to initial therapy information. Theranostic risk stratification is essentially based on genomic and molecular features of the patient's individual tumor, investigated perioperatively and associated or correlated with radioactive iodine theranostics. This approach allows a more rational selection of the extent of the initial surgical treatment and subsequent radioactive iodine treatment.

Abstract: Theranostics define diagnostic evaluations directing patient-specific therapeutic decisions. Molecular theranostics involves genomic, transcriptomic, proteomic, metabolomic and finally phenonic definitions thyroid cancer differentiation. It is the functional differentiation that determines the sensitivity and accuracy of RAI imaging as well as the effectiveness of RAI treatment. Total thyroidectomy is performed to empower an anticipated RAI treatment. A preoperative determination of the genomic and transcriptomic profile of the tumor is a strong predictor of response to therapeutic interventions. This article discusses the oncopathophysiologic basis of the theranostic risk stratification approach.

Keywords: theranostics; radioactive iodine theranostics; differentiated thyroid cancer; mis-differentiated thyroid cancer; radioactive iodine refractory; radioactive iodine indifferent; redifferentiation; genomics; molecular theranostics; risk stratification

1. Prologue

The practice of oncology has entered a personalized medicine paradigm with molecular theranostics. Cancer oncobiology is now defined based on genomic and epigenomic expressions. A clinical catalogue for genetic alterations associated with cancer has been created using next-generation sequencing and bioinformatics. The approach to clinical issues, thus, has moved beyond conventional diagnostics and therapeutic interventions. The molecular landscape of thyroid cancer is fairly well elucidated. In this new paradigm of genomics and molecular pathology, the risk stratification systems for thyroid cancer, based on traditional parameters, are challenged. The standard clinico-pathologic indicators of risk are gradually vacating their role to clear molecular markers [1].

2. Clinical Goals and Models for Risk Stratification

Risk stratification, like in all malignancies, is paramount in the management of thyroid cancer. The basic objective of risk stratification for thyroid cancer is to obtain prognostic information. The American Joint Committee on Cancer/tumor node metastasis (AJCC/TNM) staging guide is an established system that is used to predict disease-specific mortality [2].

Unlike many cancers, the risk of recurrence does not parallel mortality in differentiated thyroid cancer, the risk of recurrence far exceeding the risk of disease-specific mortality [3]. The staging systems designed to predict mortality in thyroid cancer are not predictive of disease recurrence. To address this issue, a three-tier risk stratification model was developed and first instituted in the ATA 2009 guidelines [3]. This model was further adapted in the ATA 2015 guidelines [4]. Although initially conceived as a three-category model of risk assessment [low, intermediate, or high risk], the ATA risk stratification system is now visualized as a continuum of risk, ranging from very low to very high risk of disease recurrence. This model is largely based on clinico-pathologic data provided in the surgical pathology appraisal. The risk stratification models of the ATA guidelines, though clinically useful to predict disease-specific mortality or overall survival, is suboptimal for long-term outcome predictions for an individual patient. A dynamic model was introduced by Tuttle et al. [5]. This model defined a process where the initial treatment stratification (based on preoperative and postoperative data) was modified over time as new data (response to treatment) became available. The dynamic risk stratification model adds a response-to-therapy re-evaluation and has more predictive value. The integration of response-to-therapy re-evaluations to the initial risk assessments provides more reliable outcome predictors.

A theranostic risk stratification system, beyond being predictive of disease-specific survival and the risk of recurrence, offers an evidence-based process that can govern treatment decisions, specifically for, but not limited to, the extent of initial surgical treatment and appropriate utilization of radioactive iodine (RAI). Currently, a "high-risk" disease designation typically triggers a strategy to "maximize" therapeutic interventions. The ideal strategy, however, should be *optimizing*, but not necessarily "maximizing" the strategies. Neither "less is more" nor "more for more" motto is appropriate. Theranostic risk stratification is patient-specific and is based on the elucidation of molecular markers that predict the therapeutic role and power of the RAI treatment, which is intimately linked to the indication and the clinical value of total thyroidectomy.

3. Theranostic Risk Stratification Model in Thyroid Cancer Management

Theranostic risk stratification is perioperatively initiated and dynamically updated throughout the clinical follow-up [6]. Perioperative risk stratification is a composite term referring to assembling patient-specific disease information to include preoperative, intraoperative, and postoperative data. In the perioperative, dynamic, theranostic model, the risk stratification information is extracted from preoperative imaging, cytology, molecular profiling, surgical exploration, surgical pathology, and postoperative imaging. In the theranostic model, the risk stratification begins prior to surgical treatment, with the molecular profiling of a suspicious nodule. Tumor biology information encrypted in the molecular profile determines the extent of initial surgical treatment (lobectomy vs. total thyroidectomy) beyond the size criterion, which clearly is far from being adequate. It is the molecular profile that ascribes a theranostic value to the nodule work-up. Clinical outcomes are directly linked to the mutational profile and the composition of the transcriptomic alterations. The effect of patient age and tumor size on the prognosis could merely be the reflection of a protracted time frame that allows for the accumulation of genomic and molecular alterations. The identification of clinico-pathologic or molecular predictors of recurrence or mortality does not and should not translate into a need to maximize interventions such as performing more extensive operations, expanding indications of RAI treatment, rigorous TSH suppression, or targeted therapies, but to select the appropriate interventions in the appropriate sequence.

Molecular theranostics defines a new paradigm in thyroid cancer risk stratification. New classification schemes, based on genomics and its phenotypic expressions are being formulated. Genomics with molecular pathology and molecular imaging reflect the true biologic nature of the different cancer types currently defined by conventional morphologic features. The tumor differentiation/de-differentiation and clinical behavior for each individual cancer are now being defined by molecular markers, in addition to standard morpho-pathology. Since the initiation of the cancer genome program in 2006, a large number of cancer types have been molecularly characterized under the Cancer Genome Atlas (TCGA) project [7]. In 2014 the first comprehensive study on a genomic characterization of thyroid cancer was published, compiling a large volume of data on morphologic and molecular features of papillary thyroid cancer [8]. "The integrated genomic characterization of papillary thyroid carcinoma" study marks the beginning of the new paradigm for thyroid cancer diagnosis and management. This study elucidated the pathways of thyroid cancer onco-physiology, and their impact on iodine metabolism. Correlations between morphology and driver genetic mutations as well as thyroid differentiation were first clearly described in a systematic fashion with this study (Figure 1). It since has become obvious that the traditional postoperative risk stratification criteria are insufficient to resolve the "***equipoise***" over the indications of total thyroidectomy and appropriate use of RAI treatment. There are always selection biases involved in the design of retrospective studies and the statistical "underpowering" or "overpowering" in the data analysis for prospective trials. The core matter, in truth, is the biological and functional heterogeneity of the "differentiated" thyroid cancers.

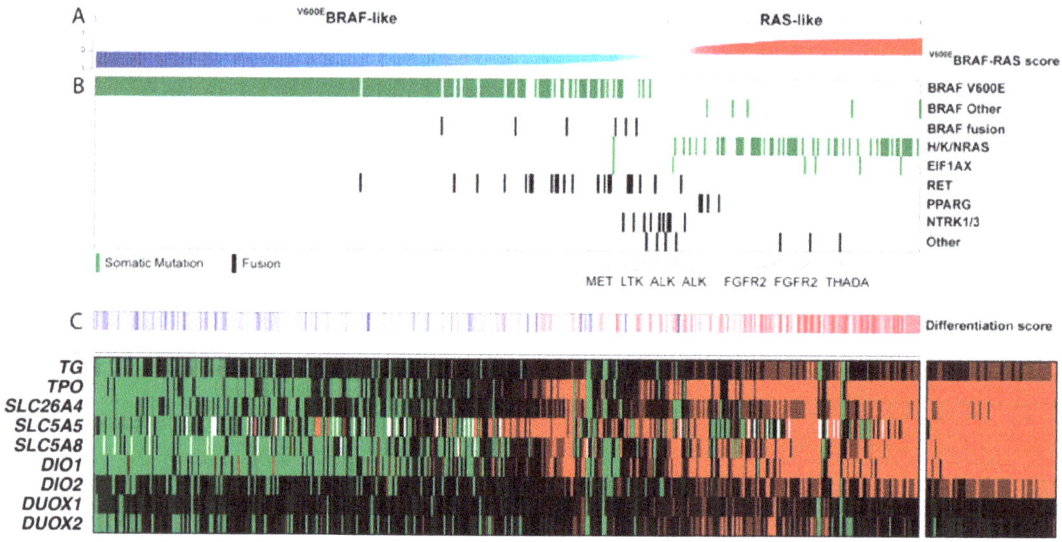

Figure 1. Genomic and transcriptomic layout of papillary thyroid cancer and their correlations with the thyroid differentiation score (TDS) and clinical risk stratification (modified from [8]). (**A**) The TCGA study developed a BRAF-RAS score to quantify an individual tumor's gene expression profile. The numerical scale of this score is a range between [−1] and [+1]. BRAF-like PTCs are in negative and RAS-like PTCs are in positive polar direction with a strong separation of the BRAFV600E- and RAS-mutant tumors. (**B**) The expression profiles of the other less common mutations have been tabulated on the BRAF-RAS scale. (**C**) TDS and RAI theranostic transcriptome pattern correlates with BRAF-RAS score. The theranostic transcriptome is depicted as a heat map. Green and red colors indicate depressed and preserved gene expressions respectively.

3.1. Mis-Differentiated Thyroid Cancer

The term "well-differentiated" thyroid cancer was originally intended to refer to a distinct morphologic architecture and nuclear morphology, but not to imply a functional differentiation. The term was introduced to the literature by Selvyn Taylor in 1962, to stress the significant differences in the clinical course of undifferentiated thyroid cancer and the differentiated varieties (papillary and follicular patterns) of thyroid cancer [9]

This convenient, yet overly simplistic classification changed the philosophy of thyroid cancer treatment drastically. The term "differentiated" was adopted to indicate a functional attribute, thus leading to a plausible conclusion that all "differentiated" thyroid cancers can most effectively be treated with RAI. Evidently, the high degree of variation in transcriptomic expressions for so-called differentiated thyroid cancers were not known at the time. The theranostic power of RAI is in fact dependent on the full expression of genes of iodine metabolism, involved in uptake, organification, and transportation.

The 2022 WHO classification of thyroid neoplasms stratify follicular cell-derived cancers based on molecular profiles and aggressiveness [10]. This classification aims to identify, diagnose, and group thyroid carcinomas from a clinical outcome and prognosis perspective. A major problem with this approach is that it continues to propagate the *misuse* of the term "differentiated" in the context of function and theranostics. The term "differentiated", in fact, should be used more judiciously to indicate distinct morphologic types and subtypes where the follicular architecture is preserved to a degree. The interpretation of the molecular data in the context of functional differentiation and theranostics indicate that the majority of PTCs and some of the FTCs are *"mis-differentiated"*.

3.2. RAI-Indifference and RAI-Refractoriness

The mis-differentiated thyroid cancers have variable degrees of depressed iodine transcriptome and metabolomics depending on the genomic signature. The "mis-differentiated" cancers exhibit variable degrees of ***"RAI-indifference"***. "Indifference" implies a lack of avidity or responsiveness to engage in RAI processing by the malignant tissue. Simply, the malignant tissue is not metabolically equipped to take up and process RAI as much as its non-neoplastic counterpart. The theranostic power of RAI is significantly diminished, the restoration of which requires a modulation of molecular pathways.

The functional "mis-differentiation" is a consequence of the constitutive activation of the MAPK signal transduction pathway due to oncoprotein mutations. The value of theranostic risk stratification is to connect the clinical efficacy of RAI molecular imaging and therapy to the cancer's transcriptomics and metabolomics. The transcriptional, translational, and post-translational regulatory mechanisms of thyroid oncogenesis and their impact on morphologic and functional differentiation have been largely characterized. Molecular theranostics is a surrogate for RAI theranostics. The link involves the MAPK pathway signaling. The term "RAI-refractoriness" is a clinical term that defines biologically RAI-indifferent mis-differentiated thyroid cancers. A ***"redifferentiation"*** can be attained by the modulation of the MAPK pathway [11–16].

4. MAPK Signal Dysregulation and Functional De-Differentiation

PTC and FTC are driven by oncoproteins that signal, for the most part, through the MAPK pathway, though other signaling pathways such as PI3K/AKT are also associated with the oncogenesis of thyroid cancers. The MAPK signal dysregulation and feedback control mechanism constitute the biologic basis of differences in the oncogenic progression and therapeutic manipulations of the two most common mutations, i.e., BRAFv600E and RAS [6]. Oncocytic carcinomas have a different genomic profile. They are characterized by copy-number alterations and mitochondrial DNA mutations [8,17]. The poorly differentiated and undifferentiated cancers arise from papillary and follicular cancers as a result of a sequential accumulation of genetic mutations and transcriptomic and metabolic aberrations [18]. A constitutive activation of the MAPK pathway results in an enhanced ERK output. The ERK-mediated transcriptional program disrupts follicular morphologic differentiation and interrupts the expression of genes associated with thyroid functional differentiation. Different driver mutations are associated with different histologic variants of papillary thyroid carcinoma and confer distinct patterns of gene expression, signaling, and clinical characteristics [19–21]. BRAF-mutated classical or tall-cell-variant papillary thyroid carcinomas have a dampened RAI metabolism.

MAPK pathway dysregulation and feedback control are different in BRAF vs. RAS initiated tumors. Those driven by BRAFV600E do not respond to the negative feedback from ERK to RAF, resulting in high MAPK signaling [20]. RAS-driven tumors, on the other hand, signaling via RAF dimers, do respond to ERK feedback, resulting in a lower MAPK output. This differential signaling results in profound phenotypic differences. The expression of genes responsible for iodine uptake and metabolism are greatly reduced in BRAFV600E tumors, in contrast to the "RAF-dimer" tumors, and the expression of these genes is preserved to a degree. The oncobiology, oncopathophysiology of tumor progression, and therapeutic responsiveness to MAPK pathway modulation strategies are categorically different for these two primary drivers [21].

5. Thyroid Differentiation Score (TDS) and Decreased RAI Theranostic Power

TCGA studied the expression levels of 16 genes associated with thyroid metabolism and function designated as the TDS, which articulates a correlation between the mutational status of the tumors and their differentiation state (Figure 2). TDS show a strong correlation with the BRAF-RAS Score. The RAS-like PTCs have relatively high TDS values. The *BRAF*-like PTCs, however, show a wide range of TDS values, maintaining a consistent correlation with the BRAF-RAS Score, albeit to a lesser degree. TDS is also associated with architectural changes and correlates with tumor grade and prognostic risk, as expressed with the MACIS clinical risk score [8]. TDS is an integrated quantity conveying the relative expression of iodine-handling proteins. However, the TDS, as defined in the TCGA study, cannot be used for theranostic purposes because the patient gene expressions are compared to a diseased cohort median. In a study performed at our research center, we evaluated the fold change (FC) of mRNA expressions of thyroid-specific proteins between thyroid tumor and normal thyroid tissue. Our results (unpublished data) demonstrated more than 2-fold depression in the transcriptome of genes involved in the RAI theranostic circuit. Developing a TDS-theranostic (TDS-T) based on molecular cytology may have an impact on clinical decision making as to the extent of thyroidectomy and postoperative RAI therapy.

There is a significant variation in transcriptomics, proteomics, and metabolomics in patients with BRAFV600E mutated tumors. This may account for the range in functional and biological differentiation observed in this category and may explain the uncertainty regarding the prognostic, predictive, and theranostic power of the BRAFV600E mutation. Papillary mis-differentiation is associated with functional de-differentiation and a dampening of the theranostic power of RAI. The BRAF-RAS score has a predictive value that is not a precise indicator of the theranostic power of RAI. The development of a theranostic TDS score has a strong potential to become a predictive measure for the theranostic power of RAI.

The theranostic risk stratification model assigns preoperative molecular profiling a critical role for initial treatment planning. In the theranostic paradigm, a total thyroidectomy decision is not independent of the preoperative molecular profiling. A molecular profile indicating a low TDS may not be amenable to an "effective" adjuvant RAI treatment. This group, thus, may not benefit from total thyroidectomy with or without RAI treatment, unless the MAPK cascade is blocked. Current schemas of blockage involve MEK inhibitors, BRAF inhibitors, and the combination of both [12–14]. BRAF-induced MAPK activation cannot be controlled with MEK inhibition only and requires combined MEK and BRAF inhibition, whereas the activation can be controlled reasonably well in RAS mutation-initiated cancers [15,16,22]. Oncocytic carcinomas (OCs), formerly named Hürthle cell cancers, and considered a variant of follicular thyroid carcinoma, are shown to be a genomically distinct entity and classified as a separate cancer type [19]. OCs are traditionally considered to be refractory to radioactive iodine. The transcriptomic profile of OCs shows significant heterogeneity. Most OCs, particularly those with aggressive biology and clinical courses, have a low TDS. The molecular mechanisms connecting the primary genomic aberrations in OCs to a depressed TDS profile are not clear. Whether the depressed TDS can be reverted in OCs is open to investigation.

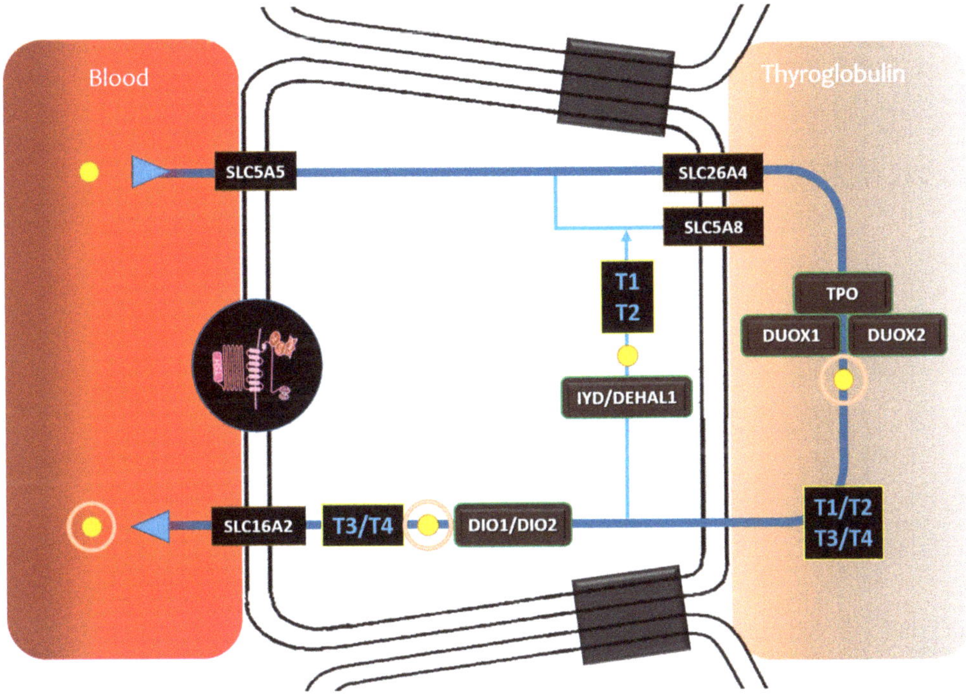

Figure 2. RAI theranostic circuit involving all the steps from uptake, transport, organification, and thyroid hormone release. Gene expressions critical for theranostic TDS. SLC5A5 (solute carrier family 5 (sodium/iodide cotransporter), member 5): sodium–iodide symporter activity, responsible for the uptake of iodine in the thyroid. SLC26A4 (solute carrier family 26 (anion exchanger), member 4): iodide transmembrane transporter activity. TPO (thyroid stimulating hormone receptor): iodination of tyrosine residues in thyroglobulin and phenoxy-ester formation between pairs of iodinated tyrosines to generate the thyroid hormones, thyroxine, and triiodothyronine. DUX01 (dual oxidase 1): involved in the synthesis of thyroid hormone. DUX02 (dual oxidase 2): involved in the synthesis of thyroid hormone. DIO1 (deiodinase, iodothyronine, type I): activates thyroid hormone by converting the prohormone thyroxine (T4) by outer ring deiodination (ORD) to bioactive 3,3′,5-triiodothyronine (T3). DIO2 (deiodinase, iodothyronine, type II): activates thyroid hormone by converting the prohormone thyroxine (T4) by outer ring deiodination (ORD) to bioactive 3,3′,5-triiodothyronine (T3). IYD (iodotyrosine deiodinase): encodes an enzyme that catalyzes the oxidative NADPH-dependent deiodination of mono- and diiodotyrosine, which are the halogenated byproducts of thyroid hormone production. SLC5A8 (solute carrier family 5 (sodium/monocarboxylate cotransporter), member 8): transport iodide by a passive mechanism. SLC16A2 (solute carrier family 16 member 2): encoded protein facilitates the cellular importation of thyroxine (T4), triiodothyronine (T3), reverse triiodothyronine (rT3), and diidothyronine (T2). TG (thyroglobulin): substrate for the synthesis of thyroxine and triiodothyronine as well as the storage of the inactive forms of thyroid hormone and iodine. TSHR (thyroid stimulating hormone receptor): receptor for thyrothropin and a major controller of thyroid cell metabolism.

The true index of functional differentiation is an orderly preservation of iodine metabolic machinery–iodine uptake to organification. This function can be interrogated at genomic/transcriptomic (next-generation sequencing), proteomic (immunohistochemistry), metabolomic (autoradiography), and finally phenomic (RAI imaging) levels (Figure 3). Functional differentiation can be quantitated in vivo and in vitro by the TDS, that is, determined by a molecular analysis and by RAI imaging after a complete removal of thyroid gland. The TDS is a transcriptomic surrogate for the theranostic power of RAI and can be determined by molecular cytology. This signifies a paradigmatic change in initial surgical treatment planning for thyroid cancers.

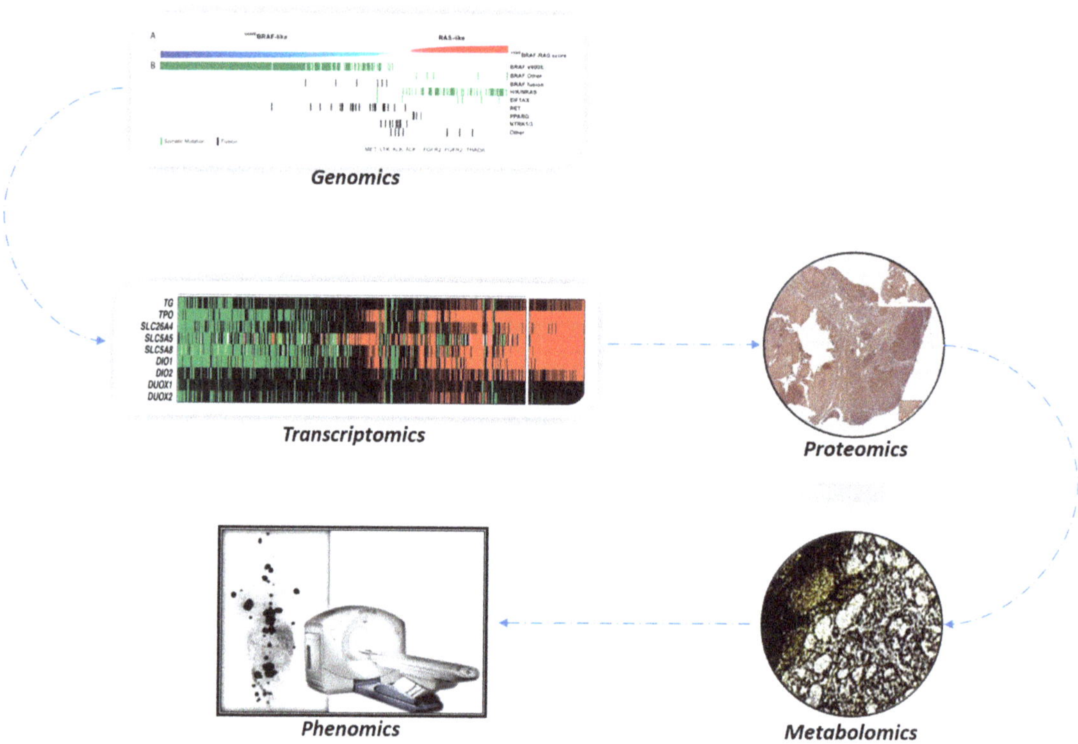

Figure 3. Genomics is predictive of transcriptomics, and transcriptomics is predictive of proteomics. Both genomics and transcriptomics can be conveniently determined by next-generation sequencing of fine needle aspiration biopsy material. Proteomics, by immunohistochemistry, demonstrates tissue expression and a functional orientation of the determinants of thyroid differentiation. RAI metabolomics implies the distribution pattern of RAI in normal and malignant neoplastic tissue. The suppressed RAI uptake can be demonstrated by autoradiography. This technique is currently not in practical clinical use. The in-vivo ultimate theranostic power of RAI is expressed as phenomics and most decisively determined by RAI imaging and dosimetry.

6. The Role for Molecular Theranostics in Determining the Extent of Initial Surgical and RAI Treatments

Total thyroidectomy is performed to facilitate the subsequent RAI treatment. The dynamic–theranostic stratification system includes molecular markers identified preoperatively. One could then evaluate the potential value/benefit of RAI on an individual basis and plan a "coupled" surgery–RAI treatment strategy. This new system revives the surgery–RAI coupling based on clear clinical indications of RAI treatment derived from molecular predictors as obtained from preoperative molecular/genomic profiling of the nodules and from imaging performed in the postoperative and post-RAI treatment period.

The traditional initial treatment protocol advocates total thyroidectomy for high-risk (larger than 4 cm) tumors, and adjuvant RAI treatment for high-risk cancers based on surgical pathology findings. The coupling of surgery and RAI treatments is based on the assumption that all "differentiated" thyroid cancers have adequate RAI avidity. The impact of initial surgical treatment to overall outcome of differentiated thyroid cancer in an independent (uncoupled) role is much less clear than its collective value with RAI treatment. In all reality, surgical treatment is tightly coupled with postoperative RAI treatment. Total thyroidectomy does not have an intrinsic power to improve clinical outcomes. This is best demonstrated with two powerful studies reported by the MSKCC group 30 years apart [23,24]. Other large-scale retrospective studies that are frequently quoted in the equipoise years have significant shortcomings in their design and analyses [25–27]. To reemphasize, the main purpose of total thyroidectomy is to remove the functioning thyroid tissue to divert the RAI toward the malignant tissue with depressed RAI avidity [28]. This RAI biokinetics-based initial treatment strategy, over the years, lost its original purpose, and total thyroidectomy became a standard procedure for the management of thyroid cancer. In the last decade, in an attempt to better define the role for total thyroidectomy–RAI treatment, prognostic risk stratification systems were developed. As a result, the patients who were deemed to have high-risk disease were recommended to receive the most intense treatment schedule. However, a major oversight is that it is this group of patients who have the most profound thyroid functional depression and cannot possibly directly benefit from the RAI treatment other than the remnant ablation intent. In the high-risk group, total thyroidectomy–RAI treatment planning should include a redifferentiation strategy.

The traditional paradigm was built upon vigilant clinical data analysis without having the benefit of molecular and genomic information. There is a bias towards more aggressive treatments combining surgery and RAI treatments based on deductive reasoning and retrospective data. The principles of RAI treatment were first systematized for clinical practice by Bierwaltes [29,30] and further refined by Mazzaferri, who generously contributed to the thyroid cancer literature with his meticulous analyses of retrospective data [25,31]. The Beirwaltes–Mazzaferri paradigm dominated the field including the ATA 2009 guidelines. The second period is represented in the ATA guidelines of 2015 and is marked by a trend to a "highly selective" use of RAI treatment based on a postoperative risk assessment model. The ATA low-, intermediate-, and high-risk categories were defined. RAI treatment was discouraged in the low-risk category and largely reserved for the high-risk category. The intermediate category was left in equipoise. Ironically, what was clearly demonstrated by the thyroid cancer genomics data was that the true high-risk "differentiated" thyroid cancers were functionally not differentiated.

7. Molecular Cytology and Theranostics

It is imperative to identify the indications for the potential to enhance the efficacy of RAI treatment prior to the initial surgical treatment. An appropriate choice of initial surgical treatment option is adherent to the a priori determination of the potential value of RAI treatment. This includes the value of RAI both as an ablative tool and its adjuvant power. The advances in the oncobiologic characterization of thyroid nodules and thyroid cancer allow one to make these deductions and decisions. A major advance in risk stratification is the implementation of the "perioperative dynamic–theranostic model".

Molecular theranostics has the potential to identify different disease categories than the traditional clinico-pathologic diagnostics. A minimalistic approach may be appropriate for papillary microcarcinomas, with a low-risk molecular profile. Nodules identified as such can be addressed with local ablative procedures or may even be safely followed using a deferred intervention [active surveillance] plan. On the other end of the spectrum, those papillary microcarcinomas with high-risk molecular profiles, may warrant a total thyroidectomy. The complete surgical removal of disease may not necessarily require total thyroidectomy. There is no clear evidence that total thyroidectomy, in the absence of nodal disease and tumor confined to one lobe and without the adjuvant benefit of radioactive iodine treatment, improves disease outcome. Complete surgical removal of the thyroid gland, however, is a prerequisite for a radioactive iodine treatment to prevent normal thyroid tissue from diverting RAI away from the neoplastic tissue. Surgical treatment, therefore, is tightly coupled with the radioactive iodine treatment potential. When the initial choice is a lobectomy, there is no role for radioactive iodine treatment in the management unless surgical pathology of the lobectomy specimen indicated risk factors that obviated a completion of the thyroidectomy. For total thyroidectomy to have a therapeutic benefit, the tumor molecular profile should allow an adequate response to RAI. Those tumors with unfavorable molecular profile for RAI may need a molecular therapeutic modulation prior to surgery–RAI treatment plan.

8. Epilogue

"Completeness" in oncologic surgery is defined as an R0 resection. Clinically apparent nodal metastases are addressed with therapeutic lymph node dissection. If an RAI treatment for ablation or adjuvant purposes is not planned preoperatively, a total thyroidectomy may not be required for an R0 resection, even for tumors >4 cm. Total thyroidectomy is surgically indicated when anatomically, there is contralateral lobe involvement, and oncologically, when a benefit from an RAI treatment is anticipated. Complete thyroidectomy, in the most precise sense, can only be accomplished by surgical total/near-total thyroidectomy followed by RAI treatment. One should be prepared to deal with structural artefacts originating from remnant tissue identified by ultrasound or RAI imaging during the surveillance and elevated but diagnostically inconclusive thyroglobulin (Tg) levels. The incidence of regional lymph node (LN) metastatic involvement and the fate [natural course] of the "latent" metastatic lymph nodes are not known. Although the regional nodal basin represents the most common site of disease recurrence, a prophylactic lymph node dissection has never been shown to have an impact on clinical outcomes.

RAI treatment following total or near-total thyroidectomy is performed with three intentions: (1) for the elimination of normal thyroid remnant; (2) for the coverage of presumed occult (or better termed as synchronous metastatic/latent disease, typically nodal) disease, and (3) for the treatment of known residual or metastatic disease (therapy). The terms remnant ablation, adjuvant treatment, and therapy are used for these specific indications, respectively. Theranostic risk stratification plays a role in guiding the latter two. The ablation of a thyroid remnant is merely performed to facilitate Tg follow-up and by the elimination of potential structural artefacts to allow easier surveillance with anatomic and functional imaging. RAI remnant ablation completes surgical total thyroidectomy.

MAPK pathway modulation to revert the indifference to RAI prior to an RAI treatment in both the adjuvant treatment setting and the treatment for metastatic disease is emerging as a new strategy [32]. It can be regarded as a "neoadjuvant" intervention to render occult or overt disease responsive to RAI therapy. The theranostic power of RAI can be improved with new and evolving redifferentiation strategies.

9. Conclusions

Existing risk stratification systems can and should be refined, by the incorporation of patient- and tumor-specific molecular markers that have theranostic value, to optimize patient-specific (individualized) treatment decisions. Appropriate interventions can be employed in an appropriate sequence. A limited number of molecular markers (mutations) have been included in the ATA risk stratification model, but their theranostic value has not been explored. A full integration of molecular theranostics in a risk stratification model is needed to improve patient care. An ideal risk stratification model should provide tumor biology data and connect these biologic data to therapeutic decisions, serving as a theranostic instrument.

Author Contributions: S.A.G.: conceptualization, investigation, data curation, original draft preparation, review and editing, visualization. E.M.: investigation, review and editing, visualization. All authors have read and agreed to the published version of the manuscript.

Funding: This research received no external funding.

Acknowledgments: The thyroid oncology translational research at MCRC is supported by MB Koenig Funding.

Conflicts of Interest: The authors have no conflicts of interest with any commercial entity.

References

1. Fagin, J.A.; Nikiforov, Y.E. Progress in Thyroid Cancer Genomics: A 40-year Journey. *Thyroid* **2023**, *33*, 1271–1285. [CrossRef] [PubMed]
2. Tuttle, R.M.; Haugen, B.; Perrier, N.D. Updated American Joint Committee on Cancer/Tumor-Node-Metastasis Staging System for Differentiated and Anaplastic Thyroid Cancer (Eighth Edition): What Changed and Why? *Thyroid* **2017**, *27*, 751–756. [CrossRef] [PubMed]
3. Cooper, D.S.; Doherty, G.M.; Haugen, B.R.; Kloos, R.T.; Lee, S.L.; Mandel, S.J.; Mazzaferri, E.L.; McIver, B.; Pacini, F. Revised American Thyroid Association management guidelines for patients with thyroid nodules and differentiated thyroid cancer. *Thyroid* **2009**, *19*, 1167–1214. [CrossRef] [PubMed]
4. Haugen, B.R.; Alexander, E.K.; Bible, K.C.; Doherty, G.M.; Mandel, S.J.; Nikiforov, Y.E.; Pacini, F.; Randolph, G.W.; Sawka, A.M.; Schlumberger, M.; et al. 2015 American Thyroid Association Management Guidelines for Adult Patients with Thyroid Nodules and Differentiated Thyroid Cancer: The American Thyroid Association Guidelines Task Force on Thyroid Nodules and Differentiated Thyroid Cancer. *Thyroid* **2016**, *26*, 1–133. [CrossRef] [PubMed]
5. Tuttle, R.M.; Alzahrani, A.S. Risk Stratification in Differentiated Thyroid Cancer: From Detection to Final Follow-Up. *J. Clin. Endocrinol. Metab.* **2019**, *104*, 4087–4100. [CrossRef] [PubMed]
6. Gulec, S.A.; Ahuja, S.; Avram, A.M.; Bernet, V.J.; Bourguet, P.; Draganescu, C.; Elisei, R.; Giovanella, L.; Grant, F.D.; Greenspan, B.; et al. A Joint Statement from the American Thyroid Association, the European Association of Nuclear Medicine, the European Thyroid Association, the Society of Nuclear Medicine and Molecular Imaging on Current Diagnostic and Theranostic Approaches in the Management of Thyroid Cancer. *Thyroid* **2021**, *31*, 1009–1019. [CrossRef]
7. Available online: https://www.cancer.gov/ccg/research/genome-sequencing/tcga (accessed on 27 January 2024).
8. Cancer Genome Atlas Research Network. Integrated genomic characterization of papillary thyroid carcinoma. *Cell* **2014**, *159*, 676–690. [CrossRef] [PubMed]
9. Taylor, S. Thyroid Carcinoma and Its Treatment. *Postgrad Med. J.* **1968**, *44*, 404–410. [CrossRef] [PubMed]
10. Baloch, Z.W.; Asa, S.L.; Barletta, J.A.; Ghossein, R.A.; Juhlin, C.C.; Jung, C.K.; LiVolsi, V.A.; Papotti, M.G. Overview of the 2022 WHO classification of thyroid neoplasms. *Endocr. Pathol.* **2022**, *33*, 27–63. [CrossRef]
11. Chakravarty, D.; Santos, E.; Ryder, M.; Knauf, J.A.; Liao, X.-H.; West, B.L.; Bollag, G.; Kolesnick, R.; Thin, T.H.; Rosen, N.; et al. Small-molecule MAPK inhibitors restore radioiodine incorporation in mouse thyroid cancers with conditional BRAF activation. *J. Clin. Investig.* **2011**, *121*, 4700–4711. [CrossRef]
12. Ho, A.L.; Grewal, R.K.; Leboeuf, R.; Sherman, E.J.; Pfister, D.G.; Deandreis, D.; Pentlow, K.S.; Zanzonico, P.B.; Haque, S.; Gavane, S.; et al. Selumetinib-enhanced radioiodine uptake in advanced thyroid cancer. *N. Engl. J. Med.* **2013**, *368*, 623–632. [CrossRef] [PubMed]
13. Rothenberg, S.M.M.; Fadden, G.D.; Pamer, E.L.; Daniels, G.H.; Wirth, L.J. Redifferentiation of Iodine-Refractory BRAF V600E-Mutant Metastatic Papillary Thyroid Cancer with Dabrafenib. *Clin. Cancer Res.* **2015**, *21*, 1028–1035. [CrossRef] [PubMed]
14. Dunn, L.A.; Sherman, E.J.; Baxi, S.S.; Tchekmedyian, V.; Grewal, R.K.; Larson, S.M.; Pentlow, K.S.; Haque, S.; Tuttle, R.M.; Sabra, M.M.; et al. Vemurafenib Redifferentiation of *BRAF* Mutant, RAI-Refractory Thyroid Cancers. *J. Clin. Endocrinol. Metab.* **2019**, *104*, 1417–1428. [CrossRef] [PubMed]
15. Leboulleux, S.; Do Cao, C.; Zerdoud, S.; Attard, M.; Bournaud, C.; Lacroix, L.; Benisvy, D.; Taïeb, D.; Bardet, S. A Phase II Redifferentiation Trial with Dabrafenib-Trametinib and 131I in Metastatic Radioactive Iodine Refractory BRAF p.V600E-Mutated Differentiated Thyroid Cancer. *Clin. Cancer Res.* **2023**, *29*, 2401–2409. [CrossRef] [PubMed]
16. Leboulleux, S.; Benisvy, D.; Taieb, D.; Attard, M.; Bournaud, C.; Terroir-Cassou-Mounat, M.; Lacroix, L.; Anizan, N.; Schiazza, A.; Garcia, M.E.; et al. MERAIODE: A Phase II Redifferentiation Trial with Trametinib and ^{131}I in Metastatic Radioactive Iodine Refractory *RAS* Mutated Differentiated Thyroid Cancer. *Thyroid* **2023**, *33*, 1124–1129. [CrossRef]
17. Ganly, I.; Makarov, V.; Deraje, S.; Dong, Y.; Reznik, E.; Seshan, V.; Nanjangud, G.; Eng, S.; Bose, P.; Kuo, F.; et al. Integrated Genomic Analysis of Hürthle Cell Cancer Reveals Oncogenic Drivers, Recurrent Mitochondrial Mutations, and Unique Chromosomal Landscapes. *Cancer Cell.* **2018**, *34*, 256–270. [CrossRef] [PubMed]
18. Landa, I.; Ibrahimpasic, T.; Boucai, L.; Sinha, R.; Knauf, J.A.; Shah, R.H.; Dogan, S.; Ricarte-Filho, J.C.; Krishnamoorthy, G.P.; Xu, B.; et al. Genomic and transcriptomic hallmarks of poorly differentiated and anaplastic thyroid cancers. *J. Clin. Investig.* **2016**, *126*, 1052–1066. [CrossRef] [PubMed]
19. Bouccai, L.; Saqcena, M.; Fengshen, K.; Ryder, M.; Ho, A.L.; Ghossein, R.A.; Morris, L.G.T.; Seshan, V.; Fagin, J.A. Genomic and transcriptomic Characteristics of metastatic thyroid cancers with exceptional responses to radioactive iodine therapy. *Clin. Cancer Res.* **2023**, *329*, 1620–1630.
20. Fagin, J.; Krishnamoorthy, G.P.; Landa, I. Pathogenesis of cancers derived from thyroid follicular cells. *Nat. Rev. Cancer* **2023**, *23*, 631–650. [CrossRef]

21. Landa, I. Cabanillas ME Genomic alterations in thyroid cancer: Biologic and clinical insights. *Nat. Rev. Endocrinol.* **2024**, *20*, 93–110. [CrossRef]
22. Ho, A.L.; Dedecjus, M.; Wirth, L.J.; Tuttle, R.M.; Iii, W.B.I.; Tennvall, J.; Vaisman, F.; Bastholt, L.; Gianoukakis, A.G.; Rodien, P.; et al. Selumetinib Plus Adjuvant Radioactive Iodine in Patients with High-Risk Differentiated Thyroid Cancer: A Phase III, Randomized, Placebo-Controlled Trial (ASTRA). *J. Clin. Oncol.* **2022**, *40*, 1870–1878. [CrossRef]
23. Shah, J.P.; Loree, T.R.; Dharker, D.; Strong, E.W. Lobectomy versus total thyroidectomy for differentiated carcinoma of the thyroid: A matched-pair analysis. *Am. J. Surg.* **1993**, *166*, 331–335. [CrossRef]
24. Matsuura, D.; Yuan, A.; Harris, V.; Shaha, A.R.; Tuttle, R.M.; Patel, S.G.; Shah, J.P.; Ganly, I. Surgical Management of Low-/Intermediate-Risk Node Negative Thyroid Cancer: A Single-Institution Study Using Propensity Matching Analysis to Compare Thyroid Lobectomy and Total Thyroidectomy. *Thyroid* **2022**, *32*, 28–36. [CrossRef]
25. Mazzaferri, E.L.; Jhiang, S.M. Long-term impact of initial surgical and medical therapy on papillary and follicular thyroid cancer. *Am. J. Med.* **1994**, *97*, 418–428. [CrossRef]
26. Hay, I.D.; Grant, C.S.; Bergstralh, E.J.; Thompson, G.B.; van Heerden, J.A.; Goellner, J.R. Unilateral total lobectomy: Is it sufficient surgical treatment for patients with AMES low-risk papillary thyroid carcinoma? *Surgery* **1998**, *124*, 958–964; discussion 964–966. [CrossRef]
27. Bilimoria, K.Y.; Bentrem, D.J.; Ko, C.Y.; Stewart, A.K.; Winchester, D.P.; Talamonti, M.S.; Sturgeon, C. Extent of surgery affects survival for papillary thyroid cancer. *Ann. Surg.* **2007**, *246*, 375–384. [CrossRef]
28. Beierwaltes, W.H. Indication and contraindications for treatment of thyroid cancer with radioactive iodine. *Ann. Intern. Med.* **1952**, *37*, 23–30. [PubMed]
29. Beierwaltes, W.H. The treatment of thyroid carcinoma with radioactive iodine. *Semin. Nucl. Med.* **1978**, *8*, 79–94. [CrossRef] [PubMed]
30. Beierwaltes, W.H.; Rabbani, R.; Dmuchowski, C.; Lloyd, R.V.; Eyre, P.; Mallette, S. An analysis of "ablation of thyroid remnants" with I-131 in 511 patients from 1947–1984: Experience at University of Michigan. *J. Nucl Med.* **1984**, *25*, 1287–1293. [PubMed]
31. Mazzaferri, E.L. Papillary thyroid carcinoma: Factors influencing prognosis and current therapy. *Semin Oncol.* **1987**, *14*, 315–332.
32. Boucai, L.; Zafero, M.; Cabanillas, M.E. Thyroid cancer. *JAMA* **2024**, *331*, 425–435. [CrossRef] [PubMed]

cancers

MDPI

Review

Advances in the Development of Positron Emission Tomography Tracers for Improved Detection of Differentiated Thyroid Cancer

Hannelore Iris Coerts [1,2], Bart de Keizer [2] and Frederik Anton Verburg [1,*]

1 Erasmus Medical Center, Department of Radiology and Nuclear Medicine, 3015 GD Rotterdam, The Netherlands; h.coerts@erasmusmc.nl
2 Department of Nuclear Medicine and Radiology, University Medical Center Utrecht, 3584 CX Utrecht, The Netherlands; b.dekeizer@umcutrecht.nl
* Correspondence: f.verburg@erasmusmc.nl; Tel.: +31-010-7040704

Simple Summary: This review discusses new radiotracers for diagnosing and treating thyroid cancer. It focuses on PSMA-based tracers, FAPI-based tracers, RGD-based tracers, and 18F-TFB. These tracers show promise in detecting thyroid cancer, especially in challenging cases. They offer better accuracy and help in choosing the right treatment. Further research is needed, especially on the promising 18F-TFB and FAP-targeting tracers, to improve thyroid cancer staging and treatment outcomes.

Abstract: Thyroid cancer poses a significant challenge in clinical management, necessitating precise diagnostic tools and treatment strategies for optimal patient outcomes. This review explores the evolving field of radiotracers in the diagnosis and management of thyroid cancer, focusing on prostate-specific membrane antigen (PSMA)-based radiotracers, fibroblast activation protein inhibitor (FAPI)-based radiotracers, Arg-Gly-Asp (RGD)-based radiotracers, and ^{18}F-tetrafluoroborate (^{18}F-TFB). PSMA-based radiotracers, initially developed for prostate cancer imaging, have shown promise in detecting thyroid cancer lesions; however, their detection rate is lower than ^{18}F-FDG PET/CT. FAPI-based radiotracers, targeting fibroblast activation protein highly expressed in tumors, offer potential in the detection of lymph nodes and radioiodine-resistant metastases. RGD-based radiotracers, binding to integrin $\alpha v\beta 3$ found on tumor cells and angiogenic blood vessels, demonstrate diagnostic accuracy in detecting radioiodine-resistant thyroid cancer metastases. ^{18}F-TFB emerges as a promising PET tracer for imaging of lymph node metastases and recurrent DTC, offering advantages over traditional methods. Overall, these radiotracers show promise in enhancing diagnostic accuracy, patient stratification, and treatment selection in differentiated thyroid cancer, warranting further research and clinical validation. Given the promising staging capabilities of 18F-TFB and the efficacy of FAP-targeting tracers in advanced, potentially dedifferentiated cases, continued investigation in these domains is justified.

Keywords: positron emission tomography; thyroid cancer; PSMA; FAPI; RGD; TFB

1. Introduction

Thyroid cancer is a common type of cancer that accounts for 3% of all cancer cases worldwide. Proper diagnosis and staging are important for determining the best treatment options and improving patient outcomes. Traditional imaging techniques like ultrasound and computed tomography (CT) have been useful for evaluating thyroid nodules and assessing thyroid cancer. However, using PET tracers like ^{18}F-FDG PET/CT can provide more accurate results in detecting and characterizing thyroid cancer lesions. According to the American Thyroid Association (ATA) guidelines, advanced imaging studies like CT and MRI with intravenous contrast should be used alongside ultrasound for preoperative assessment in patients with suspected advanced thyroid disease [1]. The European Association of Nuclear Medicine (EANM) recommends ^{18}F-FDG PET/CT for differentiated thyroid cancer (DTC) patients with rising Tg levels to aid in detecting recurrent/metastatic disease and determining the tumor's biological behavior [2].

Follow-up DxWBS in combination with Tg measurement is useful for evaluating therapy response and identifying patients with iodine-avid metastatic disease. Brain MRI is recommended in advanced DTC cases due to the potential presence of brain metastases, especially in the absence of neurological signs or symptoms, as ^{18}F-FDG PET/CT is not reliable in the brain due to high glucose metabolism. The most commonly used PET tracers are ^{18}F-FDG and iodine-124 (^{124}I). Iodine-124 is a radionuclide that emits positrons, making it suitable for NIS imaging with PET. However, ^{124}I has some limitations: (1) its 4.2-day half-life and low positron yield lead to high radiation exposures, making it less desirable for diagnostic imaging; (2) its high-energy single photon emissions (0.6–1.7 MeV) can compromise image quality; and (3) its high positron emission energy results in maximum tissue travel of >6 mm before annihilation, negatively impacting imaging resolution. In clinical settings, ^{18}F-FDG PET/CT proves valuable as a prognostic factor for RAI treatment response in metastatic DTC patients, with high ^{18}F-FDG uptake serving as an independent negative prognostic factor for overall survival.

In recent times, much effort has been spent on trying out numerous new tracers for imaging in various clinical stages of DTC in order to advance imaging sciences, especially where ultrasound and ^{18}F-FDG PET/CT are not sufficient. This has resulted in numerous publications on various situations, without a good overview of the performance of different tracers in similar situations currently available in the literature. Hence, this review aims to comprehensively evaluate the literature on new tracers for different clinical indications in thyroid cancer, such as detecting lymph node metastases, TENIS (thyroglobulin elevation/negative iodine scintigraphy) syndrome, recurrent or persistent disease, and distant metastases in DTC.

2. Prostate-Specific Membrane Antigen-Based Radiotracers for Differentiated Thyroid Cancer

Prostate-specific membrane antigen (PSMA) is a protein that was first discovered to be overproduced in prostate cancer cells. Recently, the United States Food and Drug Administration approved ^{68}Ga-PSMA-11 PET imaging to detect the potential spread or recurrence of prostate cancer in patients. ^{68}Ga-PSMA PET/CT is now being used in clinical practice and trials for prostate cancer diagnosis. Although PSMA expression has been reported in the tumor-associated endothelium of various malignancies, including colon, breast, and adrenocortical cancers, its expression in thyroid tumors has not been systematically studied. Recently, several studies found unexpected PSMA radiotracer uptake by thyroid tumors, including radioiodine-refractory (RAI-R) DTC, which has led to an interest in studying ^{68}Ga-PSMA PET/CT for thyroid cancer.

PSMA is a type 2 transmembrane protein, and it facilitates endothelial cell invasion through the extracellular matrix by interacting with the cytoskeleton via integrin signaling and actin-binding protein Filamin A. Therefore, it is overexpressed on the endothelial cells of the tumor neovasculature in several solid [3]. It has been found through functional studies that PSMA plays a role in tumor angiogenesis and is part of a self-regulating loop that involves β1-integrin and p21-activated kinase 1 (PAK1). This has led to the hypothesis that ^{68}Ga-PSMA PET/CT could be useful in detecting thyroid cancer. ^{68}Ga-PSMA PET/CT could aid in detecting a recurrence in RAI-R patients, identifying metastases in TENIS patients, and selecting patients who could benefit from PSMA-targeted radionuclide therapy (^{177}Lu-PSMA-617), particularly those with metastatic dedifferentiated thyroid cancer.

Several preclinical studies have examined the expression of PSMA in thyroid tissue, various types of thyroid cancer, lymph node metastases, in vivo small animal models, its potential role as a biomarker for tumor aggressiveness, and its correlation with patients' RAI positivity or negativity. Bychkov et al. (2017) conducted a study of 267 individuals and found that PSMA expression was commonly present in thyroid tumor microvessels, but absent in benign tissue [4]. PSMA expression varied significantly, ranging from 19% in benign tumors to over 50% in thyroid cancer, with a high degree of heterogeneity. PSMA expression was not found to be directly associated with endothelial cell proliferation, as confirmed by immunostaining with the endothelial marker CD105. Heitkotter and colleagues also reported similar outcomes, where overall PSMA expression was significantly higher in malignant tumors (57.1%; $n = 36/63$) than in benign diseases (13.2%; $n = 5/38$).

Research findings indicate that the expression of PSMA varies across different types of thyroid cancer. According to the study by Bychkov et al., the expression of PSMA was reported to be 19% in follicular adenomas, 46% ($n = 24/52$) in follicular thyroid carcinoma (FTC), and 51% in papillary thyroid carcinoma (PTC) ($n = 61/120$) [4]. These percentages were consistent with another study, revealing 40% ($n = 4/10$) in FTC and 58% ($n = 18/31$) in PTC. Santhanam et al. investigated the expression of PSMA in local metastatic thyroid cancer in lymph nodes. All three lymph node samples investigated stained positive for PSMA expression in the neovasculature [5].

In their exploration of PSMA expression as a biomarker for DTC aggressiveness and outcome prediction, Sollini et al. conducted a study involving 59 cases [6]. The study found that PSMA expression varied among the cases analyzed. The percentage of PSMA expression was $\leq$10% in 17 cases, 11 to 79% in 31 cases, and $\geq$80% in 11 cases. The multivariate analysis identified several significant predictors of distant metastases, including age, sex, histotype, vascular invasion, T and N parameters, and PSMA positivity. The final multivariate model that predicted RAI-R included the stage, high PSMA expression ($\geq$80%), and the interaction between moderate PSMA expression (11 to 79%) and the stage. Ciappucino's findings complemented this research by indicating that patients aged $\geq$ 55 years, and those with large primary tumors (>40 mm) or aggressive subtypes, had a higher mean immunoreactive score (IRS), which correlated with structural disease at the last follow-up [7]. Strong PSMA expression (IRS $\geq$ 9) was associated with a shorter progression-free survival (PFS). Bychkov et al. reported PSMA expression's correlation with tumor size ($p = 0.02$) and vascular invasion in FTC ($p = 0.03$), while no significant associations were observed with other baseline histological and clinical parameters [4].

Feng et al. conducted a comprehensive investigation employing Western blot, PCR, and [68Ga]Ga-PSMA uptake experiments on cell lines, complemented by in vivo small animal imaging [8]. Their study revealed a significant correlation between ^{68}Ga-PSMA imaging and tumor burden, as evidenced by correlations with ^{18}F-FDG PET/CT (8.08 $\pm$ 7.74 and 5.67 $\pm$ 4.23, $p = 0.01$) and thyroglobulin (Tg) levels (307.1 $\pm$ 183.4 vs. 118.0 $\pm$ 116.1, $p = 0.002$). Notably, the research indicated an association between increasing PSMA expression and decreasing thyroid cancer differentiation. However, the ^{68}Ga-PSMA uptake in thyroid cancer patients was not significantly linked solely to the degree of thyroid cancer differentiation but also demonstrated associations with the metabolic activity and tumor burden, as reflected by the ^{18}F-FDG PET/CT and Tg levels. In a parallel study, Ciappuccini et al. investigated PSMA expression in neck persistent/recurrent disease (PRD) utilizing immunohistochemistry and its correlation with RAI or ^{18}F-FDG uptake, along with patient outcomes in a cohort of 44 individuals [7]. The quantification of PSMA expression using the immunoreactive score (IRS) revealed that 68% of patients exhibited at least one PSMA-positive lesion (IRS $\geq$ 2), with comparable proportions in RAI-positive and RAI-negative patients (75% vs. 66%). In RAI-negative patients, however, the prevalence of PSMA-positive disease (79% vs. 25%, $p < 0.01$) and the mean IRS (4.0 vs. 1.0, $p = 0.01$) were notably higher in ^{18}F-FDG-positive compared to ^{18}F-FDG-negative patients.

Several imaging studies have been conducted using PSMA-based radiotracers such as ^{68}Ga-PSMA-11 (68Ga-HBED-CC-PSMA) and ^{18}F-DCFPyL (as shown in Tables 1 and 2). The efficacy of ^{68}Ga-PSMA-11 has been studied for various purposes such as detecting DTC metastases, identifying patients suitable for PSMA-targeted radionuclide therapy, diagnosing patients with RAI-R DTC, for patients with TENIS, and detecting patients with elevated Tg or anti-Tg antibodies.

In a case report by Verburg et al., strong uptake was seen in the cervical lymph nodes and pulmonary metastases in a patient with RAI-R DTC [9]. In a study by Verma et al. (2018) focusing on patients with iodine-avid metastatic disease, substantial PSMA uptake was observed in all the cases [10]. ^{68}Ga-PSMA PET/CT detected 93.75% (n = 30/32) of the total lesions, with a median SUVmax of 31.35, outperforming ^{18}F-FDG PET/CT, which was positive in 81.85% (n = 23/32) of the lesions. Notably, 70% of the lesions with PSMA expression were localized to the bones (n = 21/30).

A prospective study was conducted on patients with iodine-negative and FDG-positive metastasized DTC [11]. The study found that ^{68}Ga-PSMA-11 PET/CT was able to successfully identify metastatic disease in five out of six patients, with all 42 lesions confirmed by ^{18}F-FDG PET/CT or conventional CT imaging. Using the ^{68}Ga-PSMA-11 PET/CT, all the tumor lesions identified with the ^{18}F-FDG PET/CT imaging could be visualized in three of the five patients. In two patients, only the most prominent lesions detected with the ^{18}F-FDG PET/CT imaging were visualized by the ^{68}Ga-PSMA-11 PET/CT.

In a prospective pilot study by Verma et al., PSMA expression was detected in two TENIS patients using ^{68}Ga-PSMA-11 PET/CT [10]. The lesions were found in the bones and lungs, and the ^{68}Ga-PSMA PET/CT localized a lesion in each patient similar to the ^{18}F-FDG PET/CT results. In a later study, PSMA expression was found in five out of nine patients with TENIS [12]. A total of fourteen lesions were detected on the CT scan, and the ^{68}Ga-PSMA PET/CT detected nine of them (64.28%), with SUVmax ranging from 10.1 to 45.67 and median SUVmax of 16.31. On the other hand, ^{18}F-FDG PET/CT was positive in 11 out of 14 lesions (78.57%). The lesions that showed PSMA uptake were localized in bones (five out of nine) and lungs (four out of nine). Two lesions localized in the iliac crest and acetabulum were missed on the ^{18}F-FDG PET/CT but were seen on CT and the ^{68}Ga-PSMA PET/CT. In a case study with one patient, ^{68}Ga-PSMA-11 PET/CT was used to detect metastases in TENIS [13]. Intense radiotracer uptake was found in mediastinal and left supraclavicular lymph nodes, brain metastases, bilateral lung nodules, and skeletal sites. The patient also underwent ^{18}F-FDG PET/CT, which demonstrated similar findings; however, the number of lesions detected in the brain was fewer compared to ^{68}Ga-PSMA PET/CT. In the investigation of ^{68}Ga-PSMA-11 for detecting DTC metastases, Lawhn-Heath et al. (n = 7) found a detection rate of 93.8% for 18F-FDG PET/CT and 53.1% for ^{68}Ga-PSMA PET/CT [14]. The median lesion SUVmax was 9.0 for the ^{18}F-FDG PET/CT (range 3.5–28.4) and 9.2 for the ^{68}Ga-PSMA PET/CT (range 2.0–27.8). The ^{68}Ga-PSMA PET/CT had the highest detection rate for FTC, reaching 80.0%. In another study (n = 10), ^{68}Ga-PSMA-11 PET/CT successfully identified all 64 lesions, each of which was also confirmed by CT [15]. In contrast, ^{131}I SPECT/CT detected 55 out of the 64 lesions, with discrepant lesions localized in the lung (44.4%), brain (22.2%), postoperative thyroid bed (11.1%), lymph nodes (11.1%), and bone (11.1%). The degree of agreement among the observers was notably high for both radiotracers. For the ^{68}Ga-PSMA-11, the agreement had a κ of 0.98 (95% CI, 0.80–0.91), whereas for the ^{131}I, it was slightly lower (κ = 0.86; 95% CI, 0.71–0.76).

In their study on RAI-R DTC, de Vries et al. (n = 5) observed tracer uptake suggestive of distant metastases in all ^{68}Ga-PSMA-11 PET/CT scans [16]. Three patients underwent comparative imaging with ^{18}F-FDG PET/CT, revealing additional lesions on ^{68}Ga-PSMA PET/CT in two patients. Shi et al. prospectively enrolled 23 DTC and 17 RAI-R DTC patients [17]. The study found that the detection rates of DTC and RAI-R DTC were lower with ^{68}Ga-PSMA-11 PET/CT than with 18F-FDG PET/CT (60.00% vs. 90.00% for DTC and 59.38% vs. 96.88% for RAI-R DTC). Immunohistochemistry also revealed that RAI-R DTC had significantly higher PSMA expression levels than DTC, but this difference did not correlate significantly with the SUVmax on ^{68}Ga-PSMA-11 PET/CT.

In a separate study, Santhanam et al. (2020) investigated the localization of metastases with ^{18}F-DCFPyL PET/CT in three patients with metastatic RAI-R DTC [5]. The following are the results of two patient scans using 18F-DCFPyl: In the first patient, the scan picked up activity in the retropharyngeal CT contrast-enhancing lymph node. The ^{18}F-DCFPyl scan showed a greater SUV (3.1) compared to the ^{18}F-FDG PET/CT (1.8). In the second patient, the ^{18}F-DCFPyl scan showed intense uptake in the L3 vertebra, which was not visible on the post-treatment ^{131}I whole-body scan or the ^{18}F-FDG PET/CT. An MRI scan of the lumbar spine confirmed the presence of a sclerotic–lytic lesion in that location, indicating metastatic disease. Singh et al. also presented a case study, in which ^{18}F-DCFPyl PET/CT was able to detect PTC [18].

3. Fibroblast Activation Protein Inhibitor-Based Radiotracers for Differentiated Thyroid Cancer

Fibroblast activation protein inhibitor (FAPI) is a relatively new tracer. In the pioneering study of Kratochwil (2019), ^{68}Ga-FAPI-04 showed tracer uptake in 28 different kinds of cancer [19]. In recent years, ^{68}Ga-FAPI imaging has been explored for various purposes in different clinical settings with promising results [20].

Fibroblast activation protein (FAP) is a type II transmembrane serine protease and is highly expressed in more than 90% of epithelial tumors; it is closely associated with tumor invasion and metastasis [21]. Using FAP as a target, different FAP inhibitors (FAPIs) have been developed. FAP is highly expressed on the cancer-associated fibroblasts' membrane but not in normal tissue. It is thus associated with tumor invasion, metastasis, angiogenesis, and prognosis [22]. Its use has been investigated in the setting of detecting metastases for patients with RAI-R and patients with TENIS syndrome.

In the preclinical study conducted by Sun et al., it was observed that the presence of the BRAFV600E mutation correlated with heightened expression of cancer-associated fibroblast membrane proteins, including FAP [23]. Consequently, the use of FAPI may offer enhanced accuracy compared to ^{18}F-FDG PET/CT, especially in patients with more aggressive disease manifestations.

Clinical studies have assessed the diagnostic accuracy of different FAPi-based radiotracers for different thyroid cancer indications. These tracers include ^{68}-FAPI (not further specified), ^{68}Ga-DOTA.SA.FAPi, ^{18}F-FAPI-42, ^{18}F-FAPI-46, and ^{68}Ga-DOTA-FAPI-04 for indication of RAI-R metastatic lesions, TENIS syndrome, and DTC with elevated Tg or anti-Tg antibodies (Tables 1 and 2).

Two case studies report on ^{68}Ga-FAPI PET/CT for diagnosing metastases in patients with TENIS syndrome. One case study presents the first case of TENIS syndrome with FAPI-avid metastatic lesions. The ^{68}Ga-FAPI PET/CT localized abnormal foci at the laryngeal mass and bilateral pulmonary nodules [24]. The second case study compares ^{18}F-FDG PET/CT with FAPi: Compared with ^{18}F-FDG PET/CT, the ^{68}Ga-FAPI PET/CT showed more and higher metabolic lesions, including lesions in the liver, bones, and abdominal lymph nodes [25].

The study with the most patients included is a retrospective study (n = 117) focused on comparing ^{68}Ga-DOTA.SA.FAPi and ^{18}F-FDG PET/CT in patients' RAI-R DTC. The ^{68}Ga-DOTA.SA.FAPi exhibited a superior detection rate for lymph nodes, liver, bowel, and brain metastases compared to the ^{18}F-FDG PET/CT [26].

Mu et al. investigated ^{18}F-FAPI-42 in patients with biochemical elevations in Tg or anti-Tg antibodies (n = 42) [27]. FAPI-positive local recurrence showed the highest uptake intensity, followed by lymphatic, other site-associated (bone and pleura), and pulmonary lesions. All the positive lesions showed statistically higher uptake of ^{18}F-FDG PET/CT than that of ^{18}F-FAPI-42 (SUVmax, 2.6 versus 2.1; $p = 0.026$). However, the SUVmax of the ^{18}F-FAPI-42 was higher than that of the ^{18}F-FDG PET/CT in local recurrences and lymphatic lesions (SUVmax, 4.2 versus 2.9 and 3.9 versus 3.4, respectively; $p > 0.05$).

In a study by Nourbakhsh et al. (2024) involving 14 patients with TENIS syndrome, the performance of ^{18}F-FAPI-46 was compared to ^{18}F-FDG PET/CT imaging [28]. All the patients exhibited active lesions in both scans, with significantly lower SUVmax values in the liver and blood pool for the FAPI compared to the ^{18}F-FDG PET/CT ($p = 0.001$). Notably, the standard SUV of the hottest lesion to the liver exceeded three in all FAPI scans but only in half of the ^{18}F-FDG PET/CT scans, highlighting FAPI's consistent identification of high metabolic activity lesions. In one case, the FAPI detected pulmonary nodules (SUVmax = 3.8) missed by the ^{18}F-FDG PET/CT (SUVmax = 0.9), resulting in a 20% upstaging of patients.

In a study (n = 24) investigating ^{68}Ga-DOTA-FAPI-04 PET/CT, positive lesions were identified in 87.5% of patients, particularly in lung and lymph node metastases [29]. In a case report, ^{68}Ga-DOTA-2P(FAPI)2 was also able to detect PTC in a patient with diffuse lymph node metastases after total thyroidectomy and multiple cycles of RIT [30]. The tumor lesion became clearly visible with a good tumor-to-background ratio.

4. Arg-Gly-Asp-Based Radiotracers for Differentiated Thyroid Cancer

The tripeptide Arg-Gly-Asp (RGD) acid sequence has a high affinity and specificity for integrin $\alpha v\beta 3$, a receptor found in various malignant tumors. RGD-based tracers have been developed for diverse imaging modalities, such as positron emission tomography, single photon emission computed tomography (SPECT), molecular magnetic resonance imaging, optical fluorescence, optical bioluminescence, photoacoustic imaging, and targeted contrast-enhanced ultrasound. RGDs have undergone testing in multiple cancer types, including melanoma, brain tumors, sarcoma, squamous cell carcinoma of the head and neck, glioblastoma multiforme, breast cancer, and rectal cancer. The versatility of RGD-based tracers reflects their potential utility across a spectrum of imaging strategies and cancer types.

The Arg-Gly-Asp (RGD) sequence has been identified for its ability to attach to the $\alpha v\beta 3$ integrin found on the surface of angiogenic blood vessels or tumor cells. Integrin $\alpha v\beta 3$ is essential for cell migration and invasion and plays an important role in tumor angiogenesis. Integrin $\alpha v\beta 3$ expression is high on the surface of activated endothelial cells in newly formed blood vessels but is low in both resting endothelial cells and most normal organ systems, thus representing an interesting molecular marker for angiogenesis imaging. The RGD motif can be used to bind radiolabeled analogs. Thus, various radiolabeled derivatives of RGD peptides have been developed for angiogenesis imaging. Based on RNA-seq data from The Cancer Genome Atlas, the expression of αv and $\beta 3$ integrin subunits is particularly high in thyroid cancer. Integrin $\alpha v\beta 3$ overexpression in thyroid cancer is likely due to its presence on both the activated endothelial cells of the cancer neovasculature and the cancer cell surface, as shown by several reports documenting $\alpha v\beta 3$ integrin expression in thyroid cancer cell lines [31]. For DTC, RGD-based radiotracers have been investigated for the detection of DTC lymph node metastases, RAI-R patients, and patients with a negative post-therapy ^{131}I-scan.

The preclinical study of Cheng et al. (2016) investigated the antagonism of Arg-Gly-Asp (RGD)-binding integrin activity in three PTC cell lines (BCPAP, K1, and TPC1) [32]. The research revealed that all three cell lines exhibited moderate-to-high expression of RGD-binding integrin heterodimers $\alpha v\beta 3$ and $\alpha v\beta 5$. Antagonizing these integrins resulted in a significant inhibitory effect on cell viability, stronger apoptotic responses in TPC1 cells, and substantial inhibition of migration and invasion across all three PTC cell lines.

There are two clinical studies investigating the diagnostic accuracy of RGD-based radiotracers for the detection of DTC. These are ^{18}F-AIF-NOTA-PRGD2 and ^{68}Ga-DOTA-RGD2.

Cheng et al. (2014) (n = 20) compared ^{18}F-AIF-NOTA-PRGD2 with ^{18}F-FDG PET/CT for the detection of lymph node metastases of DTC, revealing that although ^{18}F-AIF-NOTA-PRGD2 exhibited abnormal uptake in most DTC lymph node metastases, its diagnostic value was inferior to ^{18}F-FDG PET/CT [33]. For all malignant lesions, the mean SUV for the ^{18}F-FDG PET/CT was significantly higher than that for the ^{18}F-AIF-NOTA-PRGD2 ($p < 0.05$). Another study aimed to compare the diagnostic accuracy of ^{68}Ga-DOTA-RGD2 PET/CT with ^{18}F-FDG PET/CT in RAI-R patients [34]. In a prospective enrollment of 44 RAI-R DTC patients, the ^{68}Ga-DOTA-RGD2 PET/CT demonstrated an overall sensitivity of 82.3%, specificity of 100%, and accuracy of 86.4%, while the ^{18}F-FDG PET/CT showed a sensitivity of 82.3%, specificity of 50%, and accuracy of 75%.

5. [^{18}F]Tetrafluoroborate

In 2017, a new PET tracer was tested in healthy human subjects for the imaging of DTC: ^{18}F-tetrafluoroborate (^{18}F-TFB). This study showed promising results of using ^{18}F-TFB PET/CT for noninvasive NIS imaging, as ^{18}F-TFB can mimic iodide transport. ^{18}F-TFB can go through the NIS receptor and gets trapped in thyroid cells.

^{18}F-TFB has diagnostic potential in detecting (recurrent) differentiated thyroid cancer and cervical lymph node metastases. One indication for an ^{18}F-TFB PET/CT scan is the detection of pre-operative cervical lymph node metastases to avoid a second surgery. Another indication is to predict whether radioiodine therapy will be successful in a patient. ^{18}F-TFB PET/CT has three advantages over ^{123}I- or ^{131}I-scintigraphy. First of all, ^{18}F-TFB is a positron emitter detected by PET, which is more sensitive than a gamma camera. Second, the scan takes place on the same day as the administration of the tracer, so patients do not have to attend an extra day (as is the case in iodine-123(131) scintigraphy). Third, it has a lower radiation dose.

Pre-clinical studies have been performed in xenograft mice and cell lines. These studies concluded that ^{18}F-TFB has specific uptake by the sodium/iodide symporter. Jarugeui-Osoro et al. showed a rapid accumulation of ^{18}F-TFB in FRTL-5 rat thyroid cells and in vivo in the thyroid and stomach [35]. This was confirmed by Weeks et al. and Khoshnevisan et al. in NIS-expressing human colon cell [36,37]. Diocou et al. found that ^{18}F-TFB was superior to I-123 due to better pharmacokinetics (faster tumor uptake and faster and more complete clearance from circulation) [38]. Niu et al. illustrated the possibilities of ^{18}F-TFB in NIS-expressing cell lines for the diagnosis of stomach cancer [39]. Goetz et al. provided further information on the time–activity curves and fitted kinetics for ^{18}F-TFB in mice [40]. Jiang et al. assessed the influence of specific activity on tumor uptake in NIS-expressing C6-glioma xenograft tumors [41]. Marti-Clement et al. conducted whole-body PET imaging in two non-human primates. It concluded that it is a very useful radiotracer in primates, with a characteristic biodistribution in organs expressing NIS [42].

In four clinical phase I studies with a total of 47 patients, ^{18}F-TFB PET/CT proved to be safe and effective in humans [43,44]. In these clinical trials, the safety, pharmacokinetics, metabolism, biodistribution, and dosimetry were assessed [44]. ^{18}F-TFB has a short half-life of 110 min, low-energy (Emax = 0.634 MeV), and high-yield (97%) positron emission [43]. In human subjects, it showed rapid renal clearance and no uptake in bone and joints, meaning that ^{18}F-fluoride was not released in vivo after IV administration [43]. Next to this, ^{18}F-TFB imaging was compared to ^{124}I PET/CT, ^{18}F-FDG PET/CT, and ^{131}I scintigraphy [43,45]. The ^{18}F-TFB PET/CT showed higher sensitivity and accuracy than ^{131}I in whole-body scintigraphy and SPECT-CT. The ^{18}F-TFB PET/CT was not inferior to the ^{124}I PET/CT in detecting thyroid cancer and was able to detect metastases that were not found on the ^{124}I PET/CT [43].

6. Discussion

Studies have suggested that PSMA PET/CT is better than ^{18}F-FDG PET/CT in detecting lesions in bones and lungs. These radiotracers have also been linked to radioiodine-refractory thyroid cancer. Additionally, PSMA expression levels have been explored as potential biomarkers for predicting distant metastases and radioiodine therapy (RIT) outcomes, and their inclusion in multivariate models for predicting RAI-R highlights their significance in risk stratification. FAPI-based radiotracers have also shown potential in predicting and assessing RAI-R, with higher detection rates in specific metastatic sites like lymph nodes and the liver compared to ^{18}F-FDG PET/CT. This demonstrates their value as a complementary tool in evaluating refractory disease. Furthermore, RGD-based radiotracers have shown diagnostic accuracy in patients with RAI-R-differentiated thyroid cancer (DTC), with their sensitivity and specificity indicating their potential role in predicting and confirming RAI-R, particularly when compared to ^{18}F-FDG PET/CT. ^{18}F-TFB is proving to be a promising PET tracer for noninvasive NIS imaging in DTC. Its ability to mimic iodide transport and provide diagnostic potential for detecting cervical lymph node metastases offers advantages over traditional scintigraphy methods. The development of targeted radionuclide therapies based on these tracers shows promise in advancing the management of refractory disease. Future research should focus on larger clinical trials, the standardization of imaging protocols, and head-to-head comparisons to establish the most effective and reliable tracers for specific clinical scenarios.

Several limitations should be acknowledged in this study. Firstly, the scope of the available literature concerning the tracers and indications under review is constrained by a limited number of studies and the limited number of inclusion of patients within these studies. Secondly, despite efforts to comprehensively review the English literature, it is possible that some relevant studies may have been missed. Moreover, the heterogeneity observed within the included studies poses a significant challenge. The variability in patient populations, study designs, imaging protocols, and outcome measures across different studies hinders the possibility of performing a meta-analysis and thus limits the establishment of definitive conclusions.

In conclusion, the use of various radiotracers in differentiated thyroid cancer is a rapidly evolving field with promising potential for improving diagnostic accuracy, patient stratification, and treatment selection. The current evidence underscores the preferential utility of select tracers. Notably, ^{18}F-TFB demonstrates promise in enhancing imaging resolution for DTC staging. Conversely, in the context of advanced potentially dedifferentiated DTC, tracers targeting FAP display encouraging preliminary efficacy. PSMA and RGD, in contrast, show a comparatively disappointing outcome. Hence, for future research, the authors recommend investigating FAP-targeting tracers in the advanced setting and ^{18}F-TFB for staging DTC, rather than further investigating PSMA and RGD.

Table 1. Imaging Studies.

Tracer Group	Tracer	Study	Indication	Number of Patients
PSMA	^{68}Ga-PSMA-11	Verburg et al. (2015) [9]	RAI-R	1
		Taywade et al. (2016) [13]	TENIS	1
		Lutje et al. (2017) [11]	Iodine-negative and FDG-positive metastasized DTC	6
		Verma et al. (2018) [12]	DTC metastases + find patients suitable for PSMA-targeted radionuclide therapy	10
		Lawhn-Heath et al. (2020) [46]	Metastatic DTC	7
		De Vries et al. (2020) [16]	RAI-R	5
		Verma et al. (2021) [12]	TENIS, find metastatic lesions	9
		Pitalua-Cortes et al. (2021) [15]	Metastatic DTC	10
		Shi et al. (2023) [17]	RAI-R	40
	^{18}F-DCFPyL	Singh et al. (2018) [18]	NS	1
		Santhanam et al. (2020) [5]	Elevated Tg	2
FAPI	^{68}Ga-FAPI	Fu et al. (2021) [24]	RAI-R metastatic lesions	1
		Fu et al. (2021) [24]	TENIS syndrome	1
		Wu et al. (2021) [25]	TENIS syndrome	1
	^{68}Ga-DOTA.SA.FAPi	Ballal et al. (2022) [26]	RAI-R metastatic lesions	117
	^{18}F-FAPI-42,	Mu et al. (2023) [27]	DTC with elevated Tg or anti-Tg antibodies	27
	^{18}F-FAPI-46	Nourbakhsh et al. (2024) [28]	TENIS syndrome	14
	^{68}Ga-DOTA-FAPI-04	Chen et al. (2022) [29]	RAI-R metastatic lesions	24
		Tatar et al. (2023) [30]	DTC metastases	1
	^{68}Ga-DOTA-2P(FAPI)2	Zhao et al. (2022) [47]	PTC with LNM	1
RGD	^{18}F-AlF-NOTA-PRGD2	Cheng et al. (2014) [33]	Lymph node metastases of DTC	20
	^{68}Ga-DOTA-RGD2	Parihar et al. (2020) [34]	RAI-R, patients with negative post-therapy 131I-scan.	44
TFB	^{18}F-TFB	O'Doherty et al. (2017) [48]	DTC	5
		Samnick et al. (2018) [43]	DTC + LNM	9
		Dittmann et al. (2020) [45]	Local recurrence + metastases	25

Table 2. Detection Rate of Different Tracers for Thyroid Cancer Indications.

Indication Thyroid Cancer	Tracer	Results	Conclusions
Recurrent DTC	^{18}F-TFB	52% detection rate (^{131}I WBS detection rate = 12%) [45]	^{18}F-TFB PET detected local recurrence or metastases of DTC in significantly more patients than conventional 131I-dxWBS and SPECT-CT.
Detection of DTC metastases	^{68}Ga-PSMA-11	53.1% detection rate (FDG = 93.8% detection rate) [46]; 100% detection rate (Pitalua-Cortes, Garcia-Perez et al., 2021); 100% detection rate [10]; 60% detection rate (FDG = 90% detection rate) [17]	^{68}Ga-PSMA-11 PET/CT can detect thyroid cancer metastases, but its detection rate is lower than that of 18F-FDG PET/CT.
	^{68}Ga-DOTA.SA.FAPi	95.4% detection rate lymph nodes (FDG = 86.6%) [49]	^{68}Ga-DOTA.SA.FAPi can detect lymph nodal, liver, bowel, and brain metastases better than ^{18}F-FDG in patients with RAI-R DTC.
	^{68}Ga-DOTA-FAPI-04	87.5% detection rate [29]	^{68}Ga-DOTA-FAPI-04 PET/CT has a promising detection rate for RAI-R DTC metastasis.
	^{68}Ga-DOTA-RGD2	86.4% diagnostic accuracy (FDG = 75% diagnostic accuracy) [34]	^{68}Ga-DOTA-RGD2 PET/CT showed similar sensitivity to, but higher specificity and overall accuracy than ^{18}F-FDG PET/CT in detection of lesions in RAI-R DTC.
TENIS	^{68}Ga-FAPI	100% detection rate [50]	First case of TENIS with FAPI-avid metastatic lesions.
	^{68}Ga-PSMA-11	100% detection rate [13]; 64.28% detection rate (FDG = 78.57% detection rate) [12]	^{68}Ga-PSMA-11 PET/CT demonstrates PSMA expression in TENIS patients with lesions being localized to the bones, lungs, mediastinal, and left supraclavicular lymph nodes, brain, and bilateral lung nodules.
Lymph node metastases of DTC	^{18}F-AIF-NOTA-PRGD2	FDG > RGD [33]	No correlation was found between the uptake of ^{18}F-AIF-NOTA-PRGD2 and 18F-FDG, which may suggest the two tracers provide complementary information in DTC lesions.
	^{18}F-DCFPyL	100% detection rate [5]	^{18}F-DCFPyl may prove useful for the localization of metastases in patients with metastatic RAI-refractory DTC.
	^{18}F-TFB	100% detection rate [43]	^{18}F-TFB PET was not inferior to ^{124}I-PET in detecting thyroid cancer and its metastases and was able to detect ^{124}I-PET-negative viable differentiated thyroid cancer metastases.

Author Contributions: H.I.C. reviewed the literature, drafted the manuscript, and gave final approval. B.d.K. conceptualized the review, reviewed the literature, performed a critical review of the manuscript, and gave final approval. F.A.V. conceptualized the review, did a review of the literature, conducted a critical review of the manuscript, and gave final approval. All authors have read and agreed to the published version of the manuscript.

Funding: This work was supported by the Dutch Cancer Society (Koningin Wilhelmina Fonds/Alpe d'Huzes; grant no. 14129).

Conflicts of Interest: The authors declare no conflict of interest.

References

1. Haugen, B.R.; Alexander, E.K.; Bible, K.C.; Doherty, G.M.; Mandel, S.J.; Nikiforov, Y.E.; Pacini, F.; Randolph, G.W.; Sawka, A.M.; Schlumberger, M. 2015 American Thyroid Association management guidelines for adult patients with thyroid nodules and differentiated thyroid cancer: The American Thyroid Association guidelines task force on thyroid nodules and differentiated thyroid cancer. *Thyroid* **2016**, *26*, 1–133. [CrossRef]
2. Avram, A.M.; Giovanella, L.; Greenspan, B.; Lawson, S.A.; Luster, M.; Van Nostrand, D.; Peacock, J.G.; Ovčariček, P.P.; Silberstein, E.; Tulchinsky, M. SNMMI Procedure Standard/EANM Practice Guideline for Nuclear Medicine Evaluation and Therapy of Differentiated Thyroid Cancer: Abbreviated Version. *Soc. Nucl. Med.* **2022**, *63*, 15N–35N.

3. Heitkötter, B.; Steinestel, K.; Trautmann, M.; Grünewald, I.; Barth, P.; Gevensleben, H.; Bögemann, M.; Wardelmann, E.; Hartmann, W.; Rahbar, K. Neovascular PSMA expression is a common feature in malignant neoplasms of the thyroid. *Oncotarget* **2018**, *9*, 9867. [CrossRef]
4. Bychkov, A.; Vutrapongwatana, U.; Tepmongkol, S.; Keelawat, S. PSMA expression by microvasculature of thyroid tumors—Potential implications for PSMA theranostics. *Sci. Rep.* **2017**, *7*, 5202. [CrossRef]
5. Santhanam, P.; Russell, J.; Rooper, L.M.; Ladenson, P.W.; Pomper, M.G.; Rowe, S.P. The prostate-specific membrane antigen (PSMA)-targeted radiotracer 18F-DCFPyL detects tumor neovasculature in metastatic, advanced, radioiodine-refractory, differentiated thyroid cancer. *Med. Oncol.* **2020**, *37*, 98. [CrossRef] [PubMed]
6. Sollini, M.; di Tommaso, L.; Kirienko, M.; Piombo, C.; Erreni, M.; Lania, A.G.; Erba, P.A.; Antunovic, L.; Chiti, A. PSMA expression level predicts differentiated thyroid cancer aggressiveness and patient outcome. *EJNMMI Res.* **2019**, *9*, 93. [CrossRef] [PubMed]
7. Ciappuccini, R.; Saguet-Rysanek, V.; Giffard, F.; Licaj, I.; Dorbeau, M.; Clarisse, B.; Poulain, L.; Bardet, S. PSMA expression in differentiated thyroid cancer: Association with radioiodine, 18FDG uptake, and patient outcome. *J. Clin. Endocrinol. Metab.* **2021**, *106*, 3536–3545. [CrossRef]
8. Feng, Y.Y.; Shi, Y.R.; Xia, Z.; Xu, L.; Li, W.B.; Pang, H.; Wang, Z.J. The clinical signification and application value of [68Ga] Ga-PSMA imaging in thyroid malignancy. *Endocrine*, 2023; *Online ahead of print.* [CrossRef]
9. Verburg, F.A.; Krohn, T.; Heinzel, A.; Mottaghy, F.M.; Behrendt, F.F. First evidence of PSMA expression in differentiated thyroid cancer using [68 Ga] PSMA-HBED-CC PET/CT. *Eur. J. Nucl. Med. Mol. Imaging* **2015**, *42*, 1622–1623. [CrossRef] [PubMed]
10. Verma, P.; Malhotra, G.; Agrawal, R.; Sonavane, S.; Meshram, V.; Asopa, R.V. Evidence of Prostate-Specific Membrane Antigen Expression in Metastatic Differentiated Thyroid Cancer Using 68Ga-PSMA-HBED-CC PET/CT. *Clin. Nucl. Med.* **2018**, *43*, e265–e268. [CrossRef] [PubMed]
11. Lutje, S.; Gomez, B.; Cohnen, J.; Umutlu, L.; Gotthardt, M.; Poeppel, T.D.; Bockisch, A.; Rosenbaum-Krumme, S. Imaging of Prostate-Specific Membrane Antigen Expression in Metastatic Differentiated Thyroid Cancer Using 68Ga-HBED-CC-PSMA PET/CT. *Clin. Nucl. Med.* **2017**, *42*, 20–25. [CrossRef]
12. Verma, P.; Malhotra, G.; Meshram, V.; Chandak, A.; Sonavane, S.; Lila, A.R.; Bandgar, T.R.; Asopa, R.V. Prostate-specific membrane antigen expression in patients with differentiated thyroid cancer with thyroglobulin elevation and negative iodine scintigraphy using 68Ga-PSMA-HBED-CC PET/CT. *Clin. Nucl. Med.* **2021**, *46*, e406–e409. [CrossRef] [PubMed]
13. Taywade, S.K.; Damle, N.A.; Bal, C. PSMA Expression in Papillary Thyroid Carcinoma: Opening a New Horizon in Management of Thyroid Cancer? *Clin. Nucl. Med.* **2016**, *41*, e263–e265. [CrossRef] [PubMed]
14. Lawhn-Heath, C.; Yom, S.S.; Liu, C.; Villanueva-Meyer, J.E.; Aslam, M.; Smith, R.; Narwal, M.; Juarez, R.; Behr, S.C.; Pampaloni, M.H.; et al. Gallium-68 prostate-specific membrane antigen ([68Ga]Ga-PSMA-11) PET for imaging of thyroid cancer: A feasibility study. *EJNMMI Res.* **2020**, *10*, 128. [CrossRef] [PubMed]
15. Pitalua-Cortes, Q.; Garcia-Perez, F.O.; Vargas-Ahumada, J.; Gonzalez-Rueda, S.; Gomez-Argumosa, E.; Ignacio-Alvarez, E.; Soldevilla-Gallardo, I.; Torres-Agredo, L. Head-to-Head Comparison of 68Ga-PSMA-11 and 131I in the Follow-Up of Well-Differentiated Metastatic Thyroid Cancer: A New Potential Theragnostic Agent. *Front. Endocrinol.* **2021**, *12*, 794759. [CrossRef] [PubMed]
16. De Vries, L.H.; Lodewijk, L.; Braat, A.; Krijger, G.C.; Valk, G.D.; Lam, M.; Borel Rinkes, I.H.M.; Vriens, M.R.; de Keizer, B. 68Ga-PSMA PET/CT in radioactive iodine-refractory differentiated thyroid cancer and first treatment results with 177Lu-PSMA-617. *EJNMMI Res.* **2020**, *10*, 18. [CrossRef] [PubMed]
17. Shi, Y.; Feng, Y.; Xu, L.; Li, W.; Guan, L.; Zuo, R.; Liu, S.; Pang, H.; Wang, Z. The value of Gallium-68 prostate-specific membrane antigen ([68Ga] Ga-PSMA-11) PET/CT and 2-[18F] fluoro-2-deoxy-D-glucose (2-[18F] FDG) PET/CT in the detection of thyroid cancer lesions: A prospective head-to-head comparison. *Br. J. Radiol.* **2023**, 20230291. [CrossRef] [PubMed]
18. Singh, D.; Horneman, R.; Bsci, N.K.N. More than the prostate: Intrapancreatic accessory spleen 18 and papillary thyroid cancer detected with F-PSMA PET/CT. *Hell. J. Nucl. Med.* **2018**, *21*, 145–147. [PubMed]
19. Kratochwil, C.; Flechsig, P.; Lindner, T.; Abderrahim, L.; Altmann, A.; Mier, W.; Adeberg, S.; Rathke, H.; Röhrich, M.; Winter, H. 68Ga-FAPI PET/CT: Tracer uptake in 28 different kinds of cancer. *J. Nucl. Med.* **2019**, *60*, 801–805. [CrossRef] [PubMed]
20. Sollini, M.; Kirienko, M.; Gelardi, F.; Fiz, F.; Gozzi, N.; Chiti, A. State-of-the-art of FAPI-PET imaging: A systematic review and meta-analysis. *Eur. J. Nucl. Med. Mol. Imaging* **2021**, *48*, 4396–4414. [CrossRef] [PubMed]
21. Huang, R.; Pu, Y.; Huang, S.; Yang, C.; Yang, F.; Pu, Y.; Li, J.; Chen, L.; Huang, Y. FAPI-PET/CT in Cancer Imaging: A Potential Novel Molecule of the Century. *Front. Oncol.* **2022**, *12*, 854658. [CrossRef] [PubMed]
22. Piscopo, L.; Volpe, F. PET/CT imaging with radiolabeled FAPI: New opportunities for diagnosis and treatment of thyroid cancer. *Eur. J. Nucl. Med. Mol. Imaging* **2024**, *51*, 800–802. [CrossRef] [PubMed]
23. Sun, W.-Y.; Jung, W.-H.; Koo, J.S. Expression of cancer-associated fibroblast-related proteins in thyroid papillary carcinoma. *Tumor Biol.* **2016**, *37*, 8197–8207. [CrossRef] [PubMed]
24. Fu, H.; Fu, J.; Huang, J.; Pang, Y.; Chen, H. 68Ga-FAPI PET/CT versus 18F-FDG PET/CT for detecting metastatic lesions in a case of radioiodine-refractory differentiated thyroid cancer. *Clin. Nucl. Med.* **2021**, *46*, 940–942. [CrossRef] [PubMed]
25. Wu, J.; Wang, Y.; Liao, T.; Rao, Z.; Gong, W.; Ou, L.; Chen, Y.; Zhang, C. Comparison of the Relative Diagnostic Performance of [68Ga]Ga-DOTA-FAPI-04 and [18F]FDG PET/CT for the Detection of Bone Metastasis in Patients With Different Cancers. *Front. Oncol.* **2021**, *11*, 737827. [CrossRef] [PubMed]

26. Ballal, S.; Yadav, M.; Roesch, F.; Bal, C.; Moon, E. Comparison of diagnostic performance between [68ga]ga-dota.sa.fapi and [18f]f-fdg pet/ct in the diagnosis of various radioiodine resistant thyroid cancers of follicular cell origin. *Thyroid* **2022**, *32*, A88–A89. [CrossRef]
27. Mu, X.; Huang, X.; Jiang, Z.; Li, M.; Jia, L.; Lv, Z.; Fu, W.; Mao, J. [18F] FAPI-42 PET/CT in differentiated thyroid cancer: Diagnostic performance, uptake values, and comparison with 2-[18F] FDG PET/CT. *Eur. J. Nucl. Med. Mol. Imaging* **2023**, *50*, 1205–1215. [CrossRef] [PubMed]
28. Nourbakhsh, S.; Salehi, Y.; Farzanehfar, S.; Ghaletaki, R.; Kashi, M.B.; Abbasi, M. FAPI PET/CT provides higher uptake and better target to back ground in recurrent and metastatic tumors of patients with Iodine refractory papillary thyroid cancer compared with FDG PET CT. *Nukl. Nucl.* **2024**. [CrossRef] [PubMed]
29. Chen, Y.; Zheng, S.; Zhang, J.; Yao, S.; Miao, W. 68Ga-DOTA-FAPI-04 PET/CT imaging in radioiodine-refractory differentiated thyroid cancer (RR-DTC) patients. *Ann. Nucl. Med.* **2022**, *36*, 610–622. [CrossRef] [PubMed]
30. Tatar, G.; Alçın, G.; Fenercioğlu, Ö.E.; Şahin, R.; Çermik, T.F. Findings of I-131 SPECT/CT, 18F-FDG, and 68Ga-FAPI-04 PET/CT Imaging in a Patient Treated with Radioiodine Therapy for Metastatic Papillary Thyroid Carcinoma. *Mol. Imaging Radionucl. Ther.* **2023**, *32*, 57. [CrossRef] [PubMed]
31. Klubo-Gwiezdzinska, J.; Chen, X. Targeting Integrins with Radiolabeled RGD Analogues for Radiotheranostics of Metastatic Radioactive Iodine Nonresponsive Thyroid Cancer: New Avenues in Personalized Medicine. *Thyroid* **2020**, *30*, 476–478. [CrossRef] [PubMed]
32. Cheng, W.; Feng, F.; Ma, C.; Wang, H. The effect of antagonizing RGD-binding integrin activity in papillary thyroid cancer cell lines. *OncoTargets Ther.* **2016**, *9*, 1415–1423. [CrossRef]
33. Cheng, W.; Wu, Z.; Liang, S.; Fu, H.; Wu, S.; Tang, Y.; Ye, Z.; Wang, H. Comparison of 18F-AIF-NOTA-PRGD2 and 18F-FDG uptake in lymph node metastasis of differentiated thyroid cancer. *PLoS ONE* **2014**, *9*, e100521. [CrossRef] [PubMed]
34. Parihar, A.S.; Mittal, B.R.; Kumar, R.; Shukla, J.; Bhattacharya, A. 68Ga-DOTA-RGD2 Positron Emission Tomography/Computed Tomography in Radioiodine Refractory Thyroid Cancer: Prospective Comparison of Diagnostic Accuracy with 18F-FDG Positron Emission Tomography/Computed Tomography and Evaluation Toward Potential Theranostics. *Thyroid* **2020**, *30*, 557–567. [CrossRef] [PubMed]
35. Jauregui-Osoro, M.; Sunassee, K.; Weeks, A.J.; Berry, D.J.; Paul, R.L.; Cleij, M.; Banga, J.P.; O'Doherty, M.J.; Marsden, P.K.; Clarke, S.E.; et al. Synthesis and biological evaluation of [(18)F]tetrafluoroborate: A PET imaging agent for thyroid disease and reporter gene imaging of the sodium/iodide symporter. *Eur. J. Nucl. Med. Mol. Imaging* **2010**, *37*, 2108–2116. [CrossRef] [PubMed]
36. Khoshnevisan, A.; Jauregui-Osoro, M.; Shaw, K.; Torres, J.B.; Young, J.D.; Ramakrishnan, N.K.; Jackson, A.; Smith, G.E.; Gee, A.D.; Blower, P.J. [18 F] tetrafluoroborate as a PET tracer for the sodium/iodide symporter: The importance of specific activity. *EJNMMI Res.* **2016**, *6*, 34. [CrossRef]
37. Weeks, A.J.; Jauregui-Osoro, M.; Cleij, M.; Blower, J.E.; Ballinger, J.R.; Blower, P.J. Evaluation of [18F]-tetrafluoroborate as a potential PET imaging agent for the human sodium/iodide symporter in a new colon carcinoma cell line HCT116 expressing hNIS. *Nucl. Med. Commun.* **2011**, *32*, 98. [CrossRef]
38. Diocou, S.; Volpe, A.; Jauregui-Osoro, M.; Boudjemeline, M.; Chuamsaamarkkee, K.; Man, F.; Blower, P.J.; Ng, T.; Mullen, G.E.D.; Fruhwirth, G.O. [18F] tetrafluoroborate-PET/CT enables sensitive tumor and metastasis in vivo imaging in a sodium iodide symporter-expressing tumor model. *Sci. Rep.* **2017**, *7*, 946. [CrossRef] [PubMed]
39. Niu, M.; Qin, J., Wang, L.; He, Y.; Tian, C.; Chen, Y.; Huang, P.; Peng, Z. Evaluation of [18F] tetrafluoroborate as a Potential PET Imaging Agent in a Sodium Iodide Symporter-Transfected Cell Line A549 and Endogenous NIS-Expressing Cell Lines MKN45 and K1. *Mol. Imaging* **2022**, *2022*, 2676260. [CrossRef] [PubMed]
40. Goetz, C.; Podein, M.; Braun, F.; Weber, W.A.; Choquet, P.; Constantinesco, A.; Mix, M. Influence of Animal Heating on PET Imaging Quantification and Kinetics: Biodistribution of (18)F-Tetrafluoroborate and (18)F-FDG in Mice. *J. Nucl. Med.* **2017**, *58*, 1162–1166. [CrossRef]
41. Jiang, H.; Bansal, A.; Pandey, M.K.; Peng, K.W.; Suksanpaisan, L.; Russell, S.J.; DeGrado, T.R. Synthesis of 18F-Tetrafluoroborate via Radiofluorination of Boron Trifluoride and Evaluation in a Murine C6-Glioma Tumor Model. *J. Nucl. Med.* **2016**, *57*, 1454–1459. [CrossRef] [PubMed]
42. Marti-Climent, J.M.; Collantes, M.; Jauregui-Osoro, M.; Quincoces, G.; Prieto, E.; Bilbao, I.; Ecay, M.; Richter, J.A.; Peñuelas, I. Radiation dosimetry and biodistribution in non-human primates of the sodium/iodide PET ligand [18F]-tetrafluoroborate. *EJNMMI Res.* **2015**, *5*, 70. [CrossRef] [PubMed]
43. Samnick, S.; Al-Momani, E.; Schmid, J.S.; Mottok, A.; Buck, A.K.; Lapa, C. Initial Clinical Investigation of [18F]Tetrafluoroborate PET/CT in Comparison to [124I]Iodine PET/CT for Imaging Thyroid Cancer. *Clin. Nucl. Med.* **2018**, *43*, 162–167. [CrossRef] [PubMed]
44. Jiang, H.; Schmit, N.R.; Koenen, A.R.; Bansal, A.; Pandey, M.K.; Glynn, R.B.; Kemp, B.J.; Delaney, K.L.; Dispenzieri, A.; Bakkum-Gamez, J.N.; et al. Safety, pharmacokinetics, metabolism and radiation dosimetry of (18)F-tetrafluoroborate ((18)F-TFB) in healthy human subjects. *EJNMMI Res.* **2017**, *7*, 90. [CrossRef] [PubMed]
45. Dittmann, M.; Gonzalez Carvalho, J.M.; Rahbar, K.; Schafers, M.; Claesener, M.; Riemann, B.; Seifert, R. Incremental diagnostic value of [(18)F]tetrafluoroborate PET-CT compared to [(131)I]iodine scintigraphy in recurrent differentiated thyroid cancer. *Eur J. Nucl. Med. Mol. Imaging* **2020**, *47*, 2639–2646. [CrossRef] [PubMed]

46. Lawhn-Heath, C.; Flavell, R.; Chuang, E.; Liu, C. Failure of iodine uptake in microscopic pulmonary metastases after recombinant human thyroid-stimulating hormone stimulation. *World J. Nucl. Med.* **2020**, *19*, 61–64. [CrossRef] [PubMed]
47. Zhao, L.; Niu, B.; Fang, J.; Pang, Y.; Li, S.; Xie, C.; Sun, L.; Zhang, X.; Guo, Z.; Lin, Q.; et al. Synthesis, preclinical evaluation, and a pilot clinical PET imaging study of68Ga-labeled FAPI dimer. *J. Nucl. Med.* **2022**, *63*, 263016. [CrossRef] [PubMed]
48. Ballal, S.; Yadav, M.P.; Bal, C.; Roesch, F.; Rajput, S.; Moon, E.S.; Wakade, N.; Tripathi, M.; Agarwal, S.; Sahoo, R.K. [177Lu]Lu-DOTAGA.(SA.FAPi)2 therapy in advanced stage radioiodine-resistant thyroid cancers of follicular and parafollicular cell origins. *Eur. J. Nucl. Med. Mol. Imaging* **2022**, *49*, S233–S234. [CrossRef]
49. Ballal, S.; Yadav, M.P.; Roesch, F.; Satapathy, S.; Moon, E.S.; Martin, M.; Wakade, N.; Sheokand, P.; Tripathi, M.; Chandekar, K.R.; et al. Head-to-head comparison of [(68)Ga]Ga-DOTA.SA.FAPi with [(18)F]F-FDG PET/CT in radioiodine-resistant follicular-cell derived thyroid cancers. *Eur. J. Nucl. Med. Mol. Imaging* **2023**, *51*, 233–244. [CrossRef] [PubMed]
50. Fu, H.; Fu, J.; Huang, J.; Su, X.; Chen, H. 68Ga-FAPI PET/CT in thyroid cancer with thyroglobulin elevation and negative iodine scintigraphy. *Clin. Nucl. Med.* **2021**, *46*, 427–430. [CrossRef] [PubMed]

cancers

MDPI

Review

Integrated Diagnostics of Thyroid Nodules

Luca Giovanella [1,2,*], Alfredo Campennì [3], Murat Tuncel [4] and Petra Petranović Ovčariček [5,6]

[1] Department of Nuclear Medicine, Gruppo Ospedaliero Moncucco SA, Clinica Moncucco, 6900 Lugano, Switzerland
[2] Clinic for Nuclear Medicine, University Hospital Zürich, 8004 Zürich, Switzerland
[3] Nuclear Medicine Unit, Department of Biomedical and Dental Sciences and Morpho-Functional Imaging, University of Messina, 98100 Messina, Italy; alfredo.campenni@unime.it
[4] Department of Nuclear Medicine, Hacettepe University, 06230 Ankara, Turkey; murat.tuncel@hacettepe.edu.tr
[5] Department of Oncology and Nuclear Medicine, University Hospital Center Sestre Milosrdnice, 10 000 Zagreb, Croatia; p.petranovic@gmail.com
[6] School of Medicine, University of Zagreb, 10 000 Zagreb, Croatia
* Correspondence: luca.giovanella.md@gmail.com

Simple Summary: Thyroid nodules are commonly detected in daily clinical practice, and their diagnosis and therapy usually involve different specialists and various diagnostic and therapeutic methods. Thyroid nodule management requires the integration of laboratory, imaging, and pathology examinations to achieve a proper diagnosis. It enables the elimination of unnecessary therapeutic procedures in many individuals and the timely identification of patients who require specific therapies. Furthermore, bioinformatics may change the current management of clinical data, enabling more personalized diagnostic approaches for patients with thyroid nodules. The clinical impact of artificial intelligence needs to be determined in further large-sample studies, especially in indeterminate cytology findings, that require "diagnostic surgery" to provide a definitive diagnosis.

Abstract: Thyroid nodules are common findings, particularly in iodine-deficient regions. Our paper aims to revise different diagnostic tools available in clinical thyroidology and propose their rational integration. We will elaborate on the pros and cons of thyroid ultrasound (US) and its scoring systems, thyroid scintigraphy, fine-needle aspiration cytology (FNAC), molecular imaging, and artificial intelligence (AI). Ultrasonographic scoring systems can help differentiate between benign and malignant nodules. Depending on the constellation or number of suspicious ultrasound features, a FNAC is recommended. However, hyperfunctioning thyroid nodules are presumed to exclude malignancy with a very high negative predictive value (NPV). Particularly in regions where iodine supply is low, most hyperfunctioning thyroid nodules are seen in patients with normal thyroid-stimulating hormone (TSH) levels. Thyroid scintigraphy is essential for the detection of these nodules. Among non-toxic thyroid nodules, a careful application of US risk stratification systems is pivotal to exclude inappropriate FNAC and guide the procedure on suspicious ones. However, almost one-third of cytology examinations are rendered as indeterminate, requiring "diagnostic surgery" to provide a definitive diagnosis. ^{99m}Tc-methoxy-isobutyl-isonitrile ([^{99m}Tc]Tc-MIBI) and [^{18}F]fluoro-deoxy-glucose ([^{18}F]FDG) molecular imaging can spare those patients from unnecessary surgeries. The clinical value of AI in the evaluation of thyroid nodules needs to be determined.

Keywords: thyroid; ultrasonography; thyroid stimulating hormone; nuclear medicine; cytopathology

1. Introduction

Thyroid nodules are more common in countries with iodine-deficient populations, and in women compared to men (ratio 4:1), and their prevalence increases with age and body mass index [1–5].

Luckily, most thyroid nodules (90% to 95%) are benign [6]. Risk factors for thyroid cancer include ionizing radiation (e.g., from cancer treatments, occupational exposure, or nuclear fallout, especially when the exposure occurs at a young age), rapid growth, hoarseness, and a family history of thyroid cancer or cancer syndromes (e.g., multiple endocrine neoplasia type 2, familial adenomatous polyposis) [7]. Notably, while thyroid nodules can be detected in up to 10% of healthy subjects by palpation, neck ultrasonography (US) may detect nodules in up to 68% of them, respectively [8–10]. Additionally, most thyroid nodules are currently detected incidentally (i.e., thyroid incidentalomas) when imaging procedures (i.e., computed tomography (CT), magnetic resonance imaging (MRI), and vascular Doppler) are performed for different indications [11]. Considering the high prevalence of thyroid nodules compared to the very low prevalence of thyroid malignancies, screening of thyroid cancer with neck US is discouraged as it results in overdiagnosis and overtreatment without improving patient outcomes [12]. Consequently, attending physicians are required to decide which nodules carry a significant risk of malignancy and require further diagnostic workup. Thyroid US scoring systems need to be integrated into daily clinical practice, complemented with the use of thyroid scintigraphy when indicated to avoid FNAC of low-risk and autonomously functioning nodules [13]. Furthermore, molecular imaging with [^{99m}Tc]Tc-MIBI and [^{18}F]FDG is not widely used nowadays, although its usefulness is clearly demonstrated in many studies [14–17]. It is highly recommended in indeterminate cytology findings to spare patients from "diagnostic" surgeries, improve their quality of life, and reduce total hospital costs caused by unnecessary procedures and their potential complications [14–16].

Our present narrative review aims to analyze the available literature concerning the diagnostic approach to thyroid nodules and provide an updated synopsis on the role of different procedures, including advanced molecular imaging. For this document, the authors volunteered to prepare the text for each section. A review of the literature was performed in PubMed, Web of Science, and Scopus without time or language restrictions through the use of one or more fitting search criteria and terms as well as through screening of references in relevant selected papers. The body of literature up to and including November 2023 was considered. Screening of titles/abstracts and removal of duplicates were performed and the full texts of the remaining potentially relevant articles that met the inclusion and exclusion criteria were retrieved and reviewed. Any disagreement was discussed until a consensus decision was reached.

Key learning points:

- Initial assessment of patients with thyroid nodules should be based on clinical history, clinical examination, and measurement of TSH level.
- Thyroid US and its scoring systems are important for the risk stratification of thyroid nodules.
- Thyroid scintigraphy is generally performed in patients with low to low-normal TSH value and nodules >1 cm in size.
- FNAC is performed for non-autonomous thyroid nodules, according to US scoring systems.
- [^{99m}Tc]Tc-MIBI and [^{18}F]FDG PET/CT are recommended in cytologically indeterminate thyroid nodules to reduce "diagnostic" surgeries.
- The clinical value of AI in the evaluation of thyroid nodules needs to be determined.

2. Clinical History and Clinical Examination

The initial assessment of individuals with thyroid nodules detected by palpation or during radiologic procedures includes clinical history and examination, measurement of serum TSH level, US of thyroid nodules and neck lymph nodes, thyroid scintigraphy (Na[^{99m}Tc]TcO_4 or Na[^{123}I]I) in cases of suppressed or low-normal TSH values, and FNAC if indicated according to US findings and thyroid scintigraphy.

2.1. Clinical History

Clinical history suggestive of increased risk of malignancy includes rapid nodule enlargement, head and neck external beam radiation therapy (particularly during childhood), whole-body irradiation (e.g., before bone marrow transplantation), and family history of thyroid cancer or thyroid cancer syndromes [18]. Familial occurrence of DTC is demonstrated in 5–10% of cases [19–21]. Some studies revealed that DTC occurs earlier [19,22], in a more advanced stage and more aggressive [23] with a worse outcome in the next generation [19]. Park et al. demonstrated a higher DTC recurrence rate in familial cases compared with sporadic ones and the second generation had more aggressive clinical features compared with the first one [24]. Therefore, patients with familial DTC need a careful clinical history evaluation. Thyroid cancer syndromes should be considered as they demand screening of different components of the syndrome in first-degree relatives. They include multiple endocrine neoplasia type 2 (MEN 2), Cowden syndrome, familial adenomatous polyposis, Werner syndrome, and Carney complex. Approximately 0.1% of all DTC cases are associated with these syndromes, except MEN2A and MEN2B, where the rates are 0.3% and 0.2%, respectively [25].

2.2. Clinical Examination

Thyroid gland palpation is usually the first clinical examination; however, it has low sensitivity (2–6%) for detecting thyroid nodules [26] and, in some cases, the physical examination may be limited by body habitus [27]. Most malignant thyroid nodules are asymptomatic, and a great majority of patients are euthyroid. However, there are several clinical examination findings harboring a higher risk of cancer, i.e., fixed and firm nodules, nodules larger than 4 cm in size (19% incidence of malignancy) [28], cervical lymphadenopathy, symptoms of obstruction, dysphonia, and vocal cord paralysis [6,27]. Furthermore, a combination of a solitary nodule, cervical lymphadenopathy (>1 cm), and vocal cord paralysis has a positive predictive value (PPV) of almost 100% for malignancy [29].

3. Thyroid Laboratory, Imaging, and Cytopathology

3.1. Laboratory Medicine

Thyroid function can be accurately assessed by measuring TSH and free thyroid hormones (i.e., free thyroxine, FT4; free tri-iodo-thyronine, fT3). TSH and FT4 have a complex, non-linear, inverse relationship resulting in relatively large changes in TSH compared to small changes in FT4 concentrations, respectively [30–32]. Accordingly, except in some rare conditions (i.e., central hypothyroidism, resistance to thyroid hormones, TSH-secreting pituitary adenoma, hyperthyroidism under treatment, and euthyroid sick syndrome), TSH measurement is a sensitive and the most accurate test for thyroid dysfunction [33,34]. As a consequence, different guidelines endorse the measurement of TSH alone at the front line while restricting FT4 (and rarely FT3) measurement in cases with abnormal TSH results (i.e., TSH reflex strategy) [35–38]. The same strategy is recommended in patients with thyroid nodules where TSH measurement is unanimously recommended as the first-line functional test by available clinical guidelines.

In patients with thyroid nodules, low TSH levels may be related to autonomously functioning thyroid nodule(s) and thyroid scintigraphy is indicated. A normal TSH excludes a clinically significant autonomy but, especially in countries with low iodine intake, cannot exclude compensated autonomy: in those regions, thyroid scintigraphy may properly exclude such nodules (frequently suspicious at neck US) from inappropriate FNAC [13,39]. Routine measurement of serum anti-thyroid peroxidase (TPO) antibodies is not necessary for thyroid nodule evaluation [10,40] and routine measurement of serum thyroglobulin (Tg) is strongly discouraged as it may be elevated in different thyroid diseases, including benign ones, and is aspecific and relatively insensitive for thyroid cancer [41]. Calcitonin is the standard biochemical tumor marker for medullary thyroid carcinoma (MTC) diagnosis and follow-up [42]. However, the value of routine testing in patients with thyroid nodules remains questionable due to the low prevalence, which results in a low PPV of basal calcitonin testing. Indeed, whether routine calcitonin testing improves prognosis in MTC patients remains unclear [43].

3.2. Thyroid Ultrasound

Since the 1970s, thyroid US has progressively gained a central role in assessing thyroid diseases. High-resolution US examinations are widely used worldwide, being radiation-free, relatively cheap, easy to learn, and versatile compared to other imaging modalities. Ultrasound devices are equipped with transducer probes with variable frequency (i.e., 2–20 Mega Hertz (MHz)). High-resolution linear transducers with a 7–15 MHz frequency are currently employed for thyroid examination. Since the thyroid gland is superficially located with its posterior border generally situated less than 4 cm from the skin, high-resolution (≥12 MHz) probes provide excellent image quality. High-resolution conventional B-mode (i.e., gray-scale ultrasound) evaluation is now integrated with multiparametric ultrasound (MPUS), including vascularization assessment (spectral Doppler, SD; color Doppler, CD; power Doppler ultrasound, PD; superb microvascular imaging, SMI; contrast-enhanced ultrasound, CEUS) and tissue stiffness assessment (sonoelastography), respectively [13].

In clinical practice, US is the first-line imaging method for the examination of thyroid morphology and structure. The main indications of thyroid US are summarized in Table 1.

Table 1. Thyroid ultrasound: clinical indications.

Indications
▪ To evaluate thyroid nodules and differentiate between benign and malignant ones
▪ To evaluate diffuse changes in the thyroid
▪ To differentiate thyroid nodules from cervical cysts, thyroglossal duct, and cervical masses
▪ To monitor patients with thyroid malignancies and detect recurrent/metastatic disease
▪ To guide interventional procedures (FNAC, PEI, TA)

Legend: FNAC, fine-needle aspiration cytology; PEI, percutaneous ethanol injection; TA, thermal ablation.

Although US is critical for the evaluation of diffuse thyroid disease, differentiating between benign and malignant nodules is the main application area. Despite several ancillary techniques like elastography and Doppler that were proposed to differentiate malignant nodules from benign ones, the most commonly used parameters are the high-resolution B-mode ultrasound characteristics of thyroid nodules. Sonographic findings, including assessment of the nodule echogenicity, internal composition, calcification, and border regularity, are commonly used for differential diagnosis. Briefly, solid, hypoechoic nodules, taller-than-wide shape, and irregular borders with microcalcifications have the highest chance of being malignant [44].

Today, thyroid US allows an accurate evaluation of morphologic features, which have been used to propose a standardized risk stratification for thyroid nodules (i.e., Thyroid Imaging And Data Reporting Systems (TI-RADS)) attempting to reduce the admittedly high inter-operator variability [13]. Among these, the American College of Radiology (ACR)-TI-RADS, European (EU)-TI-RADS, Korean (K)-TI-RADS, British Thyroid Association (BTA), American Thyroid Association (ATA) classification and American Association of Clinical Endocrinologists (AACE), American College of Endocrinology (ACE), and Associazione Medici Endocrinologi (AME) classification systems are commonly used [18,45–49]. The rationale of these classification systems is that the risk of malignancy rises in parallel with the increase in the number of suspicious US features and the lack of benign findings. Risk classification aims to identify the most clinically significant malignancies and decrease the number of unnecessary FNACs on benign nodules. Reviewing all the classification systems is beyond the article's scope, but we will briefly mention the most commonly used ACR-TIRADS, EU-TIRADS, and ATA thyroid ultrasound risk stratification systems (RSS).

American College of Radiology (ACR)-TI-RADS [45] is based on the assessment of different US features of thyroid nodules: composition (spongiform, mixed cystic, and solid), echogenicity (anechoic, hyperechoic/isoechoic hypoechoic and very hypoechoic), shape (wider than tall or taller than wide), margin (smooth, ill-defined, lobulated or irregular, extra-thyroidal), and echogenic foci (none or large comet-tail artifacts, macrocalcifications, peripheral (rim) calcification, and punctate echogenic foci). It associates each of these features with a score ranging from 0 to 3 points. The sum of the assigned points defines the risk of malignancies according to five grades, with each grade corresponding to benign (TR1: 0 points), not suspicious (TR2: 2 points), mildly suspicious (TR3: 3 points), moderately suspicious (TR4: 4–6 points), or highly suspicious for malignancy (TR5: ≥7 points). This system does not include subcategories or a TR0 group to indicate a normal thyroid. EU-TIRADS is one of the most commonly used TI-RADS systems across Europe. EU-TIRADS 1 defines a normal thyroid gland without nodules. EU-TIRADS 2 is defined as a benign category, whereas EU-TIRADS 3 defines a nodule with a low risk of malignancy. Nodules with EU-TIRADS 4 have an intermediate risk, and with EU-TIRADS 5 have a high risk of malignancy. Detailed EU-TIRADS categories, risks of malignancy, and recommendations are explained in Table 2.

Table 2. EU-TIRADS categories, risks of malignancy, and recommendations [46].

Category	US Features	Malignancy Risk, %	Recommendations
EU-TIRADS 1: Normal	No nodules	None	None
EU-TIRADS 2: benign	Pure cyst, Entirely spongiform	0	No FNA required (unless for therapeutic purposes/to relieve compression)
EU-TIRADS 3: low risk	Ovoid, smooth isoechoic/hyperechoic No features of high suspicion	2–4	>20 mm FNA
EU-TIRADS 4: intermediate risk	Ovoid, smooth, mildly hypoechoic No features of high suspicion	6–17	>15 mm FNA
EU-TIRADS 5: high risk	At least 1 of the following features of high suspicion: – Irregular shape – Irregular margins – Microcalcifications – Marked hypoechogenicity (and solid)	26–87	>10 mm FNA, <10 mm: consider FNA or active surveillance

Legend: EU-TIRADS, European Thyroid Imaging Reporting and Data System; US, ultrasound.

The American Thyroid Association (ATA) guidelines for assessing thyroid nodules are meant to improve inter- and intra-reader consistency when reporting thyroid nodules on ultrasound and facilitate communication with referring physicians. The 2015 guideline emphasizes the importance of the sonographic pattern of the nodule for risk stratification. This system does not include scoring but categorizes the risk of malignancy from very low risk to high. The malignancy risk as well as the size of the nodule are the two main criteria for FNA (Table 3).

Comparison of thyroid ultrasound RSS is an ongoing debate in the literature. This is understandable; each society deems its RSS to be the preferred system. Endocrinologists from Europe prefer EU-RADS, endocrinologists from the USA uses ATA guidelines, and radiologists and nuclear medicine physicians prefer the ACR-TIRADS system [50,51] (Figure 1).

Table 3. ATA sonographic patterns, estimated risk of malignancy, and fine-needle aspiration guidance for thyroid nodules [18].

Sonographic Pattern	US Features	Estimated Risk of Malignancy, %	FNA Size Cutoff (Largest Dimension)
High suspicion	Solid hypoechoic nodule or solid hypoechoic component of a partially cystic nodule *with* one or more of the following features: irregular margins (infiltrative, micro-lobulated), microcalcifications, taller-than-wide shape, rim calcifications with small extrusive soft tissue component, evidence of extrathyroidal extension	>70–90	Recommend FNA at ≥1 cm
Intermediate suspicion	Hypoechoic solid nodule with smooth margins *without* microcalcifications, ETE, or taller-than-wide shape	10–20	Recommend FNA at ≥1 cm
Low suspicion	Isoechoic or hyperechoic solid nodule, or partially cystic nodule with eccentric solid areas, *without* microcalcification, irregular margin or ETE, or taller-than-wide shape	5–10	Recommend FNA at ≥1.5 cm
Very low suspicion	Spongiform or partially cystic nodules *without* any of the sonographic features described in low-, intermediate-, or high-suspicion patterns	<3	Consider FNA at ≥2 cm Observation without FNA is also a reasonable option
Benign	Purely cystic nodules (no solid component)	<1	No biopsy

Legend: US, ultrasound; FNA, fine-needle aspiration; ETE, extrathyroidal extension.

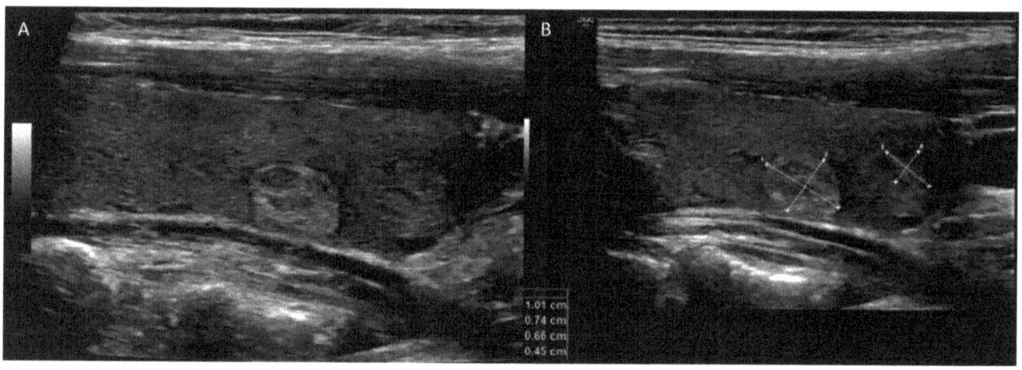

Figure 1. A 56-year-old woman with small hyperechoic and isoechoic nodules with regular borders ((**A**) longitudinal-plane US image) and size equal to and less than 1 cm ((**B**) labeled longitudinal-plane image). Thyroid US risk evaluations were reported using ACR TIRADS 3, EU-TIRADS 3, ATA classifications: low suspicion. Considering the size and risk of the nodules, no biopsy was recommended.

In a multicentric German trail, EU-TIRADS was proved to be inferior when compared to other RSSs with diagnostic accuracies of 0.70 vs. 0.79, 0.78, 0.82, and 0.79 for Kwak-TIRADS, ACR-TI-RADS, Korean-TIRADS, and American Thyroid Association (ATA) Guidelines, respectively [52]. In another study, authors found that ACR TI-RADS, American Association of Clinical Endocrinologists/American College of Endocrinology/Associazione Medici Endocrinologi guidelines, European TI-RADS, ATA guidelines, and Korean TI-RADS would have avoided FNA for 34.7%, 31%, 25.7%, 20%, and 6% of nodules with false-negative rates (FNRs) of 24%, 28.5%, 22%, 7.2%, and 1.9%, respectively. In this study, ATA guidelines had the highest area under the curve and a low FNR, whereas ACR TI-RADS would have spared more patients from FNA with a high FNR [53]. So far, no uniform, worldwide accepted RSS has been established because of the controversy in the literature, and the differences in the expertise and preferences of ultrasonographers (Figure 2). Also, there are limitations of RSS like insufficient sensitivity for the diagnosis of follicular thyroid carcinoma and follicular subtypes of PTC and insufficient specificity to rule out autonomously functioning thyroid nodules from FNAC. However, work has recently begun on a new international US-based RSS for thyroid nodules. With the participation of several scientific societies, an International TIRADS (I-TIRADS) will be proposed and established internationally as a uniform evidence-based system. Currently, several working groups are investigating ultrasound criteria. In addition, promising data already exist regarding the use of AI to identify US patterns. This technique could significantly reduce interobserver variability and may be associated with improvements in specificity and accuracy, without significantly sacrificing sensitivity for malignancy detection [54].

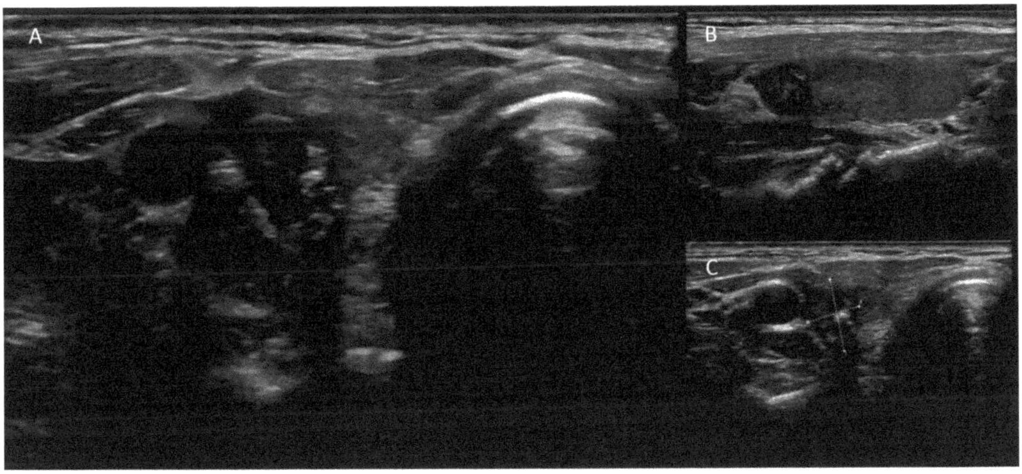

Figure 2. A 45-year-old woman with a family history of thyroid cancer. US showed ((**A**) transverse-plane image, (**B**) longitudinal-plane image, (**C**) labeled longitudinal-plane image) hypoechoic nodule with microcalcifications, taller-than-wide shape, irregular borders, and size > 1 cm. Thyroid US risk evaluations were reported using ACR TIRADS 5, EU-TIRADS 5, and ATA classifications: high suspicion. Considering the size and risk of the nodules, FNAC was performed; they were reported to be malignant, and total thyroidectomy revealed papillary thyroid carcinoma.

3.3. *Nuclear Medicine*

Thyroid scintigraphy performed with functional tracers is used to map the global and regional activity of sodium iodide transporter (NIS) within the thyroid gland. Nowadays, it is commonly performed by using Na[^{99m}Tc]TcO$_4$, preferred over iodine tracers (Na[^{131}I]I or Na[^{123}I]I) due to its shorter physical half-life (6 h), pure gamma emission (140 keV), low radiation burden, wide availability, and significantly lower costs [55]. Na[^{99m}Tc]TcO$_4$ is caught within thyrocytes through NIS located on the basolateral membrane, like radioiodine tracers. On the contrary, as the main difference, it is not organified and leaves thyrocytes with an effective half-life (6 h) shorter than that of Na[^{123}I]I (about 13 h) and Na[^{131}I]I (about 8 days). However, Na[^{99m}Tc]TcO$_4$ uptake is representative of thyroid hormone biosynthesis and provides relevant clinical information on the global and regional function of thyroid cells (Figure 3).

Figure 3. A 65-year-old man affected by overt hyperthyroidism (TSH 0.00 μIU/mL (0.35–4.94), FT3 9.61 pg/mL (1.58–3.91), FT4 2.25 ng/dL (0.70–1.48)) associated with tachycardia, insomnia, and irritability. Thyroid ultrasonography showed a large-sized nodule (38 × 34 × 20 mm) in the right thyroid lobe, isoechoic with a hypoechoic ring. Moderately increased intra-nodular blood flow was also noted. Thyroid scintigraphy was performed 20 min after Na[^{99m}Tc]TcO$_4$ administration (111 MBq). Image (anterior view; magnification: 1.4; matrix: 256 × 256; time frame: 100 Kcs) demonstrated a well-defined hyperfunctioning area located in the middle–lower part of the right thyroid lobe. In this latter, tracer uptake/distribution was quite intense and homogeneous, respectively. On the contrary, mild tracer uptake was noted in the remaining right lobe (upper part), isthmus, and left lobe. Thus, a toxic nodular goiter with severe functional inhibition of the remaining thyroid parenchyma was diagnosed.

In physiological conditions, NIS activity is positively regulated by TSH and, as a consequence, Na[^{99m}Tc]TcO$_4$ uptake in the gland can be properly interpreted in light of TSH values (ideally performed before thyroid scintigraphy). The activity of NIS is inversely regulated by the intrathyroidal iodine pool that reflects the iodine intake.

Although almost all thyroid cancers are non-functioning, most of these nodules are benign (i.e., 90–95%), which greatly reduces the specificity of a thyroid scan. Accordingly, a thyroid scan is generally performed when nodules occur in people with low or low-to-normal TSH levels. The relationship between thyroid autonomy and TSH levels, however, is affected by the degree of iodine sufficiency and varies widely regionally [31,32,34]. Therefore, although autonomous nodules are almost invariably accompanied by decreased TSH levels (i.e., <0.1–0.4 mUI/L) when the iodine supply is adequate, the bulk of autonomous tissue may be insufficient to suppress the TSH level in iodine-depleted thyroids, especially in the early phases of autonomy. As a consequence, different indications are given in current clinical guidelines with a thyroid scan recommended when the TSH level is low or low to normal in the USA (iodine-repleted country), whereas a Na[^{99m}Tc]TcO$_4$ scan is recommended in all people with a nodule greater than 10 mm, independently of the TSH level in Germany (iodine-deficient country) [5,39,55,56]

Consequently, high iodine concentrations (e.g., regular use of products rich in iodine) may reduce the quality of a functional image. For this reason, any "excess" iodine intake should be avoided before scintigraphy or it should be postponed for several (i.e., 1–3) to many (i.e., 6 or more) months in patients with severe iodine contamination due to radiological contrast media administration or amiodarone therapy, respectively [55]. [^{99m}Tc]Tc-MIBI is a lipophilic cation able to cross the cell membrane, reversibly penetrating the cytoplasm and then irreversibly moving through the membrane of the mitochondria using a different electrical gradient caused by a high negative electric potential of the inner membrane. It is regularly used as a marker for myocardial perfusion and hyperfunctioning parathyroid tissue. All in all, studies reported its abnormal uptake in different tumors such as in the lungs, brain, breast, bone, and thyroid [57–60]. The role of [^{99m}Tc]Tc-MIBI thyroid scintigraphy (i.e., molecular imaging) to better assess the risk of malignancy in hypofunctioning and cytologically indeterminate thyroid nodules has been investigated for more than three decades [56]. In 2004, Hurtado-Lopez first compared intranodular [^{99m}Tc]Tc-MIBI and Na[^{99m}Tc]TcO_4 uptake and found a quite absolute NPV for nodules with a matching hypoactive pattern with both tracers [61]. More recently, the [^{99m}Tc]Tc-MIBI uptake in the thyroid nodule has been qualitatively (i.e., visual analysis) compared to the uptake in the extranodular (i.e., normal) thyroid parenchyma and classified as hyper-, iso-, and hypointense, with the latter ruling out malignancy with up to 99% NPV [62,63]. Vice versa, an increased [^{99m}Tc]Tc-MIBI uptake with respect to surrounding parenchyma or compared to a Na[^{99m}Tc]TcO_4 image conferred a higher risk of cancer [61,62,64–66]. However, a positive pattern (i.e., abnormal [^{99m}Tc]Tc-MIBI uptake in the nodule) was found in a significant proportion of histologically benign nodules (especially follicular and oxyphilic adenomas), and an unsatisfactory PPV (i.e., 27%) was reported [67]. To improve the diagnostic performance of molecular imaging in such patients, Saggiorato and colleagues proposed a semiquantitative approach using the so-called Retention Index (RI) method [68]. They concluded that [^{99m}Tc]Tc-MIBI-positive nodules with an RI value ≥ -11.94 were suspicious for malignancy, thus suggesting more aggressive clinical management. In addition, they proved a reduced accuracy of [^{99m}Tc]Tc-MIBI scintigraphy in oxyphilic nodules and discouraged its use in such a setting. More recently, a new semiquantitative method (i.e., wash-out index—WO*ind*) was proposed, taking into account the [^{99m}Tc]Tc-MIBI kinetics within the nodules, and was found able to improve the diagnostic accuracy compared to qualitative evaluation [63,64,66] (Figures 4 and 5).

Finally, Schenke and colleagues, in a recent European multicenter study, confirmed that the semiquantitative approach using the WO*ind* method could significantly improve the overall diagnostic performance of [^{99m}Tc]Tc-MIBI imaging [65]. In clinical routine, thyroid [^{99m}Tc]Tc-MIBI imaging can also be used to differentiate between amiodarone-induced hyperthyroidism (AIT) type 1 (i.e., normal or high uptake) and type 2 (low uptake), respectively [69,70].

Currently, single-photon emission computed tomography (SPECT) associated with computed tomography (SPECT/CT, hybrid imaging) is able to provide a co-registration of anatomic and functional/molecular data results for a better localization and characterization of tracer uptake [65]. [^{18}F]FDG positron emission tomography/computed tomography (PET/CT) is widely used for initial staging, restaging, recurrence detection, and assessment of treatment outcomes in a variety of malignant diseases [71]. [^{18}F]FDG uptake is related to an overexpression of the transmembrane glucose transporter proteins (GLUTs), which move the tracer into the cell, and to the overactivation of hexokinases that phosphorylate [^{18}F]FDG to [^{18}F]FDG-6-phosphate and trap the tracer in the cell [72]. Interestingly, a visually [^{18}F]FDG-negative thyroid nodule with indeterminate cytology carries a negligible risk of malignancy, making [^{18}F]FDG an accurate ruling-out biomarker. Notably, a recent blinded, randomized, controlled multicenter trial in the Netherlands consistently proved that a [^{18}F]FDG PET/CT-driven workup of cytologically indeterminate thyroid nodules may change the clinical management and safely reduce inappropriate surgical interventions by 40%. Notably, the authors warned against the use of [^{18}F]FDG PET/CT in patients with Hurthle cell nodules where a high [^{18}F]FDG is expected, even in benign ones [73].

Conversely, a positive [^{18}F]FDG PET/CT is not reliable as a rule-in test since approximately 50% of patients with positive nodules have a benign disease in the final histological report [74–76] (Figure 6).

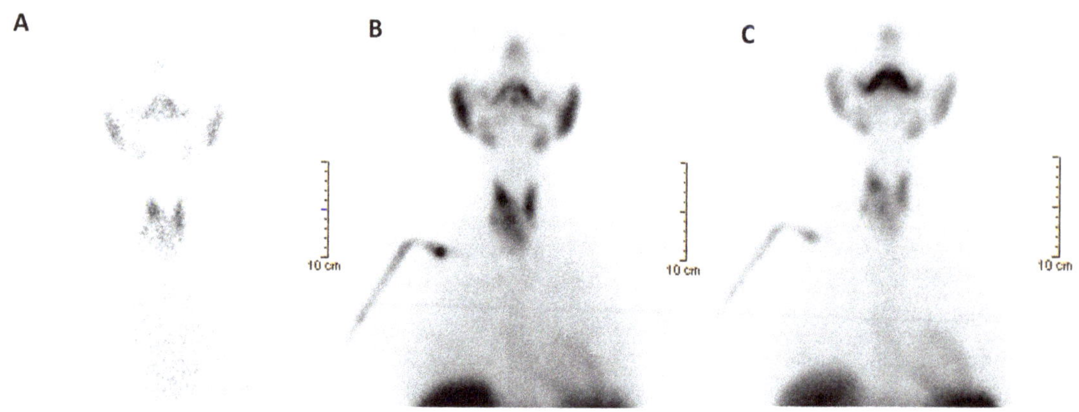

Figure 4. A 52-year-old woman affected by nodular goiter in euthyroid status (TSH 0.60 μIU/mL (0.35–5.50), FT3 3.18 pg/mL (2.30–4.20), FT4 1.17 ng/dL (0.89–1.76)). Thyroid ultrasonography showed a large-sized nodule (39 × 36 × 33 mm) in the right thyroid lobe, irregularly hypoechoic with the presence of isoechoic areas. A moderately increased intra-nodular blood flow was also noted. (**A**) Thyroid scintigraphy, performed 20 min after Na[^{99m}Tc]TcO$_4$ administration (111 MBq; anterior view; magnification: 1.4; matrix: 256 × 256; time frame: 100 Kcs), showed a well-defined hypofunctioning area located in the middle–lower part of the right thyroid lobe. Thus, a nodular goiter was diagnosed while FNAC was conclusive for a benign lesion (Tir2) according to the Italian scoring system. [^{99m}Tc]Tc-MIBI scintigraphy was obtained 10 and 120 min (**B**,**C**, respectively) after tracer administration (370 MBq). Images were acquired in anterior view, magnification 256 × 256, matrix 1.4, time frame 10 min. Increased [^{99m}Tc]Tc-MIBI uptake was noted in the hypofunctioning nodule.

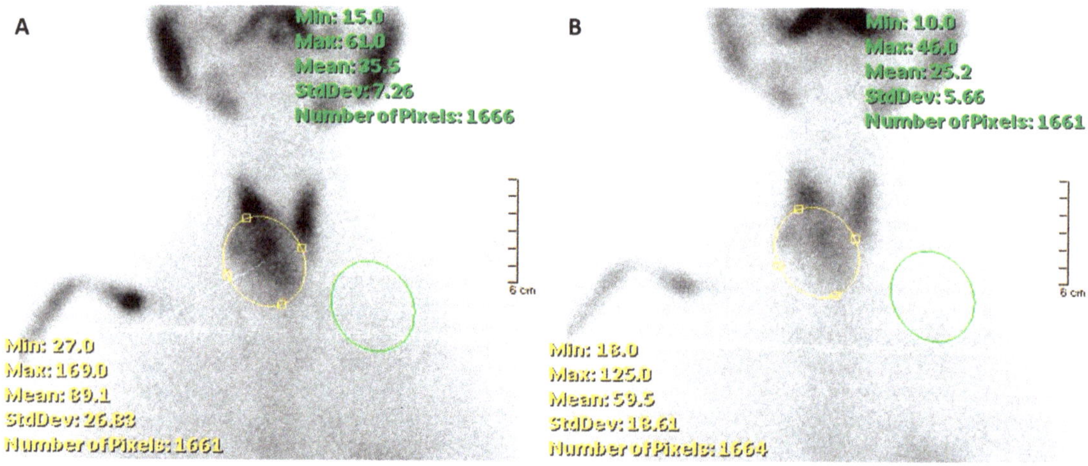

Figure 5. A 52-year-old woman affected by nodular goiter, cytologically benign (TIR2 according to the Italian scoring system). [^{99m}Tc]Tc-MIBI scintigraphy was obtained 10 and 120 min after tracer administration (**A**,**B**, respectively) using a semiquantitative approach by calculating the wash-out index (WOind). WOind value was $<-19\%$ (exactly -37%), thus consistent with a no-malignant lesion. Final histology diagnosis: follicular adenoma.

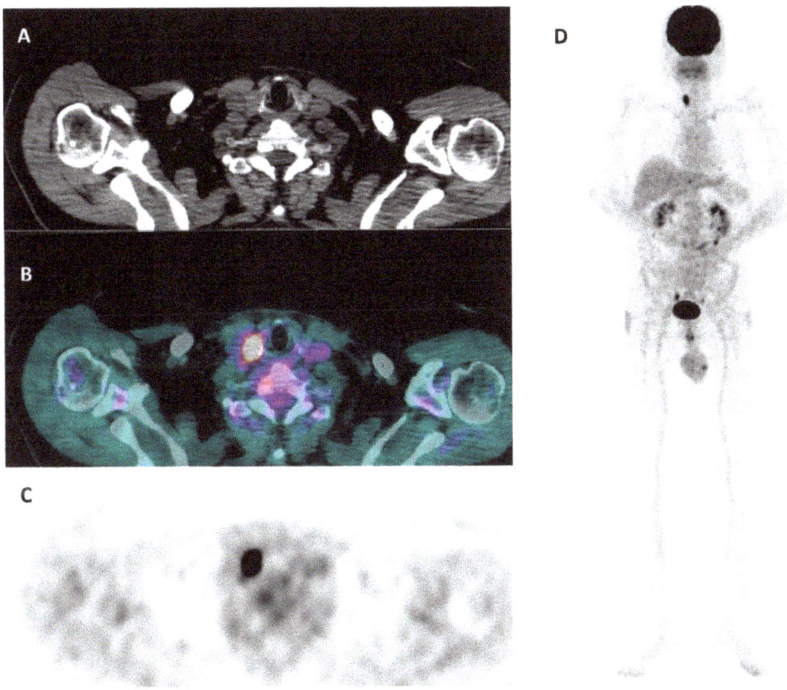

Figure 6. A 62-year-old man with a hypermetabolic thyroid nodule (SUV max = 18.3) unexpectedly discovered in the right lobe during a [^{18}F]FDG PET/CT study performed for staging in suspected paraneoplastic syndrome. (**A**) CT – axial view, (**B**) a [^{18}F]FDG PET/CT axial view, (**C**) [^{18}F]FDG PET axial view, (**D**) whole-body [^{18}F]FDG PET. A laboratory test was consistent with euthyroid status (i.e., TSH 2.1 μIU/mL (0.27–4.2), FT3 3.30 pg/mL (2.0–4.4), FT4 18.2 pmol/L (12–22)) with negative anti-thyroid antibodies (i.e., TPOAb, TgAb). Thyroid ultrasound demonstrated a multinodular goiter with a dominant hypoechoic nodule in the right lobe (maximum size: 22 mm), which was then classified as hypofunctioning at thyroid scintigraphy. Accordingly, FNAC was performed: an indeterminate lesion with a high risk of being malignant (i.e., TIR3B according to the Italian scoring system) was diagnosed. The patient underwent total thyroidectomy, and the final histological diagnosis was consistent with Hurtle cell follicular adenoma.

In summary, either [^{99m}Tc]Tc-MIBI or [^{18}F]FDG PET/CT may safely rule out inappropriate diagnostic surgeries in about half of patients with cytologically indeterminate nodules (non-Hurthle types). When adopted as a rule-out test, both [^{99m}Tc]Tc-MIBI scintigraphy and [^{18}F]FDG PET/CT also proved to be cost-effective in comparison with the standard practice (i.e., diagnostic surgery) and the use of Gene Expression Classifiers [14–17]. Their use, however, should be optimized and restricted to patients with non-Hurtle cell cytological patterns and without additional indications to surgery as multinodular goiters or large-index lesions (i.e., >40–50 mm). However, more specific rule-in biomarkers are still warranted in patients with [^{99m}Tc]Tc-MIBI- or [^{18}F]FDG-positive cytologically indeterminate nodules in order to improve the PPV.

Moreover, radiomics analysis of [^{18}F]FDG PET/CT data preliminarily proved to increase specificity and PPV in discriminating benign from malignant cytologically indeterminate nodules [77]. However, currently, available data are contrasting [78], likely due to differences in pretest probabilities and other variables. All in all, the application of radiomic analysis in this setting should be reserved for clinical studies and not performed to make clinical decisions.

3.4. Fine-Needle Aspiration Cytology and Cytopathology

Thyroid nodules are common in clinical practice, with a prevalence of up to 60% depending on age, sex, etc. [3,4,26]. The majority are benign [79], and the risk of malignancy is 7 to 15% [79], depending on the nodule size, findings of ultrasound and nuclear medicine techniques, and patient characteristics.

Several guidelines and RSSs (Table 4) recommend biopsy based on the size and imaging findings.

Table 4. Ultrasound-based recommendations for fine-needle aspiration cytology: (a) Biopsy recommendations of EU TI-RADS [46]. (b) Biopsy recommendations of ACR TI-RADS guidelines [45]. (c) Biopsy recommendations of ATA guidelines [18].

(a)

Category	Malignancy Risk, %	Recommendations
EU-TIRADS 1: Normal	None	None
EU-TIRADS 2	benign, malignancy risk 0%;	No FNA required (unless for therapeutic purposes/to relieve compression)
EU-TIRADS 3	low risk, malignancy risk 2–4%	>20 mm FNA
EU-TIRADS 4	intermediate risk, malignancy risk 6–17%	>15 mm FNA
EU-TIRADS 5	high risk, malignancy risk 26–87%	>10 mm FNA, <10 mm: consider FNA or active surveillance

(b)

Category	Points	Malignancy Risk, %	Recommendations
TR1:	0 points	benign (aggregate risk level 0.3%);	No FNA required
TR2:	2 points	not suspicious (aggregate risk level 1.5%);	No FNA required
TR3:	3 points	mildly suspicious (aggregate risk level 4.8%);	≥25 mm FNA
TR4:	4–6 points	moderately suspicious (aggregate risk level 5.9–12.8%);	≥15 mm FNA
TR5:	7 points or more	highly suspicious (aggregate risk level 20.8–68.4% for 10 points).	≥10 mm FNA,

(c)

Category	Malignancy Risk, %	Recommendations
Benign	Risk level < 1%	No FNA required
Very low suspicion	Risk level < 3%	Consider FNA at ≥2 cm Observation without FNA is also a reasonable option
Low suspicion	Risk level 5–10%	Recommend FNA at ≥1.5 cm
Intermediate suspicion	Risk level 10–20%	Recommend FNA at ≥1 cm
High suspicion	Risk level > 70–90%	Recommend FNA at ≥1 cm

The shape, margin, echogenicity, and presence of calcification are useful criteria for the discrimination of malignant from benign nodules [80].

FNAC Technique:

- *Preprocedural*

The patient should be informed that limited intra- and peri-thyroidal bleeding and mild local pain radiating to the ear may occur. Informed consent should be obtained after a detailed procedure discussion with the patient. The most significant possible complication of the procedure is the development of a neck hematoma, especially in hypervascular nodules, but this complication is fortunately rare [81] and usually resolves without intervention. A preprocedural test for coagulation is not routinely needed, but the patient should be questioned about recent or current anticoagulant therapy. To avoid excessive bleeding, anticoagulation therapy should be discontinued 4–7 days before biopsy; however, the preprocedural discontinuation of aspirin therapy is controversial [82]. Most use fine or thin (22- to 27-gauge) needles for FNAC. Thinner needles should be preferred for hypervascular nodules. The procedure can be performed with local anesthesia (lidocaine hydrochloride 1–2%, 1–2 mL) or without. Oertel and colleagues advocated using ice as an alternative for local anesthesia because it numbs the area and causes vasoconstriction, decreasing the aspirate's hemodilution [83]. Per nodule, three passes are typically obtained, particularly if rapid on-site evaluation by a cytopathologist is unavailable. Under US guidance, the needle may be introduced parallel or perpendicular to the transducer, and the needle tip should be carefully monitored during the procedure. The collected material is placed on glass slides, smeared, and fixed in 95% ethyl alcohol or left to air dry.

- *Specimen Staining*

When using the Papanicolaou staining method, the smears should be quickly placed in 95% ethyl alcohol. When Diff-Quik or Giemsa stain is used, the smear should be allowed to air dry. Papanicolaou staining is most commonly used for cytologic analysis of thyroid specimens, and it provides the most precise depiction of nuclear chromatin, ground-glass nuclei, and nuclear groove characteristics in papillary carcinoma. Diff-Quik or Giemsa stain helps visualize the characteristics of the cytoplasm and colloid [83].

- *Material Adequacy and False-Negative Results*

Appropriate specimen preparation significantly increases the likelihood of material adequacy and decreases the frequency of false-negative findings. Both may be affected by the level of operator experience, lesion localization, method of guidance (palpation or US), number of aspirations, needle gauge, sampling technique, capability for immediate on-site cytologic analysis, and many other factors. The percentage of unsatisfactory specimens should remain less than 15%, or, ideally, 10%.

- *Comparison of Aspiration and Capillary Action*

Thyroid fine-needle aspiration is a safe, simple, relatively accurate, and first-line diagnostic tool in the evaluation of thyroid nodules. However, especially in hypervascular lesions, the aspiration technique frequently leads to microscopic hemorrhages, which obscure proper cytologic interpretation. Fine-needle capillary (FNC) sampling, a technique without aspiration, was developed in the 1980s [84]. It has been suggested that this non-aspiration sampling technique could reduce the amount of blood in samples and produce superior-quality specimens. Various comparative studies showed that aspiration FNAC and FNC sampling have no statistically significant difference in sample adequacy and diagnostic accuracy. The choice of technique should be based on the operator's personal preferences and experience. However, Degirmenci and colleagues showed that selecting finer needles (24–25 G) for sonography-guided sampling of thyroid nodules and using the FNC technique increased the rate of adequate material in the cytological examination when compared to aspiration FNAC (76.9% vs. 49.4%, $p < 0.001$) [85]. Non-aspiration FNC sampling is less traumatic and causes less hemodilution of aspirate, which is critical for hypervascular lesions. Titton et al. and Oertel have suggested that the thyroid sampling should begin with non-aspiration FNC and, if the specimens collected with that technique are inadequate, should continue with aspiration FNAC [83,86].

- *Comparison with Core-Needle Biopsy*

Core-needle biopsy is performed with an 18–20-gauge needle and provides a large histologic tissue core, which may have a greater effect on surgical decision-making than cytologic diagnosis. In a separate prospective study in which FNAC was compared with core-needle biopsy performed with a spring-activated, short-throw, 18–20-gauge needle, the diagnostic yield with core-needle biopsy of thyroid nodules exceeded that with FNAC techniques by approximately 10% [87]. As can be predicted, there was also a higher complication rate with the use of the core needle and a higher need for anesthesia [88]. For these reasons, a core-needle biopsy is considered for patients in whom FNAC produces only specimens of inadequate cellularity after several passes or in patients who return for a repeat biopsy after a non-diagnostic initial FNAC.

Fine-needle aspiration cytology represents the diagnostic cornerstone because of its accuracy, reproducibility, and cost-effectiveness. However, FNAC is characterized by a grey diagnostic area in which the indeterminate cytology precludes a distinction between benign and malignant lesions. Physicians should manage the patients according to the different findings of cytology reports concerning the chance of malignancy. Several reporting systems and recommendations were proposed. Among these reporting systems, the Italian SIAPeC-AIT classification, in its latest version updated in 2014; The Bethesda System for Reporting Thyroid Cytopathology, proposed in 2007 and updated in 2017 and 2023; and the Guidance On The Reporting Of Thyroid Cytology Specimens from The UK Royal College Of Pathologists (RCPath) are among the most widely used in the world [89–92].

The Bethesda System for Reporting Thyroid Cytopathology is preferred by many centers, especially in the USA. The updated version (Table 5) also accounts for the possibility of a relatively new entity: non-invasive follicular neoplasm with papillary-like nuclear features (NIFTP).

Table 5. The 2017 Bethesda System for Reporting Thyroid Cytopathology: implied risk of malignancy and recommended clinical management [93].

Diagnostic Category	Risk of Malignancy if NIFTP ≠ CA (%)	Risk of Malignancy if NIFTP = CA (%)	Usual Management
I. Non-diagnostic or unsatisfactory	5–10	5–10	Repeat FNA with ultrasound guidance
II. Benign	0–3	0–3	Clinical and sonographic follow-up
III. Atypia of undetermined significance or follicular lesion of undetermined significance	6–18	~10–30	Repeat FNA, molecular testing, or lobectomy
IV. Follicular neoplasm or suspicious for a follicular neoplasm	10–40	25–40	Molecular testing, lobectomy
V. Suspicious for malignancy	45–60	50–75	Near-total thyroidectomy or lobectomy
VI. Malignant	94–96	97–99	Near-total thyroidectomy or lobectomy

The system includes six categories, with the most controversial being III–IV, where repeat FNAC, molecular testing, or lobectomy may be warranted. The cytological characteristics of the indeterminate categories (III–IV) can be divided into four different subgroups: qualitatively unsatisfactory specimen, cytologic atypia (mostly nuclear), architectural atypia (microfollicular), and the combination of the latter two [94]. The first case includes specimens with inadequate preparation and artifacts that may cause the appearance of nuclear enlargements suspicious for atypia. Specimens with atypical cells also belong to this category. Atypia can be epithelial, lymphoid, mesenchymal, or even non-specific and does not suggest any specific tumor by itself (Bethesda III). The second case includes cytological atypia in specimens, no matter the cell architecture. Usually, there are very few atypical cells, so the confirmation/exclusion of malignancy is not possible. The presence of oncocytes, without an adequate clinical picture, e.g., Hashimoto's thyroiditis, is also considered atypical (Bethesda III). The third case involves specimens with some or abundant microfollicular structures but without atypia of the nucleus (Bethesda III and IV). Also, samples with many oncocytes, but without colloid or lymphocytes, are in this category (Bethesda IV). The fourth case includes scarce cellularity and the presence of microfollicular structures and nuclear atypia (Bethesda III). FNAC in these cases is considered as a screening tool because it cannot confirm or exclude malignancy [94].

Although the morphologic parameters used by these various systems (Table 6) are very similar, there are differences in the criteria for inclusion in cytologically indeterminate categories which may affect the recommendations for the clinical management of patients (Table 7).

Table 6. Comparison between 2014 Italian SIAPEC-AIT classification, 2017 Bethesda, and 2016 UK RCPath reporting system for thyroid cytology.

RCPath	Bethesda	Italian SIAPEC-AIT
Thy1 Non-diagnostic for cytological diagnosis Thy1c Non-diagnostic for cytological diagnosis—cystic lesion	I. Non-diagnostic or unsatisfactory II. Virtually acellular specimen III. Other (obscuring blood, clotting artifact, etc.) IV. Cyst fluid only	TIR1 Non-diagnostic TIR1c Non-diagnostic cystic
Thy2 Non-neoplastic Thy2c Non-neoplastic, cystic lesion	Consistent with a benign follicular nodule (includes adenomatoid nodule, colloid nodule, etc.). Consistent with lymphocytic (Hashimoto) thyroiditis in the proper clinical context Consistent with granulomatous (subacute) thyroiditis	TIR2 Non-malignant
Thy3a Neoplasm possible—atypia/non-diagnostic	III. Atypia of undetermined significance or follicular lesion of undetermined significance	TIR3A Low-risk indeterminate lesion (LRIL)
Thy3f Neoplasm possible, suggesting follicular neoplasm	IV. Follicular neoplasm or suspicious for a follicular neoplasm Specify if Hürthle cell (oncocytic) type	TIR3B High-risk indeterminate lesion (HRIL)
Thy4 Suspicious of malignancy	V. Suspicious for malignancy	TIR4 Suspicious of malignancy
Thy5 Malignant	VI. Malignant	TIR5 Malignant

Table 7. "Indeterminate" diagnostic categories: comparison of risk of malignancy (ROM) and clinical management between Italian, Bethesda, and British classifications.

2014 Italian SIAPEC-AIT		2017 Bethesda		2016 RCPath Classification	
Diagnostic category (ROM %)	Management	Diagnostic category (ROM %)	Management	Diagnostic category (ROM %)	Management
TIR 3A Low-risk indeterminate lesion (12–22%)	Clinical follow up/Repeat FNA	III. AUS/FLUS (10–30%)	Repeat FNA/Molecular testing or lobectomy	Thy 3a Neoplasm possible – atypia/non-diagnostic (25%)	Multidisciplinary assessment
TIR 3B High-risk indeterminate lesion (30–55%)	Surgery	IV. Follicular neo-plasm/suspicious follicular neoplasm (25–40%)	Molecular testing, lobectomy	Thy 3f Neoplasm possible, suggesting follicular neoplasm (31%)	Multidisciplinary assessment

Legend: ROM: risk of malignancy; AUS: atypia of undetermined significance; FLUS: follicular lesion of undetermined significance.

Despite all these nuances in ultrasound RSS and cytopathology reporting systems, physicians should decide the optimal management with the help of the patient's history and preferences, the data obtained from nuclear medicine imaging findings, and molecular testing if available.

4. Molecular Biomarkers

Molecular markers may have diagnostic or prognostic purposes. Approximately 15 to 30% of thyroid nodules are classified as indeterminate in the FNAC report [95]. They include Bethesda III (atypia of undetermined significance) and Bethesda IV (follicular neoplasm) lesions, with risks of malignancy (mean, range) of 28 (11–54)% and 50 (28–100)%, respectively [92]. If excluding nodules diagnosed by surgical pathologic examination as non-invasive follicular thyroid neoplasms with papillary-like nuclear features, the risks of malignancy are 6.4 (6–20) and 7.1 (0.2–30) [92]. The principal use of molecular markers in this FNAC categories is diagnostic, i.e., ruling out or ruling in thyroid cancer, with implications for further patient management.

The Cancer Genome Atlas Research Network 2014 investigated the molecular profile of 496 papillary thyroid cancers (PTCs), mainly classical and follicular subtypes, and demonstrated two distinct molecular profiles: $BRAF^{V600E}$-like and RAS-like [96]. The first included the $BRAF^{V600E}$ mutation as well as RET/PTC and BRAF fusions, while the other one included RAS family (HRAS, NRAS, KRAS) mutations, $BRAF^{K601E}$ mutation, EIF1AX mutations, and THADA and PPARG fusions. These two molecular profiles seem to be associated with classical and follicular PTCs but are also noted in other DTC histotypes. Non-invasive follicular neoplasm with papillary-like nuclear features (NIFTP) and follicular thyroid carcinoma (FTC) are also considered RAS-like tumors [95]. Furthermore, benign lesions may also have RAS-like molecular profiles [97].

Molecular panels for indeterminate thyroid nodules range from the 7-gene panel, including BRAF, KRAS, NRAS, HRAS, RET/PTC1, RET/PTC3, and PPARG/PAX8, to 112-gene panels [95]. The small seven-gene panel includes the most common gene alterations in thyroid nodules and has a high specificity. Therefore, it may be useful as a rule-in test. According to a recent prospective study, this test can significantly increase the probability of cancer in mutated undetermined thyroid nodules, with a specificity of 95% and a PPV of 67% [98]. Commercially available panels for molecular testing of indeterminate thyroid nodules include Afirma GSC, Thyroseq v3, and ThyGeNEXT/ThyraMIR. Afirma GSC combines next-generation RNA sequencing and small genomic alterations that are not identifiable with standard methods. It is used mainly as a rule-out test with a high NPV of 96%, while the sensitivity, specificity, and PPV are 68, 91, and 47%, respectively [99]. Thyroseq v3 is a panel of 112 genes with a high NPV of 97%, and the sensitivity, specificity, and PPV are 82, 94, and 66%, respectively, and is also applicable as a rule-out test [99]. ThyGeNEXT is a next-generation sequencing panel with the purpose of sequencing gene mutations (BRAF, NRAS, HRAS, KRAS, and PIK3CA) and mRNA fusions (RET/PTC1, RET/PTC3, and PPARG/PAX8) [95]. It is combined with a miRNA risk classifier ThyraMIR, which determines the expression of growth-promoting miRNA (miR-31, -146, -222, -375, -551) and growth-suppressing miRNA (miR-29, -138, -139, -155, -204) and increases its accuracy, demonstrating sensitivity, specificity, NPV, and PPV of 90, 93, 95, and 74%, respectively [99].

In terms of prognosis, a recent study demonstrated that tumors with BRAF-like profiles positively correlate with larger tumors, higher initial tumor stage, and presence of lateral neck metastasis, compared with the RAS-like profile tumors and non-BRAF/non-RAS-like tumors which included PAX8::PPARG fusion and DICER1, EIF11AX, PTEN, and IDH1 mutations [100].

In malignant thyroid nodules (Bethesda VI), $BRAF^{V600E}$ mutation is detected in 64–76% of tumors, while TERT promoter mutations are detected in 11% of cases [101]. The presence of both mutations positively correlates with extrathyroidal extension, local and distant metastasis, tumor recurrence, and mortality [99], and predicts the development of radioiodine-refractory DTC in PTC patients [102].

5. Integrated Diagnostics of Thyroid Nodules

Even if thyroid nodules are very common, randomized clinical trials are scarce, likely due, almost partially, to the good prognosis of thyroid cancer. Instead, recommendations in clinical guidelines are largely based on observational studies and experts' opinions. Thyroid nodules mostly derive from follicular thyroid cells, and benign nodules (unifocal or multifocal) are the most common thyroid lesions. Additionally, thyroid nodules may also occur and coexist in conditions such as subacute thyroiditis, autoimmune thyroiditis, and Graves' disease, respectively. Thyroid cancer, however, occurs in 2–5% of thyroid nodules. Finally, infiltrative disorders, lymphoma, metastases from non-thyroid cancers, and paraganglioma can rarely result in a thyroid nodule. Factors related to an increased risk of cancer are summarized in Table 8.

Table 8. Thyroid nodules: factors increasing the risk of cancer.

History	▪ Childhood irradiation (head and neck) ▪ Fallout from ionizing radiation ▪ Radiation exposure ▪ Family history of thyroid cancer ▪ Enlarging nodule or rapid nodule growth ▪ Male sex ▪ Age less than 20 or more than 70 years
Clinical examination	▪ Neck lymphadenopathy ▪ Hard nodule ▪ Nodule fixed to surrounding tissues ▪ Hoarseness
Clinical investigations	▪ Suspicious ultrasound features ▪ High-risk TI-RADS classes ▪ Largest diameter > 40 mm ▪ Thyroid scintigraphy (Na[^{99m}Tc]TcO$_4$ or Na[^{123}I]I): not hot ▪ Thyroid scintigraphy ([^{99m}Tc]Tc-MIBI): high uptake, slow washout ▪ [^{18}F]FDG -avid (PET/CT) ▪ Serum calcitonin > 100 pg/mL (MTC)

Legend: TI-RADS, Thyroid Imaging-Reporting and Data System; Na[^{99m}Tc]TcO$_4$, ^{99m}Tc-pertechnetate; Na[^{123}I]I, iodine-123; PET/CT, positron emission tomography/computed tomography; MTC, medullary thyroid cancer.

As thyroid nodules are very frequent while thyroid cancers are rare and relatively indolent in most cases, the main challenge in approaching patients with thyroid nodules is to identify malignant lesions while avoiding inappropriate excess use of thyroid US, scintigraphy, FNAC, and surgery. Unfortunately, a significant lack of standardization in the preoperative characterization of thyroid nodules is reported in the literature and in guidelines, and, in turn, is commonly observed in clinical practice [103].

To further complicate the problem, a major proportion of nodules are currently detected during imaging examinations for non-thyroid issues or during so-called thyroid nodule screening. Notably, thyroid US examination is discouraged in patients without clinical evidence of thyroid enlargement or nodules, and thyroid incidentaloma, especially when <10 mm, should not be referred for additional examinations [104]. Unfortunately, such concepts are rarely incorporated into clinical practice and a plethora of non-significant nodules are detected, inducing fear and anxiety in our patients and a lot of inappropriate additional examinations [105]. Interestingly, Asian thyroid nodule practice has a more conservative approach in general, not only for indeterminate thyroid nodules [106] but also for papillary microcarcinoma [107,108].

Usually, patients experience cancer fears and anxiety during the evaluation of thyroid nodules. Accordingly, a "one-stop-shop" multidisciplinary approach represents an ideal solution. The objectives of a one-stop-shop diagnostic thyroid unit are to concentrate in one place and time all specialists required to provide a correct diagnosis and reach a clinical decision as soon as possible (ideally within 1 day). In any case, patients should be first examined by an experienced clinician (i.e., endocrinologist, nuclear medicine physician, endocrine surgeon) and a blood sample should be obtained for TSH measurement. Based on clinical examination and TSH results, most patients can be properly informed and reassured, and avoid further examinations.

Among patients with clinically relevant nodules and low-to-suppressed TSH levels, a thyroid scintigraphy with either Na[^{99m}Tc]TcO$_4$ or Na[^{123}I]I should be ordered to detect autonomously functioning nodules and exclude them from FNAC, as malignancies are exceedingly rare in such cases. In other cases, US examination should be performed and interpreted/reported according to one of the available TI-RADS systems in order to standardize the selection of nodules that need further investigation with FNAC. All in all, FNAC will be necessary for the minority of patients with non-autonomous thyroid nodules and a high-risk TIRADS score. Cytopathology examinations should be reported according to the Bethesda System for Reporting Thyroid Cytopathology and molecular imaging should be considered in selected patients with indeterminate non-Hurtle cell cytology and no additional factors in favor of surgery (i.e., multinodular goiter). Proper patient–physician communication is pivotal before any step in order to clearly explain the pros and cons of a data procedure and its impact on clinical decisions.

Finally, integrating different reports allows the coordinator physician to inform the patient about the diagnosis and formulate a tailored management plan (i.e., surgery, wait and see, thermal ablation). A diagnostic algorithm is proposed in Figure 7.

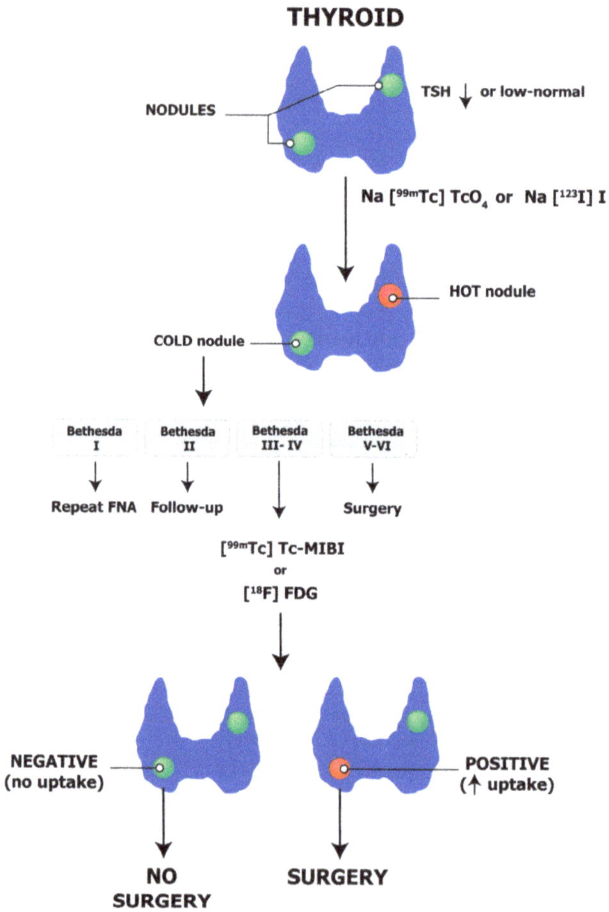

Figure 7. Thyroid nodules: integrated diagnostic flow-chart.

The implementation of this algorithm into clinical practice is mandatory to reassure patients regarding unnecessary therapeutic procedures and to identify those who need specific therapies. The value of thyroid US and its scoring systems, scintigraphy, FNAC, and molecular imaging is proven in many previously mentioned studies and requires further, more extensive, and wider integration into the national guidelines of each country to ensure widespread adoption and accessibility of integrated diagnostics of thyroid nodules.

6. Perspectives

The process presented above (i.e., clinical integration) is based on high-standing diagnostic methods and physicians' experience in interpreting and integrating different data. This is a long process requiring time and resource investment and continuous education. Artificial intelligence (AI) and machine learning (ML) can support clinicians by providing them with additional insights not routinely available in clinical practice. The high potential of AI and ML can be exploited in "integrated diagnostics", defined as the "convergence of imaging, pathology, and laboratory tests with advanced information technology" [109].

AI algorithms can be trained to analyze images from multiple modalities and detect phenotyping information that may not be obvious to the human eye. Lai and colleagues compared the diagnostic performance of artificial intelligence algorithms and radiologists with different experience levels in distinguishing benign and malignant TI-RADS 4 nodules where heterogeneity is observed in the malignancy rates. They enrolled 1117 pathologically defined TI-RADS 4 nodules and incorporated an independent external dataset of 125 TIRADS-4 nodules for testing purposes. Traditional feature-based machine learning models, deep convolutional neural network (DCNN) models, and a fusion model that integrated all prediction outcomes were used to score benign and malignant TI-RADS 4 nodules. A fivefold cross-validation approach was employed, and the diagnostic performance of each model and radiologist was compared. Briefly, in the external test, the area under the receiver operating characteristic curve (AUROC) of the three tested DCNN models ranged from 0.852 to 0.856, respectively. These values were higher than those of the three traditional ML models (0.767–0.709), respectively, and higher than that of an experienced radiologist (0.815). The fusion diagnostic model developed by the authors, with an AUROC of 0.880, outperformed the experienced radiologist in diagnosing TI-RADS 4 nodules [110]. These results demonstrate that automated clinical decision support significantly improves diagnostic accuracy, i.e., sensitivity, specificity, and AUC, and minimizes interpretation times and inter-reader variability. AI is also used in the analysis of genomic data [111].

AI algorithms analyze large amounts of data and identify genetic variations that may be associated with cancers or other common non-communicable diseases [112] or assist in the interpretation of laboratory test results, such as pathology reports, and other diagnostic data. As an example, longitudinal data analysis centered on collecting and analyzing longitudinal data, specifically cluster analysis, already showed clinical usefulness in patients with chronic renal failure for determining the required dialysis frequency [113].

Digital image analysis in pathology can identify and quantify specific cell types for quickly and accurately evaluating histological features, morphological patterns, and biologically relevant regions of interest [114]. Overall, AI is playing a growing role in the diagnosis and management of diseases through integrated diagnostics, and appears promising even in endocrine and thyroid diseases [115] (Figure 8).

However, some limitations should be considered, including the need for large amounts of data to train AI algorithms and the need for more research to validate the use of AI. Moreover, the broad implementation of AI and integrated diagnostics requires central organizations (i.e., national or international level) to ensure common structures and methodologies, standards, and data safety.

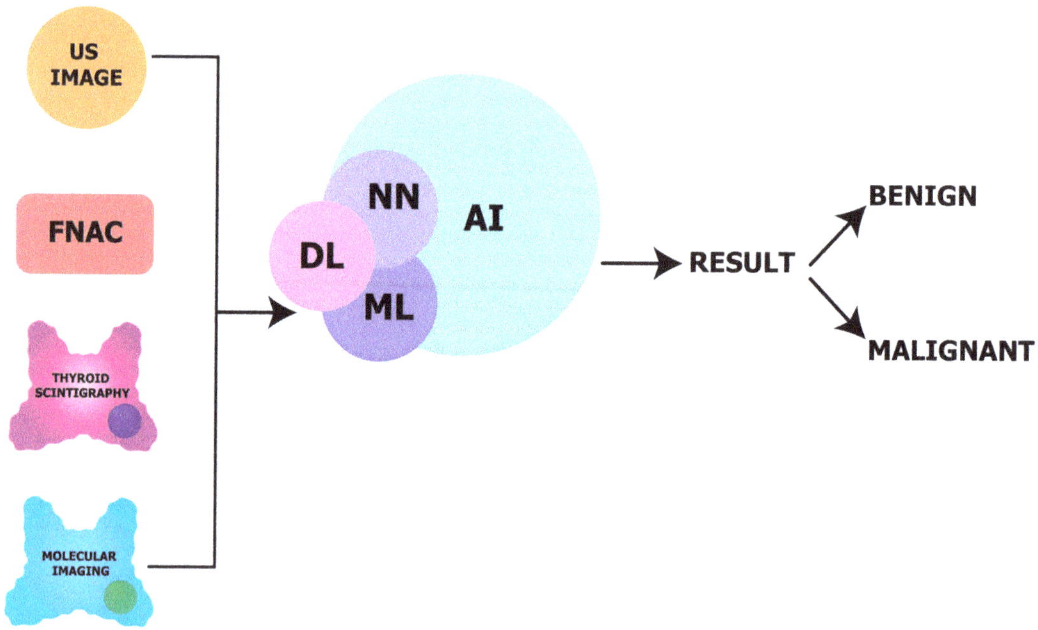

Figure 8. Potential role of deep learning, neural networks, machine learning, and artificial intelligence in thyroid nodule management. Legend: US image, ultrasonography image; FNAC, fine-needle aspiration cytology; DL, deep learning; NN, neural networks; ML, machine learning; AI, artificial intelligence.

An extensive discussion of such issues is out of the scope of our present paper; our readers are directed to a recent review by Ali MA and Mohammed MA where the inherent limitations of AI in analyzing omics data (i.e., preprocessing, datasets, validation of models, testbed applications) are illustrated while potential solutions are proposed [116].

Future research integrating deep learning, ML, and AI on US images, FNAC, thyroid scintigraphy, and specific molecular imaging is required to determine their value in discriminating benign from malignant thyroid nodules, especially in cases of indeterminate thyroid nodules where current molecular imaging is more powerful as a rule-out than rule-in test.

7. Limitations

The majority of the reported data came from retrospective studies, with inherent methodological limitations. However, the roles of US, FNAC, and thyroid scintigraphy are consolidated in clinical practice and defined in clinical guidelines. Moreover, prospective, and even randomized, studies are available for more recent molecular imaging methods as well as cost-effectiveness analysis. Accordingly, the proposed modalities and their use seem to be adequately supported by the current literature.

8. Conclusions

The current state of diagnostic medicine is well presented by the "silo metaphor", where radiology, laboratory medicine, and pathology are conceptually separate diagnostic approaches. On the other hand, progress in understanding biochemical–biological–structural interplays in human diseases, compounded with technological advances, is generating relevant multidisciplinary convergences, leading the way for a new frontier called integrated diagnostics. Thyroid nodules are commonly encountered in clinical practice and their diagnosis and therapy typically involve different specialists using different tools. Accordingly, thyroid nodules represent an ideal condition to develop and test integrated diagnostics: an appropriate integration of laboratory, imaging, and pathology data is essential to refine our diagnosis, reassure most patients with non-dangerous nodules, and quickly identify those requiring specific therapies. Furthermore, bioinformatics and computer sciences will change our current management of clinical data, allowing more personalized and tailored diagnostic approaches.

The main advantages of our proposed diagnostic flow-chart are *i.* the reduction in the number of nodules requiring any imaging procedure through use of a careful clinical examination; *ii.* the reduction in FNAC procedures by using TIRADS criteria and (selectively) functional thyroid scintigraphy; and *iii.* the reduction in inappropriate diagnostic surgeries in patients carrying cytologically indeterminate nodules through selective use of new molecular imaging procedures.

Looking forward, we believe studies concerning the management of thyroid incidentalomas are urgently needed to inform radiological reports and, hopefully, spare most patients from any further investigation. In addition, the proper use of thyroid US (i.e., avoiding "screening") should be more effectively supported by clinical societies. In such context, the selective use of more advanced methods in patients with clinically relevant, well-characterized nodules will be useful in avoiding unjustified surgeries and will be cost-effective as well.

Author Contributions: Conceptualization, L.G. and P.P.O.; writing—original draft preparation, L.G., A.C., M.T. and P.P.O.; writing—review and editing, L.G. and P.P.O.; supervision, L.G. and P.P.O. All authors have read and agreed to the published version of the manuscript.

Funding: This research received no external funding.

Institutional Review Board Statement: Not applicable.

Informed Consent Statement: Not applicable.

Data Availability Statement: Data sharing not applicable.

Conflicts of Interest: The authors declare no conflicts of interest.

References

1. Leung, A.M.; Braverman, L.E.; Pearce, E.N. History of U.S. Iodine Fortification and Supplementation. *Nutrients* **2012**, *4*, 1740–1746. [CrossRef]
2. Popoveniuc, G.; Jonklaas, J. Thyroid Nodules. *Med. Clin. N. Am.* **2012**, *96*, 329–349. [CrossRef] [PubMed]
3. Jolanta, M.D.; Bogsrud, T.V. Nuclear Medicine in Evaluation and Therapy of Nodular Thyroid. In *Thyroid Nodules*; Springer International Publishing AG: Cham, Switzerland, 2018. [CrossRef]
4. Alexander, E.K.; Cibas, E.S. Diagnosis of Thyroid Nodules. *Lancet Diabetes Endocrinol.* **2022**, *10*, 533–539. [CrossRef]
5. Schenke, S.A.; Kreissl, M.C.; Grunert, M.; Hach, A.; Haghghi, S.; Kandror, T.; Peppert, E.; Rosenbaum-Krumme, S.; Ruhlmann, V.; Stahl, A.; et al. Distribution of Functional Status of Thyroid Nodules and Malignancy Rates of Hyperfunctioning and Hypofunctioning Thyroid Nodules in Germany. *Nuklearmedizin* **2022**, *61*, 376–384. [CrossRef]
6. Hegedüs, L. Clinical Practice. The Thyroid Nodule. *N. Engl. J. Med.* **2004**, *351*, 1764–1771. [CrossRef]
7. Durante, C.; Costante, G.; Lucisano, G.; Bruno, R.; Meringolo, D.; Paciaroni, A.; Puxeddu, E.; Torlontano, M.; Tumino, S.; Attard, M.; et al. The Natural History of Benign Thyroid Nodules. *JAMA* **2015**, *313*, 926–935. [CrossRef]
8. Fisher, S.B.; Perrier, N.D. The Incidental Thyroid Nodule. *CA Cancer J. Clin.* **2018**, *68*, 97–105. [CrossRef] [PubMed]
9. Guth, S.; Theune, U.; Aberle, J.; Galach, A.; Bamberger, C.M. Very High Prevalence of Thyroid Nodules Detected by High Frequency (13 MHz) Ultrasound Examination. *Eur. J. Clin. Investig.* **2009**, *39*, 699–706. [CrossRef] [PubMed]
10. Li, L.Q.; Hilmi, O.; England, J.; Tolley, N. An Update on the Management of Thyroid Nodules: Rationalising the Guidelines. *J. Laryngol. Otol.* **2023**, *137*, 965–970. [CrossRef] [PubMed]
11. Yousem, D.M.; Huang, T.; Loevner, L.A.; Langlotz, C.P. Clinical and Economic Impact of Incidental Thyroid Lesions Found with CT and MR. *Am. J. Neuroradiol.* **1997**, *18*, 1423–1428.
12. Bibbins-Domingo, K.; Grossman, D.C.; Curry, S.J.; Barry, M.J.; Davidson, K.W.; Doubeni, C.A.; Epling, J.W.; Kemper, A.R.; Krist, A.H.; Kurth, A.E.; et al. Screening for Thyroid Cancer: US Preventive Services Task Force Recommendation Statement. *JAMA* **2017**, *317*, 1882–1887. [CrossRef] [PubMed]
13. Schenke, S.A.; Groener, D.; Grunert, M.; Stahl, A.R. Integrated Thyroid Imaging: Ultrasound and Scintigraphy. In *Integrated Diagnostics and Theranostics of Thyroid Diseases*; Giovanella, L., Ed.; Springer: Cham, Switzerland, 2023; pp. 25–62. [CrossRef]

14. de Koster, E.J.; Morreau, H.; Bleumink, G.S.; van Engen-van Grunsven, A.C.H.; de Geus-Oei, L.-F.; Links, T.P.; Wakelkamp, I.M.M.J.; Oyen, W.J.G.; Vriens, D. Molecular Diagnostics and [18F]FDG-PET/CT in Indeterminate Thyroid Nodules: Complementing Techniques or Waste of Valuable Resources? *Thyroid* 2023, *online ahead of print*. [CrossRef]
15. de Koster, E.J.; Vriens, D.; van Aken, M.O.; Dijkhorst-Oei, L.T.; Oyen, W.J.G.; Peeters, R.P.; Schepers, A.; de Geus-Oei, L.F.; van den Hout, W.B. FDG-PET/CT in Indeterminate Thyroid Nodules: Cost-Utility Analysis alongside a Randomised Controlled Trial. *Eur. J. Nucl. Med. Mol. Imaging* **2022**, *49*, 3452–3469. [CrossRef] [PubMed]
16. Wale, A.; Miles, K.A.; Young, B.; Zammit, C.; Williams, A.; Quin, J.; Dizdarevic, S. Combined (99m)Tc-Methoxyisobutylisonitrile Scintigraphy and Fine-Needle Aspiration Cytology Offers an Accurate and Potentially Cost-Effective Investigative Strategy for the Assessment of Solitary or Dominant Thyroid Nodules. *Eur. J. Nucl. Med. Mol. Imaging* **2014**, *41*, 105–115. [CrossRef]
17. Heinzel, A.; Müller, D.; Behrendt, F.F.; Giovanella, L.; Mottaghy, F.M.; Verburg, F.A. Thyroid Nodules with Indeterminate Cytology: Molecular Imaging with ^{99}mTc-Methoxyisobutylisonitrile (MIBI) Is More Cost-Effective than the Afirma Gene Expression Classifier. *Eur. J. Nucl. Med. Mol. Imaging* **2014**, *41*, 1497–1500. [CrossRef] [PubMed]
18. Haugen, B.R.; Alexander, E.K.; Bible, K.C.; Doherty, G.M.; Mandel, S.J.; Nikiforov, Y.E.; Pacini, F.; Randolph, G.W.; Sawka, A.M.; Schlumberger, M.; et al. 2015 American Thyroid Association Management Guidelines for Adult Patients with Thyroid Nodules and Differentiated Thyroid Cancer: The American Thyroid Association Guidelines Task Force on Thyroid Nodules and Differentiated Thyroid Cancer. *Thyroid* **2016**, *26*, 1–133. [CrossRef] [PubMed]
19. Capezzone, M.; Marchisotta, S.; Cantara, S.; Busonero, G.; Brilli, L.; Pazaitou-Panayiotou, K.; Carli, A.F.; Caruso, G.; Toti, P.; Capitani, S.; et al. Familial Non-Medullary Thyroid Carcinoma Displays the Features of Clinical Anticipation Suggestive of a Distinct Biological Entity. *Endocr. Relat. Cancer* **2008**, *15*, 1075–1081. [CrossRef] [PubMed]
20. Loh, K.C. Familial Nonmedullary Thyroid Carcinoma: A Meta-Review of Case Series. *Thyroid* **1997**, *7*, 107–113. [CrossRef] [PubMed]
21. Stoffer, S.S.; van Dyke, D.L.; Bach, J.V.; Szpunar, W.; Weiss, L. Familial Papillary Carcinoma of the Thyroid. *Am. J. Med. Genet.* **1986**, *25*, 775–782. [CrossRef] [PubMed]
22. Moses, W.; Weng, J.; Kebebew, E. Prevalence, Clinicopathologic Features, and Somatic Genetic Mutation Profile in Familial versus Sporadic Nonmedullary Thyroid Cancer. *Thyroid* **2011**, *21*, 367–371. [CrossRef] [PubMed]
23. Mazeh, H.; Benavidez, J.; Poehls, J.L.; Youngwirth, L.; Chen, H.; Sippel, R.S. In Patients with Thyroid Cancer of Follicular Cell Origin, a Family History of Nonmedullary Thyroid Cancer in One First-Degree Relative Is Associated with More Aggressive Disease. *Thyroid* **2012**, *22*, 3–8. [CrossRef]
24. Park, Y.J.; Ahn, H.Y.; Choi, H.S.; Kim, K.W.; Park, D.J.; Cho, B.Y. The Long-Term Outcomes of the Second Generation of Familial Nonmedullary Thyroid Carcinoma Are More Aggressive than Sporadic Cases. *Thyroid* **2012**, *22*, 356–362. [CrossRef] [PubMed]
25. Balinisteanu, I.; Panzaru, M.C.; Caba, L.; Ungureanu, M.C.; Florea, A.; Grigore, A.M.; Gorduza, E.V. Cancer Predisposition Syndromes and Thyroid Cancer: Keys for a Short Two-Way Street. *Biomedicines* **2023**, *11*, 2143. [CrossRef] [PubMed]
26. Dean, D.S.; Gharib, H. Epidemiology of Thyroid Nodules. *Best Pract. Res. Clin. Endocrinol. Metab.* **2008**, *22*, 901–911. [CrossRef] [PubMed]
27. Bomeli, S.R.; LeBeau, S.O.; Ferris, R.L. Evaluation of a Thyroid Nodule. *Otolaryngol. Clin. N. Am.* **2010**, *43*, 229. [CrossRef] [PubMed]
28. McCoy, K.L.; Jabbour, N.; Ogilvie, J.B.; Ohori, N.P.; Carty, S.E.; Yim, J.H. The Incidence of Cancer and Rate of False-Negative Cytology in Thyroid Nodules Greater than or Equal to 4 Cm in Size. *Surgery* **2007**, *142*, 837–844.e3. [CrossRef] [PubMed]
29. Raza, S.N.; Shah, M.D.; Palme, C.E.; Hall, F.T.; Eski, S.; Freeman, J.L. Risk Factors for Well-Differentiated Thyroid Carcinoma in Patients with Thyroid Nodular Disease. *Otolaryngol. Head Neck Surg.* **2008**, *139*, 21–26. [CrossRef]
30. Koulouri, O.; Moran, C.; Halsall, D.; Chatterjee, K.; Gurnell, M. Pitfalls in the Measurement and Interpretation of Thyroid Function Tests. *Best Pract. Res. Clin. Endocrinol. Metab.* **2013**, *27*, 745–762. [CrossRef]
31. D'Aurizio, F.; Kratzsch, J.; Gruson, D.; Petranović Ovčariček, P.; Giovanella, L. Free Thyroxine Measurement in Clinical Practice: How to Optimize Indications, Analytical Procedures, and Interpretation Criteria While Waiting for Global Standardization. *Crit. Rev. Clin. Lab. Sci.* **2023**, *60*, 101–140. [CrossRef]
32. Giovanella, L.; Petranović Ovčariček, P. Functional and Molecular Thyroid Imaging. *Q. J. Nucl. Med. Mol. Imaging* **2022**, *66*, 86–92. [CrossRef]
33. Kronenberg, H.M.; Melmed, S.; Larsen, P.R.; Polonsky, K.S. Principles of Endocrinology. In *Williams Textbook of Endocrinology*; Melmed, S., Polonsky, K.S., Larsen, P.R., Kronenberg, H.M., Eds.; Elsevier Saunders: Philadelphia, PA, USA, 2011; pp. 3–12.
34. Giovanella, L.; Avram, A.M.; Ovčariček, P.P.; Clerc, J. Thyroid Functional and Molecular Imaging. *Presse Med.* **2022**, *51*, 104116. [CrossRef] [PubMed]
35. Jonklaas, J.; Bianco, A.C.; Bauer, A.J.; Burman, K.D.; Cappola, A.R.; Celi, F.S.; Cooper, D.S.; Kim, B.W.; Peeters, R.P.; Rosenthal, M.S.; et al. Guidelines for the Treatment of Hypothyroidism: Prepared by the American Thyroid Association Task Force on Thyroid Hormone Replacement. *Thyroid* **2014**, *24*, 1670–1751. [CrossRef] [PubMed]
36. Demers, L.M.; Spencer, C.A. Laboratory Medicine Practice Guidelines: Laboratory Support for the Diagnosis and Monitoring of Thyroid Disease. *Clin. Endocrinol.* **2003**, *58*, 138–140. [CrossRef] [PubMed]
37. Plebani, M.; Giovanella, L. Reflex TSH Strategy: The Good, the Bad and the Ugly. *Clin. Chem. Lab. Med.* **2019**, *58*, 1–2. [CrossRef] [PubMed]

38. Sheehan, M.T. Biochemical Testing of the Thyroid: TSH Is the Best and, Oftentimes, Only Test Needed—A Review for Primary Care. *Clin. Med. Res.* **2016**, *14*, 83–92. [CrossRef]
39. Giovanella, L.; D'Aurizio, F.; Campenni', A.; Ruggeri, R.; Baldari, S.; Verburg, F.; Trimboli, P.; Ceriani, L. Searching For The Most Effective Thyrotropin (TSH) Threshold To Rule-Out Autonomously Functioning Thyroid Nodules In Iodine Deficient Regions. *Endocrine* **2016**, *54*, 757–761. [CrossRef] [PubMed]
40. Repplinger, D.; Bargren, A.; Zhang, Y.W.; Adler, J.T.; Haymart, M.; Chen, H. Is Hashimoto's Thyroiditis a Risk Factor for Papillary Thyroid Cancer? *J. Surg. Res.* **2008**, *150*, 49–52. [CrossRef]
41. Giovanella, L.; D'Aurizio, F.; Algeciras-Schimnich, A.; Görges, R.; Petranovic Ovcaricek, P.; Tuttle, R.M.; Visser, W.E.; Verburg, F.A. Thyroglobulin and Thyroglobulin Antibody: An Updated Clinical and Laboratory Expert Consensus. *Eur. J. Endocrinol.* **2023**, *189*, R11–R27. [CrossRef] [PubMed]
42. Wells, S.A.; Asa, S.L.; Dralle, H.; Elisei, R.; Evans, D.B.; Gagel, R.F.; Lee, N.; MacHens, A.; Moley, J.F.; Pacini, F.; et al. Revised American Thyroid Association Guidelines for the Management of Medullary Thyroid Carcinoma. *Thyroid* **2015**, *25*, 567–610. [CrossRef]
43. Verbeek, H.H.; de Groot, J.W.B.; Sluiter, W.J.; Kobold, A.C.M.; van den Heuvel, E.R.; Plukker, J.T.; Links, T.P. Calcitonin Testing for Detection of Medullary Thyroid Cancer in People with Thyroid Nodules. *Cochrane Database Syst. Rev.* **2020**, *3*, CD010159. [CrossRef]
44. Rago, T.; Vitti, P. Role of Thyroid Ultrasound in the Diagnostic Evaluation of Thyroid Nodules. *Best Pract. Res. Clin. Endocrinol. Metab.* **2008**, *22*, 913–928. [CrossRef]
45. Tessler, F.N.; Middleton, W.D.; Grant, E.G.; Hoang, J.K.; Berland, L.L.; Teefey, S.A.; Cronan, J.J.; Beland, M.D.; Desser, T.S.; Frates, M.C.; et al. ACR Thyroid Imaging, Reporting and Data System (TI-RADS): White Paper of the ACR TI-RADS Committee. *J. Am. Coll. Radiol.* **2017**, *14*, 587–595. [CrossRef] [PubMed]
46. Russ, G.; Bonnema, S.J.; Erdogan, M.F.; Durante, C.; Ngu, R.; Leenhardt, L. European Thyroid Association Guidelines for Ultrasound Malignancy Risk Stratification of Thyroid Nodules in Adults: The EU-TIRADS. *Eur. Thyroid J.* **2017**, *6*, 225–237. [CrossRef] [PubMed]
47. Shin, J.H.; Baek, J.H.; Chung, J.; Ha, E.J.; Kim, J.H.; Lee, Y.H.; Lim, H.K.; Moon, W.J.; Na, D.G.; Park, J.S.; et al. Ultrasonography Diagnosis and Imaging-Based Management of Thyroid Nodules: Revised Korean Society of Thyroid Radiology Consensus Statement and Recommendations. *Korean J. Radiol.* **2016**, *17*, 370–395. [CrossRef]
48. Gharib, H.; Papini, E.; Garber, J.R.; Duick, D.S.; Harrell, R.M.; Hegedüs, L.; Paschke, R.; Valcavi, R.; Vitti, P. American association of clinical endocrinologists, american college of endocrinology, and associazione medici endocrinologi medical guidelines for clinical practice for the diagnosis and management of thyroid nodules-2016 update. *Endocr. Pract.* **2016**, *22*, 622–639. [CrossRef] [PubMed]
49. Perros, P.; Boelaert, K.; Colley, S.; Evans, C.; Evans, R.M.; Gerrard Ba, G.; Gilbert, J.; Harrison, B.; Johnson, S.J.; Giles, T.E.; et al. Guidelines for the Management of Thyroid Cancer. *Clin. Endocrinol.* **2014**, *81* (Suppl. 1), 1–122. [CrossRef] [PubMed]
50. Hoang, J.K.; Asadollahi, S.; Durante, C.; Hegedüs, L.; Papini, E.; Tessler, F.N. An International Survey on Utilization of Five Thyroid Nodule Risk Stratification Systems: A Needs Assessment with Future Implications. *Thyroid* **2022**, *32*, 675–681. [CrossRef]
51. Durante, C.; Hegedüs, L.; Czarniecka, A.; Paschke, R.; Russ, G.; Schmitt, F.; Soares, P.; Solymosi, T.; Papini, E. 2023 European Thyroid Association Clinical Practice Guidelines for Thyroid Nodule Management. *Eur. Thyroid J.* **2023**, *12*, e230067. [CrossRef]
52. Seifert, P.; Schenke, S.; Zimny, M.; Stahl, A.; Grunert, M.; Klemenz, B.; Freesmeyer, M.; Kreissl, M.C.; Herrmann, K.; Görges, R. Diagnostic Performance of Kwak, EU, ACR, and Korean TIRADS as Well as ATA Guidelines for the Ultrasound Risk Stratification of Non-Autonomously Functioning Thyroid Nodules in a Region with Long History of Iodine Deficiency: A German Multicenter Trial. *Cancers* **2021**, *13*, 4467. [CrossRef]
53. Kuru, B.; Kefeli, M.; Danaci, M. Comparison of 5 Thyroid Ultrasound Stratification Systems for Differentiation of Benign and Malignant Nodules and to Avoid Biopsy Using Histology as Reference Standard. *Endocr. Pract.* **2021**, *27*, 1093–1099. [CrossRef]
54. Li, X.; Peng, C.; Liu, Y.; Hu, Y.; Yang, L.; Yu, Y.; Zeng, H.; Huang, W.; Li, Q.; Tao, N.; et al. Modified American College of Radiology Thyroid Imaging Reporting and Data System and Modified Artificial Intelligence Thyroid Imaging Reporting and Data System for Thyroid Nodules: A Multicenter Retrospective Study. *Thyroid* 2023, *online ahead of print*. [CrossRef]
55. Giovanella, L.; Avram, A.M.; Iakovou, I.; Kwak, J.; Lawson, S.A.; Lulaj, E.; Luster, M.; Piccardo, A.; Schmidt, M.; Tulchinsky, M.; et al. EANM Practice Guideline/SNMMI Procedure Standard for RAIU and Thyroid Scintigraphy. *Eur. J. Nucl. Med. Mol. Imaging* **2019**, *46*, 2514–2525. [CrossRef]
56. Giovanella, L.; Ceriani, L.; Treglia, G. Role of Isotope Scan, Including Positron Emission Tomography/Computed Tomography, in Nodular Goitre. *Best Pract. Res. Clin. Endocrinol. Metab.* **2014**, *28*, 507–518. [CrossRef] [PubMed]
57. Hetrakul, N.; Civelek, A.C.; Stagg, C.A.; Udelsman, R. In Vitro Accumulation of Technetium-99m-Sestamibi in Human Parathyroid Mitochondria. *Surgery* **2001**, *130*, 1011–1018. [CrossRef] [PubMed]
58. Karamzade-Ziarati, N.; Manafi-Farid, R.; Ataeinia, B.; Langsteger, W.; Pirich, C.; Mottaghy, F.M.; Beheshti, M. Molecular Imaging of Bone Metastases Using Tumor-Targeted Tracers. *Q. J. Nucl. Med. Mol. Imaging* **2019**, *63*, 136–149. [CrossRef] [PubMed]
59. Delmaire, C.; Savatovsky, J.; Boulanger, T.; Dhermain, F.; Le Rhun, E.; Météllus, P.; Gerber, S.; Carsin-Nicole, B.; Petyt, G. Imagerie Des Métastases Cérébrales. *Cancer/Radiothérapie* **2015**, *19*, 16–19. [CrossRef] [PubMed]
60. Liu, H.; Zhan, H.; Sun, D. Comparison of 99mTc-MIBI Scintigraphy, Ultrasound, and Mammography for the Diagnosis of BI-RADS 4 Category Lesions. *BMC Cancer* **2020**, *20*, 1–8. [CrossRef]

61. Hurtado-López, L.M.; Arellano-Montaño, S.; Torres-Acosta, E.M.; Zaldivar-Ramirez, F.R.; Duarte-Torres, R.M.; Alonso-De-Ruiz, P.; Martínez-Duncker, I.; Martínez-Duncker, C. Combined Use of Fine-Needle Aspiration Biopsy, MIBI Scans and Frozen Section Biopsy Offers the Best Diagnostic Accuracy in the Assessment of the Hypofunctioning Solitary Thyroid Nodule. *Eur. J. Nucl. Med. Mol. Imaging* **2004**, *31*, 1273–1279. [CrossRef]
62. Giovanella, L.; Campenni, A.; Treglia, G.; Verburg, F.A.; Trimboli, P.; Ceriani, L.; Bongiovanni, M. Molecular Imaging with (99m)Tc-MIBI and Molecular Testing for Mutations in Differentiating Benign from Malignant Follicular Neoplasm: A Prospective Comparison. *Eur. J. Nucl. Med. Mol. Imaging* **2016**, *43*, 1018–1026. [CrossRef]
63. Campennì, A.; Giovanella, L.; Siracusa, M.; Alibrandi, A.; Pignata, S.A.; Giovinazzo, S.; Trimarchi, F.; Ruggeri, R.M.; Baldari, S. (99m)Tc-Methoxy-Isobutyl-Isonitrile Scintigraphy Is a Useful Tool for Assessing the Risk of Malignancy in Thyroid Nodules with Indeterminate Fine-Needle Cytology. *Thyroid* **2016**, *26*, 1101–1109. [CrossRef]
64. Campennì, A.; Siracusa, M.; Ruggeri, R.M.; Laudicella, R.; Pignata, S.A.; Baldari, S.; Giovanella, L. Differentiating Malignant from Benign Thyroid Nodules with Indeterminate Cytology by 99m Tc-MIBI Scan: A New Quantitative Method for Improving Diagnostic Accuracy. *Sci. Rep.* **2017**, *7*, 6147. [CrossRef]
65. Schenke, S.A.; Campennì, A.; Tuncel, M.; Bottoni, G.; Sager, S.; Crncic, T.B.; Rozic, D.; Görges, R.; Özcan, P.P.; Groener, D.; et al. Diagnostic Performance of 99mTc-Methoxy-Isobuty-Isonitrile (MIBI) for Risk Stratification of Hypofunctioning Thyroid Nodules: A European Multicenter Study. *Diagnostics* **2022**, *12*, 1358. [CrossRef]
66. Schenke, S.A.; Campenni, A.; Tuncel, M.; Piccardo, A.; Sager, S.; Bogovic Crncic, T.; Rozic, D.; Goerges, R.; Özcan Kara, P.P.; Groener, D.; et al. A Multicenter Survey of Current Practices of 99mTc-Methoxy-Isobutyl-Isonitrile (MIBI) Imaging for the Diagnosis of Thyroid Nodules: More Standardization Is Essential. *Clin. Transl. Imaging* **2021**, *9*, 413–422. [CrossRef]
67. Giovanella, L.; Suriano, S.; Ricci, R.; Ceriani, L.; Verburg, F.A. Postsurgical Thyroid Remnant Estimation by (^{99}m) Tc-Pertechnetate Scintigraphy Predicts Radioiodine Ablation Effectiveness in Patients with Differentiated Thyroid Carcinoma. *Head Neck* **2011**, *33*, 552–556. [CrossRef] [PubMed]
68. Saggiorato, E.; Angusti, T.; Rosas, R.; Martinese, M.; Finessi, M.; Arecco, F.; Trevisiol, E.; Bergero, N.; Puligheddu, B.; Volante, M.; et al. 99mTc-MIBI Imaging in the Presurgical Characterization of Thyroid Follicular Neoplasms: Relationship to Multidrug Resistance Protein Expression. *J. Nucl. Med.* **2009**, *50*, 1785–1793. [CrossRef] [PubMed]
69. Piga, M.; Cocco, M.C.; Serra, A.; Boi, F.; Loy, M.; Mariotti, S. The Usefulness of 99mTc-SestaMIBI Thyroid Scan in the Differential Diagnosis and Management of Amiodarone-Induced Thyrotoxicosis. *Eur. J. Endocrinol.* **2008**, *159*, 423–429. [CrossRef] [PubMed]
70. Pattison, D.A.; Westcott, J.; Lichtenstein, M.; Toh, H.B.; Gunawardana, D.; Better, N.; Forehan, S.; Sivaratnam, D. Quantitative Assessment of Thyroid-to-Background Ratio Improves the Interobserver Reliability of Technetium-99m Sestamibi Thyroid Scintigraphy for Investigation of Amiodarone-Induced Thyrotoxicosis. *Nucl. Med. Commun.* **2015**, *36*, 356–362. [CrossRef]
71. Hervás Morón, A. PET-CT in Oncology. *Clin. Transl. Oncol.* **2007**, *9*, 473–474. [CrossRef]
72. Meyer, H.J.; Wienke, A.; Surov, A. Associations between GLUT Expression and SUV Values Derived from FDG-PET in Different Tumors-A Systematic Review and Meta Analysis. *PLoS ONE* **2019**, *14*, e0217781. [CrossRef]
73. de Koster, E.J.; de Geus-Oei, L.F.; Brouwers, A.H.; van Dam, E.W.C.M.; Dijkhorst-Oei, L.T.; van Engen-van Grunsven, A.C.H.; van den Hout, W.B.; Klooker, T.K.; Netea-Maier, R.T.; Snel, M.; et al. [18F]FDG-PET/CT to Prevent Futile Surgery in Indeterminate Thyroid Nodules: A Blinded, Randomised Controlled Multicentre Trial. *Eur. J. Nucl. Med. Mol. Imaging* **2022**, *49*, 1970–1984. [CrossRef]
74. Vriens, D.; De Wilt, J.H.W.; Van Der Wilt, G.J.; Netea-Maier, R.T.; Oyen, W.J.G.; De Geus-Oei, L.F. The Role of [18F]-2-Fluoro-2-Deoxy-d-Glucose-Positron Emission Tomography in Thyroid Nodules with Indeterminate Fine-Needle Aspiration Biopsy: Systematic Review and Meta-Analysis of the Literature. *Cancer* **2011**, *117*, 4582–4594. [CrossRef]
75. Wang, N.; Zhai, H.; Lu, Y. Is Fluorine-18 Fluorodeoxyglucose Positron Emission Tomography Useful for the Thyroid Nodules with Indeterminate Fine Needle Aspiration Biopsy? A Meta-Analysis of the Literature. *J. Otolaryngol. Head Neck Surg.* **2013**, *42*, 38. [CrossRef]
76. Castellana, M.; Trimboli, P.; Piccardo, A.; Giovanella, L.; Treglia, G. Performance of 18 F-FDG PET/CT in Selecting Thyroid Nodules with Indeterminate Fine-Needle Aspiration Cytology for Surgery. A Systematic Review and a Meta-Analysis. *J. Clin. Med.* **2019**, *8*, 1333. [CrossRef] [PubMed]
77. Giovanella, L.; Milan, L.; Piccardo, A.; Bottoni, G.; Cuzzocrea, M.; Paone, G.; Ceriani, L. Radiomics Analysis Improves 18FDG PET/CT-Based Risk Stratification of Cytologically Indeterminate Thyroid Nodules. *Endocrine* **2022**, *75*, 202–210. [CrossRef] [PubMed]
78. de Koster, E.J.; Noortman, W.A.; Mostert, J.M.; Booij, J.; Brouwer, C.B.; de Keizer, B.; de Klerk, J.M.H.; Oyen, W.J.G.; van Velden, F.H.P.; de Geus-Oei, L.F.; et al. Quantitative Classification and Radiomics of [18F]FDG-PET/CT in Indeterminate Thyroid Nodules. *Eur. J. Nucl. Med. Mol. Imaging* **2022**, *49*, 2174–2188. [CrossRef] [PubMed]
79. Siegel, R.L.; Miller, K.D.; Jemal, A. Cancer Statistics, 2020. *CA Cancer J. Clin.* **2020**, *70*, 7–30. [CrossRef]
80. Moon, W.J.; So, L.J.; Jeong, H.L.; Dong, G.N.; Baek, J.H.; Young, H.L.; Kim, J.; Hyun, S.K.; Jun, S.B.; Dong, H.L. Benign and Malignant Thyroid Nodules: US Differentiation--Multicenter Retrospective Study. *Radiology* **2008**, *247*, 762–770. [CrossRef] [PubMed]
81. Kim, M.J.; Kim, E.K.; Park, S.I.; Kim, B.M.; Kwak, J.Y.; Kim, S.J.; Youk, J.H.; Park, S.H. US-Guided Fine-Needle Aspiration of Thyroid Nodules: Indications, Techniques, Results. *Radiographics* **2008**, *28*, 1869–1886. [CrossRef] [PubMed]
82. Black, J.M. Anticoagulation in Elective Surgery. *Plast. Surg. Nurs.* **2004**, *24*, 8–11. [CrossRef]

83. Oertel, Y.C. Fine-Needle Aspiration of the Thyroid: Technique and Terminology. *Endocrinol. Metab. Clin. N. Am.* **2007**, *36*, 737–751. [CrossRef]
84. Santos, J.E.; Leiman, G. Nonaspiration Fine Needle Cytology. Application of a New Technique to Nodular Thyroid Disease. *Acta Cytol.* **1988**, *32*, 353–356.
85. Degirmenci, B.; Haktanir, A.; Albayrak, R.; Acar, M.; Sahin, D.A.; Sahin, O.; Yucel, A.; Caliskan, G. Sonographically Guided Fine-Needle Biopsy of Thyroid Nodules: The Effects of Nodule Characteristics, Sampling Technique, and Needle Size on the Adequacy of Cytological Material. *Clin. Radiol.* **2007**, *62*, 798–803. [CrossRef]
86. Titton, R.L.; Gervais, D.A.; Boland, G.W.; Maher, M.M.; Mueller, P.R. Sonography and Sonographically Guided Fine-Needle Aspiration Biopsy of the Thyroid Gland: Indications and Techniques, Pearls and Pitfalls. *AJR Am. J. Roentgenol.* **2003**, *181*, 267–271. [CrossRef]
87. Quinn, S.F.; Nelson, H.A.; Demlow, T.A. Thyroid Biopsies: Fine-Needle Aspiration Biopsy versus Spring-Activated Core Biopsy Needle in 102 Patients. *J. Vasc. Interv. Radiol.* **1994**, *5*, 619–623. [CrossRef] [PubMed]
88. Taki, S.; Kakuda, K.; Kakuma, K.; Annen, Y.; Katada, S.; Yamashita, R.; Kosugi, M.; Michigishi, T.; Tonami, N. Thyroid Nodules: Evaluation with US-Guided Core Biopsy with an Automated Biopsy Gun. *Radiology* **1997**, *202*, 874–877. [CrossRef] [PubMed]
89. Pusztaszeri, M.; Rossi, E.D.; Auger, M.; Baloch, Z.; Bishop, J.; Bongiovanni, M.; Chandra, A.; Cochand-Priollet, B.; Fadda, G.; Hirokawa, M.; et al. The Bethesda System for Reporting Thyroid Cytopathology: Proposed Modifications and Updates for the Second Edition from an International Panel. *Acta Cytol.* **2016**, *60*, 399–405. [CrossRef] [PubMed]
90. Nardi, F.; Basolo, F.; Crescenzi, A.; Fadda, G.; Frasoldati, A.; Orlandi, F.; Palombini, L.; Papini, E.; Zini, M.; Pontecorvi, A.; et al. Italian Consensus for the Classification and Reporting of Thyroid Cytology. *J. Endocrinol. Investig.* **2014**, *37*, 593–599. [CrossRef] [PubMed]
91. Cross, P.; Chandra, A.; Giles, T.; Johnson, S.; Kocjan, G.; Poller, D. *Guidance on the Reporting of Thyroid Cytology Specimens*; The Royal College of Pathologists: London, UK, 2016.
92. Ali, S.Z.; Baloch, Z.W.; Cochand-Priollet, B.; Schmitt, F.C.; Vielh, P.; VanderLaan, P.A. The 2023 Bethesda System for Reporting Thyroid Cytopathology. *Thyroid* **2023**, *33*, 1039–1044. [CrossRef]
93. Cibas, E.S.; Ali, S.Z. The 2017 Bethesda System for Reporting Thyroid Cytopathology. *Thyroid* **2017**, *27*, 1341–1346. [CrossRef]
94. Bongiovanni, M.; Bellevicine, C.; Troncone, G.; Sykiotis, G.P. Approach to Cytological Indeterminate Thyroid Nodules. *Gland Surg.* **2019**, *8* (Suppl. 2), S98–S104. [CrossRef]
95. Vignali, P.; Macerola, E.; Poma, A.M.; Sparavelli, R.; Basolo, F. Indeterminate Thyroid Nodules: From Cytology to Molecular Testing. *Diagnostics* **2023**, *13*, 3008. [CrossRef]
96. Agrawal, N.; Akbani, R.; Aksoy, B.A.; Ally, A.; Arachchi, H.; Asa, S.L.; Auman, J.T.; Balasundaram, M.; Balu, S.; Baylin, S.B.; et al. Integrated Genomic Characterization of Papillary Thyroid Carcinoma. *Cell* **2014**, *159*, 676–690. [CrossRef]
97. Marotta, V.; Bifulco, M.; Vitale, M. Significance of RAS Mutations in Thyroid Benign Nodules and Non-Medullary Thyroid Cancer. *Cancers* **2021**, *13*, 3785. [CrossRef]
98. Bardet, S.; Goardon, N.; Lequesne, J.; Vaur, D.; Ciappuccini, R.; Leconte, A.; Monpeyssen, H.; Saguet-Rysanek, V.; Clarisse, B.; Lasne-Cardon, A.; et al. Diagnostic and Prognostic Value of a 7-Panel Mutation Testing in Thyroid Nodules with Indeterminate Cytology: The SWEETMAC Study. *Endocrine* **2021**, *71*, 407–417. [CrossRef]
99. Alzumaili, B.; Sadow, P.M. Update on Molecular Diagnostics in Thyroid Pathology: A Review. *Genes* **2023**, *14*, 1314. [CrossRef] [PubMed]
100. Yoo, S.K.; Lee, S.; Kim, S.J.; Jee, H.G.; Kim, B.A.; Cho, H.; Song, Y.S.; Cho, S.W.; Won, J.K.; Shin, J.Y.; et al. Comprehensive Analysis of the Transcriptional and Mutational Landscape of Follicular and Papillary Thyroid Cancers. *PLoS Genet.* **2016**, *12*, e1006239. [CrossRef]
101. Labourier, E.; Fahey, T.J. Preoperative Molecular Testing in Thyroid Nodules with Bethesda VI Cytology: Clinical Experience and Review of the Literature. *Diagn. Cytopathol.* **2021**, *49*, E175–E180. [CrossRef] [PubMed]
102. Liu, J.; Liu, R.; Shen, X.; Zhu, G.; Li, B.; Xing, M. The Genetic Duet of BRAF V600E and TERT Promoter Mutations Robustly Predicts Loss of Radioiodine Avidity in Recurrent Papillary Thyroid Cancer. *J. Nucl. Med.* **2020**, *61*, 177–182. [CrossRef] [PubMed]
103. Eloy, C.; Russ, G.; Suciu, V.; Johnson, S.J.; Rossi, E.D.; Pantanowitz, L.; Vielh, P. Preoperative Diagnosis of Thyroid Nodules: An Integrated Multidisciplinary Approach. *Cancer Cytopathol.* **2022**, *130*, 320–325. [CrossRef]
104. Iglesias, P.; Acosta, M.; Sánchez, R.; Fernández-Reyes, M.J.; Mon, C.; Díez, J.J. Ambulatory Blood Pressure Monitoring in Patients with Hyperthyroidism before and after Control of Thyroid Function. *Clin. Endocrinol.* **2005**, *63*, 66–72. [CrossRef]
105. Jansen, T.; Stikkelbroeck, N.; van de Ven, A.; van Engen-van Grunsven, I.; Janssen, M.; Bonenkamp, H.; Gotthardt, M.; Netea-Maier, R.T. Clinical Characteristics, Diagnostic Approach and Outcome of Thyroid Incidental Findings vs. Clinically Overt Thyroid Nodules: An Observational Single-Centre Study. *Cancers* **2023**, *15*, 2350. [CrossRef]
106. Vuong, H.G.; Ngo, H.T.T.; Bychkov, A.; Jung, C.K.; Vu, T.H.; Lu, K.B.; Kakudo, K.; Kondo, T. Differences in Surgical Resection Rate and Risk of Malignancy in Thyroid Cytopathology Practice between Western and Asian Countries: A Systematic Review and Meta-Analysis. *Cancer Cytopathol.* **2020**, *128*, 238–249. [CrossRef]
107. Sakai, T.; Sugitani, I.; Ebina, A.; Fukuoka, O.; Toda, K.; Mitani, H.; Yamada, K. Active Surveillance for T1bN0M0 Papillary Thyroid Carcinoma. *Thyroid* **2019**, *29*, 59–63. [CrossRef] [PubMed]

108. Miyauchi, A.; Kudo, T.; Ito, Y.; Oda, H.; Sasai, H.; Higashiyama, T.; Fukushima, M.; Masuoka, H.; Kihara, M.; Miya, A. Estimation of the Lifetime Probability of Disease Progression of Papillary Microcarcinoma of the Thyroid during Active Surveillance. *Surgery* **2018**, *163*, 48–52. [CrossRef] [PubMed]
109. Plebani, M.; Lippi, G. Integrated Diagnostics: The Future of Diagnostic Medicine? In *Integrated Diagnostics and Theranostics of Thyroid Diseases*; Giovanella, L., Ed.; Springer: Cham, Switzerland, 2023; pp. 1–4. [CrossRef]
110. Lai, M.; Feng, B.; Yao, J.; Wang, Y.; Pan, Q.; Chen, Y.; Chen, C.; Feng, N.; Shi, F.; Tian, Y.; et al. Value of Artificial Intelligence in Improving the Accuracy of Diagnosing TI-RADS Category 4 Nodules. *Ultrasound Med. Biol.* **2023**, *49*, 2413–2421. [CrossRef] [PubMed]
111. Wetterstrand, M.S. The Cost of Sequencing a Human Genome. Available online: https://www.genome.gov/about-genomics/fact-sheets/Sequencing-Human-Genome-cost (accessed on 21 December 2023).
112. Dlamini, Z.; Francies, F.Z.; Hull, R.; Marima, R. Artificial Intelligence (AI) and Big Data in Cancer and Precision Oncology. *Comput. Struct. Biotechnol. J.* **2020**, *18*, 2300–2311. [CrossRef]
113. Seyala, N.; Abdullah, S.N. Cluster Analysis on Longitudinal Data of Patients with Kidney Dialysis Using a Smoothing Cubic B-Spline Model. *Int. J. Math. Stat. Comput. Sci.* **2024**, *2*, 85–95. [CrossRef]
114. Bera, K.; Schalper, K.A.; Rimm, D.L.; Velcheti, V.; Madabhushi, A. Artificial Intelligence in Digital Pathology—New Tools for Diagnosis and Precision Oncology. *Nat. Rev. Clin. Oncol.* **2019**, *16*, 703–715. [CrossRef]
115. Milan, L. Artificial Intelligence and Machine Learning in Integrated Diagnostic. In *Integrated Diagnostics and Theranostics of Thyroid Diseases*; Giovanella, L., Ed.; Springer: Cham, Switzerland, 2023; pp. 5–11. [CrossRef]
116. Ali, A.M.; Mohammed, M.A. A Comprehensive Review of Artificial Intelligence Approaches in Omics Data Processing: Evaluating Progress and Challenges. *Int. J. Math. Stat. Comput. Sci.* **2024**, *2*, 114–167. [CrossRef]

MDPI AG
Grosspeteranlage 5
4052 Basel
Switzerland
Tel.: +41 61 683 77 34

Cancers Editorial Office
E-mail: cancers@mdpi.com
www.mdpi.com/journal/cancers

www.ingramcontent.com/pod-product-compliance
Lightning Source LLC
Chambersburg PA
CBHW062051220926
51850CB00010B/2735
* 9 7 8 3 7 2 5 8 6 9 7 6 3 *